New Leadership
in Health Care Management

The
Physician
Executive

Edited by Wesley Curry

 The American College of Physician Executives

ISBN: 0-9605218-3-6

Printed in the United States of America
by Lithocolor Printing Corp., Tampa, Florida

FOREWORD

The profession of medical management has grown at a rapid pace over the past few years. Not very long ago, the American Academy of Medical Directors was more like a club. Everyone knew everyone. The numbers were small and the Academy was chummy. Much of that flavor has been maintained over the years, but the numbers are far greater. Growing at the rate of more than 100 new members each month, the Academy will reach 4,000 members in the not too distant future, and the 5,000 level is not that far away.

Probably of more importance, the reach of the membership has expanded greatly. In hospitals, group practices, health maintenance organizations, industry, and other environments, physicians are assuming more, and more responsible, management roles. Clinical experience has combined with management expertise to place physicians in chief executive officer and other key executive positions. While the bulk of physician executives are in medical director and other medical positions, medicine is no longer a constricting boundary. Physicians have moved and will continue to move into more general managerial spots as they assimilate knowledge and skills and advance in the profession of management.

Those physicians who have labored in the management vineyards for the past decade or two will notice a subtle but significant change in terms in this new book from the Academy. The general term is now "physician executive." When the Academy was formed, the term of choice was "medical director" and the most common environment was the group practice. The list of titles is now more substantial--CEO, vice president of medical affairs, associate administrator, and, yes, medical director.

Regardless of title, physician executives have assumed many executive roles. Medical staff and quality issues dominate the list of responsibilities for physician executives, but it is also common to see physician executives in business or marketing. More needs to be done to prepare both physicians and the career path for such changes in responsibilities, but the preliminary work has been done.

And that is why this book is important to the profession. It acknowledges that great progress has been made, and it sets the stage for further development of the profession. Physicians have proven that they can master the management disciplines. This book shows how the progress has been achieved and shows all physician executives, both those new to the field and those who see it as a future option, what it means to be a physician executive and what will be required to be successful in management. All physicians, even those with no known or obvious interest in the field of management could benefit from reading and understanding the concepts of this text. The ability of the medical profession to maintain a position of influence in health care, as the numbers and diversity of health care organizations increase and competition for patients and dollars places quality in a subservient position to cost containment, will depend greatly on how well physician excutives represent themselves and the profession of medical management in these competitive arenas. Mastery of the concepts in this book will go a long way in ensuring the profession's success.

Frank A. Riddick, Jr., MD, FACPE
Medical Director
Ochsner Clinic
New Orleans, Louisiana
June 1, 1988

INTRODUCTION

Just eight years ago, the American Academy of Medical Directors published its first textbook on The Physician in Management. That textbook, summarizing as it did the material that attendees used at the Academy's "Physician in Management" seminars, served the profession well. Along with the seminars, it has assisted the profession to grow in stature within the health care field.

This new textbook came from our realization that the field had changed substantially over the past eight years. This is no longer a fledgling profession. Physician executives are well established, their numbers growing rapidly. It was time to bring the text up to date. Much of the discipline of business management remains unchanged. Marketing and finance are as important now as they were in 1980. But there have been changes in the health care field itself, and in the way that physician executives must relate to that field, and this book addresses those changes.

The most important change between the two textbooks of the Academy, however, is one of authorship. In the earlier textbook, the authors were largely consultants and professors. In this new text, physician executives, members of the Academy, have assumed part of the writing responsibility. The profession has reached a stage in which its practitioners are increasingly the best judges of both the content and the needs of the profession. It is safe to predict, I think, that the next such general textbook on medical management will demonstrate a more even balance between practitioners and those outside the profession from whom physician executives can continue to learn.

Roger S. Schenke
Executive Vice President
American Academy of Medical Directors
Tampa, Florida

CONTENTS

Section I. The Context of Management

Section II. The Content of Management

Section I.

The Context of Management

The Challenges Facing American Medicine: The Search for a New Equilibrium and Its Implications for Physician Executives

by Edward F.X. Hughes, MD, MPH

O n September 28, 1984, I was a featured speaker at the annual meeting of the McMahon and Illini County Chapters of the Illinois Healthcare Financial Management Association (HFMA) in Bettendorf, Iowa. HFMA is the association of chief financial officers and their colleagues in health care institutions. The presentation was to address the future of American health care. In the months immediately preceding the address, the majority of the financial managers in attendance had seen their hospitals come under Medicare's new prospective payment system. In fact, the last two hospitals in the nation were scheduled to be subsumed under the system two days later. Illinois had recently moved to a negotiated bidding payment system in its Medicaid program, and the Health Care Financing Administration (HCFA) had, within the year, just begun to demonstrate the feasibility of enrolling Medicare beneficiaries into health maintenance organizations (HMOs) on a risk-contract basis. The speaker immediately before me on the program, representing Illinois' Blue Cross-Blue Shield program, was scheduled to describe a new type of health care plan that his organization had recently begun experimenting with on a demonstration basis in one of the state's medium-sized cities. The type of plan, new to most in the audience, was called a Preferred Provider Organization (PPO).

The anxiety in the room was palpable. The change occurring in our health care system within this year had been greater in breadth and depth than most in the room had experienced in their entire careers. My challenge was to make some sense out of it. Listening to the speaker preceding me, I literally set aside my prepared notes and began writing a new speech, attempting to explain what was going on and why. The speech carried the title: "The Future of American Medicine: The Search for a New Equilibrium." With it came a conceptual framework that enabled me to relate the seemingly disparate and, to that point, largely unappreciated forces buffeting American medicine and to suggest not only why things were happening as they were but what might be expected to happen in the future.

This conceptual framework has stood the test of time. I would like to share it with you in this chapter. I will first address, "What is going on and why?" and then, "Why now?" I will next speak to the changes that were, and are being, wrought in the way health care is paid for in this country as a result of the above, and to the goals of those creating the changes. I will then address whether these goals will be met and why. I will speak to the impact of all of the above on the principal actors in the health care industry, namely hospitals, physicians, and patients, and explore how they might be expected to be affected by the forces now driving our health care system. In so doing, I will say a word about what I see as the need for, and potential role of, physician executives in the present and future of our health care industry. I will conclude by stating where I see all this going and what I believe must be addressed at both the institutional and the societal level to ensure that a high-quality health care system is available to Americans in the future.

What Is Going on and Why?

In brief, the American people are saying: "Enough is enough! We are spending too much money on health care." They are saying this principally through their representatives in the political process--federal and state lawmakers--and their representatives in their places of employment--the vice presidents of human resources of their corporations and/or their labor union leaders.

The reason why they are saying this is that last year in the United States, by the most recent figures available, $498.9 billion was spend on health care.[1] This figure represents a $40.8 billion increase over the previous year, an increase of 8.9 percent, when the CPI increased approximately 4.4 percent. The figure, now 11.2 percent of the Gross National Product, represents a doubling, in current dollars, since 1980 and more than a tripling since 1977. Whether one agrees with the perception of the American people about the appropriateness of our current level of health care spending or not, their representatives are acting to prevent as many dollars as possible from entering our sector of the economy. They are attempting to achieve "a new equilibrium" where expenditures would be less but somehow quality would be the same or possibly even enhanced.

Why Now?

There are four principal reasons why the above perception is now being acted on with the current level of intensity rather than 15 years ago or 15 years in the future. They entail (1) the national budget deficit, (2) the solvency of the Medicare Trust Fund, (3) the financial condition of the states, and (4) the pressures health care costs are placing on private industry.

The National Budget Deficit. When President Reagan took office in

1981, the federal budget deficit was approximately $24 billion. We have seen it rise in recent years to a level of over $200 billion, and efforts such as the Gramm-Rudman-Hollings legislation have been marginally successful at best in reducing it. It is our single highest domestic priority, and it is the most important force affecting federal legislation across all domestic policy issues. Medicare Part B expenditures, covering the ambulatory care delivered in the program, are paid from general revenues. They are currently among the most rapidly growing of all categories of health expenses. Similarly, the federal portion of Medicaid expenses is also drawn from general revenues. Thus every dollar spent in these programs is one more dollar added to the budget deficit.

It generally is not realized that, even though Medicare Part A expenditures, covering hospitalizations, are drawn from a source other than general revenues, namely the Medicare Trust Fund, the balance in this fund counts in determining the size of the budget deficit.

Servicing the national debt caused by the repeated deficits has itself become the third largest category of federal expenditures. The size of the debt influences interest rates, which in turn influence the value of the dollar, our balance of trade, and the level of domestic employment. Needless to say, federal policy makers are reacting to deep-seated social concerns in their attempt to hold down publicly financed health care costs.

The Solvency of the Medicare Trust Fund. The Medicare Trust Fund is financed through a 1.45 percent payroll tax on each American worker contributing to the Social Security Program. Careful research by the Congressional Budget Office in the early 1980s showed that, at current levels of spending and receipts, the Medicare Trust Fund would go bankrupt by 1989 and by 1995 be in deficit by $250 billion.[2] This was a political outcome that could not be allowed to happen and led in part to the political consensus that gave us the Social Security Amendments of 1983. These amendments, through both expanding the number of those who had to contribute to the Fund and altering the mechanisms for paying for hospital care (to be discussed below), forestalled the insolvency of the Fund. It is now projected to remain solvent until the first decade of the Twenty-first Century.

While this prospect is encouraging, the new century is not much more than a decade away. Hence, the potential insolvency of the fund will continue in saliency as an explicitly driving political force to hold down health care costs. The generation of managers now coming into senior positions in the health care field will have to live with this political reality for the duration of their careers. Even now, there are analysts who contend that the current projections for solvency are too rosy and that the potential for insolvency could occur well before currently anticipated.

The Financial Viability of the States. In the early 1980s, the State of California found itself facing extreme budgetary pressures as a result of Proposition 13. The northern tier of states simultaneously found themselves facing similar pressure as a result of the worst recession since the 1930s. Currently, the oil states are experiencing particularly severe financial problems. The Medicaid programs of many states have grown to become their largest social programs. The dollars expended in these programs are general revenue dollars and their growth requires either increased taxes or cutbacks in other areas of state spending. The burden Medicaid programs pose for state budgets is vividly illustrated by the fact that, in 1987 alone, four states exhausted their Medicaid appropriations before the end of their fiscal years.[3] Illinois is the most recent to join this list. It has terminated all provider payments fully two months before the end of the fiscal year and will require hospitals, physicians, and other providers to wait until the next fiscal year for the resumption of payments. It is small wonder that states have added their voices to those saying costs must come down.

The Burden on Private Employers. In 1987, the typical American corporation paid an average of $1,285 in health care benefits for each employee. For many American firms, health care coverage is the single largest individual expense item beyond salaries and wages. In fact, General Motors alone spent $2.9 billion in health care benefits in 1987. It is not only the cost of the coverage of present employees that is of concern, however. Of serious consequence are the contractual obligations of many American firms to cover the health care expenses of retirees.[4] For many firms, these obligations amount to billions of dollars and for many of them these liabilities are as yet unfunded. These unfunded liabilities are seen as a serious accounting issue by the Financial Accounting Standards Board, which has issued guidelines requiring firms to begin accounting, in the near future, for these liabilities in calculating their bottom lines. These requirements could have a depressing effect on the earnings per share of many firms and further stress American business.

These health expenditures affect the price of American products and the competitiveness of American business in international markets. Thus, American business stands firmly aligned with government on the goal of reducing health care costs. In fact, I know of no time outside of war when business has stood so united with government on a social goal. The goal is also bipartisan in nature. A change in the party in the White House or that controlling Congress will not change the commitment to reducing health care costs. There may be variations in the emphasis placed on specific approaches or programs, but the overall goal will remain the same.

What Are They Doing?

Given the above consensus, the payers, both public and private, are doing five things to bring down health care costs. They all entail changes in the payment for health care. The five categories of changes are:

- Changes in *the way health care is paid for.*

- Changes in *the levels of payment.*

- Changes in *who is paid.*

- Changes in *who pays.*

- Changes in *when they pay.*

This typology can serve as a convenient way to conceptualize the many changes now under way.

Changes in the Way Health Care Is Paid for. Since the mid-1930s with the development of the "Baylor Plan" at Baylor University and its offspring, the various Blue Cross and Blue Shield plans across the United States, medical care, most specifically hospital care and increasingly ambulatory care covered by insurance, has been paid for on an after-the-fact basis. It has been reimbursed after its consumption on a cost-based, and in certain instances a cost-plus, basis. No matter what was ordered, barring flagrant fraud or abuse, it was generally paid for. Reasonable students of health economics have long pointed out that such an approach to payment is inflationary in nature. The incentives for both provider and patient/consumer are to overconsume. The marginal value of a service need not be zero for overconsumption to occur. It need only be less than the patient/consumer would be willing to pay for it if he or she were paying for the service directly and confronting its cost prior to consumption.

Payers have come to realize the inflationary nature of retrospective, cost-based reimbursement and have begun to move systematically from retrospective reimbursement for medical services to prospective pricing. This prospective pricing has generally taken three forms: (a) per case, (b) per diem, and (c) per capita.

(a) *Per Case Pricing.* The most common form of per case pricing is through the diagnosis-related groups (DRG) methodology. Under this methodology, no matter what inputs are ordered for a hospitalized Medicare beneficiary, barring an extreme outlier case, the hospital is paid a flat fee for the care of the patient based upon the diagnostic grouping of the patient. This methodology is a result of the sweeping reforms set in motion by the Tax Equity and Fiscal Responsibility Act (TEFRA) of 1982 and implemented through the Social Security Amendments of 1983, alluded to above. It changes the incentives facing providers in that it rewards hospitals for shorter stays and for reduced

Section I - The Context of Management

inputs in the provision care.

(b) *The Per Diem Methodology.* This methodology entails the payment to a hospital of a flat fee for a day of hospitalization, again regardless of the inputs into the care of the patient. There may be one rate for all cases or a small number of different rates that depend on the diagnostic/therapeutic category of the patient. This methodology was born of the California financial crisis following Proposition 13. Instituted in the state's Medicaid program by California's "Health Czar" in the early 1980s, the methodology also has the advantage of changing the incentives facing providers, though only for inputs per day as opposed to the length of stay that the DRG approach also addresses. The adoption of this methodology, within a competitive bidding framework, was responsible for the State of California's saving millions of dollars in the first year of use alone. It soon spread to other states and has been chosen by many PPOs as their preferred method of hospital payment.

(c) *Per Capita Pricing.* This methodology, commonly referred to as "capitation," is the sine qua non of HMOs. It is included in our typology because it is a form of prospective pricing. The providers are paid, in advance of care, a lump sum per head for each plan member under their care. Incentives are thus created for the efficient delivery of all care.

Although it does not fall under the category of prospective payment, the attention currently being directed at the development of a Resource-Based Relative Value Scale (RBRVS), which promises to become the basis for physician payment reform in our federal programs, is a further instance of payers exploring new ways to change how they pay for care. The interest in RBRVS is in part due to the growth of Medicare Part B expenses cited earlier.[5]

Changing the Level of Payment. Each of the three prospective pricing mechanisms discussed above changes the incentives facing providers toward more efficient delivery of care. To that extent, they represent appropriate and salutary reforms in the financing of health care. Problems arise, however, when the payment levels associated with these new mechanisms are not allowed to rise to reflect the true market increases in the costs of the inputs into care. Between 1983 and 1987, the CPI rose 17.4 percent, whereas physician fees under Medicare were allowed to rise less than 4 percent. Between 1986 and 1987, the CPI rose 4.4 percent. The inputs into hospital care, by HCFA's calculations, were up over 6 percent, yet DRGs were allowed to rise only 3 percent.[6] Following the first year of this use, they were allowed to rise only 1.15 percent.

In another variation of changing the level of reimbursement, Massachusetts has enacted legislation to prevent physicians from billing the difference between what Medicare pays (assignment rate) and their actual fee for the procedure/service. The law has been sustained by the United States Supreme Court in its refusal to hear an appeal of it. Of all the changes to be discussed in this Chapter, it is this inability to allow payments to rise with true market forces that is of most concern to the future of our health system.[7]

Changing Who Is Paid. From the late 1970s until the present--either as a result of new legislation; changes in regulations interpreting existing legislation; or, on the private side, changes in benefit design--entire classes of new providers have been enfranchised under public and private coverages. Examples are ambulatory surgery centers under Medicare and private policies, hospices in both public programs and private policies, HMOs under private coverage, HMOs under Medicare, PPOs under private coverage, home health care (although limited) public programs and under private policies, and other ambulatory modalities under private coverage. All of these delivery modalities were added in the hope of both allowing care to be rendered in a less costly setting and enhancing competition among providers to seek lower cost alternatives for care. For a while, this proliferation of organizational entities caused consternation among traditional providers. Only now does growth in the list of new entrants appear to be slowing, the current demonstration by HCFA of the latest entry, the Medicare Insured Group (MIG), not withstanding. The more flexible and aggressive among the traditional providers, adapted to these competitive threats, often developing their own versions of them and therein further enhancing the drive toward efficiency.

Changing Who Pays. Recent years have seen systematic efforts by both public and private payers to make the recipient of care pay an increasing proportion of the cost of care. Earlier this year, the monthly premiums for Medicare Part B recipients rose by over one-third.[8] Private policies have increased coinsurance and deductibles and now even General Motors' salaried employees must pay a deductible in seeking care. The net effect of these changes is to cause the recipient of care to pay for a greater proportion of it and therein reduce the cost to the third party. Well-conceived and well-executed research by the RAND Corporation has shown that deductibles and coinsurance play an important role in reducing the consumption of discretionary care.[9] The question remains, however, as to what is the socially optimal level for such coinsurance and deductibles. Many analysts state that the average Medicare beneficiary is now paying as great a proportion, if not greater, of his or her disposable income as he or she was prior to the passage of Medicare. The deductibles placed on the poor further discourage their consumption of needed care. The "Catastrophic Bill," currently wending its way through the federal legislative process, has as one of its goals the reduction of the negative financial impact of multiple deductibles and extended coinsurance on the sick Medicare beneficiary.

The surge of coinsurance and deductibles in private coverage is also a source of concern--20 percent of a $10,000 hospital bill is not a trivial amount of money, let alone such a percentage of a $100,000 bill. For

Section I - The Context of Management

reasons to be discussed below, private payers will undoubtedly attempt to keep increasing the amounts to be paid by the recipients of care. It is a trend that bears close scrutiny and that will undoubtedly become a source of increasing controversy in the workplace.

It is probably appropriate to mention at this point the employment-based "universal" coverage recently enacted in Massachusetts.[10] It is a variation on "changing who pays." Although the program requires employers of greater than six workers to provide insurance coverage for them, the costs of the program will ultimately be borne by the citizenry, who will pay for the coverage through the necessitated increased costs of goods and services they will purchase. The approach has the advantage of keeping the costs "off budget"--i.e., not readily apparent as in public programs requiring appropriations. In addition to the cost increases it will generate, it has the additional negative aspect that it will further heighten the sensitivity of the business community to health care costs and further their resolve to keep costs from rising.

Changing When They Pay. Contrary to what one may hear alleged about the federal bureaucracy, Medicare has been a very well-administered program. It paid its bills on time. HCFA told Congress a few years ago that it would no longer pay hospitals according to its customary schedule but a new more extended one--enhancing its cash flow but forcing hospitals to borrow to meet their obligations. Initially, Congress forbade the practice. It has recently, however, instructed HCFA to extend the payment schedule for hospitals out progressively over the next few years. In industry, most successful business relationships between a supplier of services and a purchaser of those services assume the characteristics of a partnership with each party looking out for the other's interests and working to the other's betterment.[11,12] The extension of Medicare's payment schedule would appear to be a poor omen for the relationship between the purchasers and suppliers in this industry. It points to the extent to which payers will go to reduce the costs of health care.

What Are They Trying to Accomplish through the Above?

I mentioned earlier that payers were attempting to reduce the flow of dollars into the health care sector. As we enter the last year of the 1980s, it may be difficult to remember that in the early to middle years of this decade, a frank reduction in the level of health care expenses was not only the goal of payers/policymakers, but an outcome felt achievable. I remember a statement to me by a HCFA official in late 1983: "Now that we have hospital costs controlled, we are going after physician costs next." The CEO of a midsized Chicago firm bet me $50 in 1985 that, because of all the reforms then under way or in place in the financing of health care, health care costs would be less in that year than in 1984. He was off by more than $30 billion dollars!

What Were They Able to Accomplish and Why?

The bulk of the reforms discussed above were able to achieve unit cost reductions--e.g., a case of congestive heart failure treated under DRGs will, on average, generate fewer hospital costs than one treated under retrospective reimbursement; an inguinal herniorrhaphy performed in a freestanding ambulatory surgical center will, on average, generate fewer direct costs than one treated on an inpatient basis. (There is some anecdotal evidence appearing that hospitals have sufficiently loaded overhead costs onto hospital-based ambulatory care facilities so that this statement may no longer apply in those settings.) The net result of these changes in unit costs was an inflection in the rate of growth of costs in the mid-1980s--a reduction in the rate of increase, not a reduc-tion in level.[5] As the number of units of service continues to grow, and the other forces to be discussed below play themselves out, health care costs will only continue to rise.

Why Health Care Costs Will Only Continue to Rise

There are at least eight reasons why heath care costs will continue to rise: (1) the aging of the population, (2) the physician "surplus," (3) the nurse shortage, (4) technology, (5) the fallacy of health insurance, (6) epidemiologic vagaries, (7) the malpractice problem, and (8) the pres-ence of the under- and uninsured.

The Aging of the Population. The changing demographics of the popu-lation of the United States are now well known to the readers of this chapter. The fastest growing segment of the population may no longer be those over 85 years of age but rather those over 100. Medical care has played a very positive role in this increased longevity. It is not so much the old-old of today who will continue to drive up costs, however, as much as the sizable proportion of the older middle-aged population now entering the age where the diseases of senescence express them-selves and the demand for care increases. The relative aging of our population will continue for a substantial period and will, in and of itself, guarantee an increase in the costs of health care.

The Physician "Surplus." Between 1970 and 1980, medical schools in the United States doubled the size of their enrollment. The result is an increase in the number of physicians per capita to historic levels. Although precincts are now beginning to report in suggesting that the physician "surplus" may not be what it was touted to be, the fact remains we have more physicians per capita than ever before.[13] The demand for the average physician's services will fall. As a result, physicians will engage in practices to counteract this falling demand. Offices will be open at hours more convenient to patients, patients will be brought back for revisits more frequently, more tests will be ordered, etc. The costs of medical care, all things being equal, will rise.

Section I - The Context of Management

The Nurse Shortage. It is generally believed we now have a nationwide nurse shortage.[14] This shortage is a result, among many factors, of more broadly based career opportunities for women, more difficult hospital working conditions owing, in part, to the post-DRG increased severity of illness of the average hospital patient, and a lack of well-defined upward mobility within the profession. One of the ways one generally cures shortages is to raise the incomes of the job categories in short supply. Any systematic effort to alleviate the nurse shortage will entail an increase in health care costs.

Technology. The readers of this chapter are again familiar with the enormous technological strides that have been made in medicine in the past 20 years--renal dialysis, kidney transplantation, coronary by-pass surgery, coronary perfusion therapies, antihypertensive therapies, magnetic imaging resonance, bone marrow transplantation, cardiac transplantion, the new positron emission tomography, etc. The list is even more startling when one realizes that these advances were made on top of an already highly efficacious technological armamentarium. Fortunately, we are learning how to more effectively use these new, and existing, technologies and thereby reduce marginal or ineffective use. The size of the investment of the United States government in the National Institutes of Health in and of itself, let alone the investments in research and development by the private firms in the health care industry, almost guarantees the continued, if not rising, introduction of efficacious technology into our health care system. A look at the new patents announced in each Saturday's *New York Times* further reinforces this belief. These new technologies will increase the demand for care and increase its costs. As has been the case in the past, it will require an even more sophisticated labor force in the health field, further raising costs.

The Fallacy of Health Insurance. Insurance is a social vehicle designed to spread the risk of low probability events over which one has no control among individuals of similar levels of risk. Tornadoes, hurricanes, and fires are examples of such low probability events one can successfully insure against. The probability of death is 100 percent. In health care, we are insuring against a certainty. One of the downsides of the above-discussed technology is that we have the means to prolong the advent of the certainty without, in certain instances, enhancing the quality of life of the individual being treated. In other words, we may be prolonging death rather than prolonging life. America as a nation does not have a very effective way to deal with death. We have chosen as the place for one's final days the most expensive institution in our society-- the acute care hospital. I quip that one could check into the most expensive hotel in town, have "Dom Perignon" I.V., and go out in far finer fashion and with less expense than occurs in our hospitals. Hospice care has made a reasonable beginning in reducing the costs and technological intensity associated with death. We have, however, a long way to go. There is a need for a resurgence of the family-centered, religious, or culturally oriented approach of an earlier day. Until that is found, the very presence of health insurance in our population will interact with technology and the aging of the population to ensure the continuing rise in health care costs.

Epidemiologic Vagaries. By this term, I mean the changing pattern of diseases in our society. Earlier in this decade, those who were talking about a possible fall in health care expenses did not appropriately perceive the magnitude of the implications of the spread of AIDS for health care costs. It is now estimated there will be 66,000 AIDS cases by 1991, costing $2.3 billion annually.

The increasing number of surviving elderly in our population also suggests we may see more cases of Alzheimer's Disease and other chronic invaliding conditions. These too will contribute to the rise in health care costs.

The Malpractice Problem. Given the threat of malpractice, physicians will order increased numbers of tests, consultations, etc. to protect themselves not only from possible suits but also within the suits that inevitably follow. These indirect costs will contribute to the increasing costs of care and war against the spread of parsimony in clinical care, an important component of any efficient health care system.

The increased premiums doctors will have to pay for malpractice coverage will necessitate their raising their fees, thus directly increasing the costs of care. Where physicians will be driven out of a specialty or geographic area by the high costs of malpractice insurance, e.g., in the field of obstetrics and gynecology, the physicians remaining will experience an increased demand for their services, leading to further increased fees, all things being equal.

The Problem of the Under- and Uninsured. Despite the widespread availability of health insurance in our society, it is estimated that as many as 37 million Americans could be without it. Any conscientious attempt to provide coverage for these individuals will raise the costs of care, both for the coverage itself and the services that otherwise would not be utilized. It has been estimated that the recently enacted Massachusetts employment-based universal coverage alluded to above will cost employers $1,680 per year per employee by the year 1992.[10] It is of concern to me that some policy makers may be motivated to increase coverage of the above individuals without appreciating the implications of such actions for the costs of care.

The Implications of the Above for the "Search for a New Equilibrium "

Given the fact that health care costs will only continue to rise, the implications for the health care industry are dire. As stated above, policy makers, not fully appreciating why costs are rising and often choosing to ascribe the trend to a virulent sort of inefficiency or "fat" in the system, will want to continue to cut back on health care costs. (In order to explain the yearly increasing costs of care, this inefficiency would have to be escalating in nature.) The implications of such efforts, if pursued in an overzealous manner, could be detrimental to the quality of care in our health system and the health and welfare of the American people.[7]

Thus, the "Search for a New Equilibrium" will be a difficult and painstaking social process. Payers will become increasingly aggressive in trying to hold down health care costs. As they see health care costs continue to rise in the face of their efforts, they will tend to conclude, barring some of the interventions to be discussed at the conclusion of this chapter, that their efforts have not been aggressive enough and intensify them.

Equilibrium is an economic concept wherein the price of a product offered for sale is accepted by a purchaser and the market clears. It is also a chemical concept in which two atoms or molecules interact to form a third chemical entity. In the process, they fall into a lower energy state, and heat is liberated. In the reaction of the payers described above, heat is being, and will continue to be, felt by all health care providers.

The next few years will be critical to the long-term future of our health system. Before addressing what I believe are the challenges that should be addressed in these years and the role that physician executives should play in that process, I would like to discuss briefly the implications of the above for the future of principal actors in the industry: (1) hospitals, (2) physicians, and (3) patients/consumers.

The Implications of the Above for the Future of the Principal Actors

Hospitals. The hospitals of the future will, on the whole, be smaller institutions caring for sicker patients. Some have gone so far as to say they will be a string of intensive care units, though I do not believe we will see things carried quite that far. All of the changes in the "ways" of reimbursement alluded to above, with the exception of the per diem approach, will serve to reduce the length of hospital stay for each admission, raising the average severity of illness of the remaining patients. Hospitals will continue to shift resources and care to the outpatient department. Ultimately, some sort of prospective pricing methodology will be implemented for hospital outpatient care, replacing the retrospective approach still in existence and challenging further the financial stability and management versatility of our hospitals.

Hospitals determined to be among the survivors in the tough days still to come have long since realized that they are no longer in the hospital business but in the health care business. The goal of such institutions is to efficiently and effectively meet the health care needs of their communities through an expanded array of services--services for which they can be either the sole proprietor or partners with their physicians.

The critical skill in the above diversification is an appropriate targeting of services. The glory days of vertical integration preached by many in recent years have been oversold, and many health care institutions, not only hospitals, now find themselves in lines of business for which they were poorly prepared, with concomitant financial losses.[16] This overexpansion having been, or soon to be, weeded out, tomorrow's hospital will remain a realistically scoped diversified enterprise.

As alluded to above, the relationship of the hospital to its physicians becomes critically important not only to the survivability of the hospital but also to the welfare of the physicians themselves. Physician referral patterns and the quality of care they provide are the lifeblood of the hospital and the hospital can assist its physicians augment their practices in countless ways--referral services, new services, advertising, etc. This hospital partnership with its physicians entails not only enhancement of each other's traditional roles, but also exploration of new services both within and external to the hospital as well as an expanded role for physicians in general within the management and governance of the hospital. This is a point to which I will return below.

Central to the survival, if not the flourishing, of tomorrow's hospitals is the primacy of management. The running of a hospital is as complex a management task as exists. In fact, Peter Drucker has recently identified the successful management of a hospital as a model American managers overall should try to emulate in their more traditionally hierarchical firms.[17] This successful management requires a solid grounding in the management sciences such as marketing, finance, and organizational behavior, as well as an ability to relate effectively to highly educated and entrepreneurial professionals--physicians. As quality of care becomes an increasingly important and more readily quantified output of institutional care (both inpatient and ambulatory), relations with physicians become even more important.[18] This fact is true not only for hospitals but also for managed care plans etc. There is a need for leadership, standard setting, and accountability.

Thus, it is my bias that, given the appropriate level of management training, a physician makes an ideal institutional health care manager. The emphasis in the last sentence is on the words: "given the appropriate level of management training." In these trying times, it is difficult, though not impossible, for one to master in a timely way the sciences needed to manage effectively through on-the-job training. We have seen many instances of physicians' failing in management positions where the job to be done was viewed as an extension of business as

Section I - The Context of Management

usual.

The successful executive in today's and tomorrow's institutions must possess the ability to understand the nuances of cost-quality tradeoffs; to communicate such nuances effectively to his/her physician colleagues; and, through this communication, to inspire in them a level of performance and achievement that might otherwise not be possible. Physician executives would appear to be especially well equipped for this critical role.

This role is especially important because one of the dual requirements for the survival of our health care system is enhanced institutional efficiency--the ability to do more, or at least as much, with possibly less. This challenge will require an understanding by hospital managers of the nature of the caregiving process as never before. Similarly, although I believe the case is overstated, there are a number of observers of the medical care industry who feel much of the process of medical care now being delivered may not be efficacious or effective. They are calling for a sustained examination of what physicians do and why--with the goal of eliminating redundant services and those with low marginal utility. Were such a mission undertaken in our health system, the physician executive would appear well poised to provide leadership.

It is because of this belief in the efficacy and effectiveness of the physician executive that we at Northwestern University two years ago initiated for medical students a five-year joint Master's of Management (MBA)/Doctor of Medicine degree program. In this collaborative effort between our management and medical schools, medical students will be able to obtain the two degrees in five years of interrelated work as opposed to the usual six.

Physicians. The years ahead for the medical profession will be difficult ones. The resources going to physicians will be squeezed through the various mechanisms described above. The average practicing physician will lose market share owing to the "surplus" mentioned above and to the growth of managed care plans. As a result, at the mean, physicians will earn less. Of greater concern than falling incomes is an attendant fall in prestige of the profession. The degree of this fall in prestige can already be gauged, in part, by the fact that applications to medical schools have now fallen to a number only 30 percent in excess of the positions available.

To counteract this loss in market share, I have advised physicians to contemplate coalition-building among their peers; the formation of partnerships and groups; the joining of managed care plans; and, where it makes sense, multiple plans. It is not sufficient simply to join a group or a managed care plan. Leadership must be provided to guide the evolution of these organizations in a manner that befits the preservation of quality of care in an era of constrained resources. Thus physician executives also have a critical role to play in the evolution of these important components of our health care system.

Another troublesome hurdle for the profession to surmount will be the effort by public payers to impose Resource-Based Relative Value Scales (RBRVS) on the profession as a means of controlling payment levels for various services and procedures both within and across specialties.[6] Though I believe RBRVS can serve to correct potential long-standing economic inequities in traditional fees, weighted in the favor of proceduralists, one can be assured on the basis of our experience with other payment reforms that, no matter how carefully researched, they will be imperfect tools, may tend to overcorrect, and will probably afford the government further opportunity to reduce physician incomes overall within an alleged goal of redistribution.

The stage is thus being set through RBRVS for interspecialty divisiveness as never before seen. It will call for a very expansive social vision to prevent this divisiveness from leading to serious harm to the profession. Some elements of what might constitute this social vision are discussed below.

Patients. I do not subscribe to the "doom and gloom" scenario of a number of observers of our health care system--provided a number of preconditions are met.[19] Thus, the "Search for the New Equilibrium" need not be detrimental to patients *in the long term.* First, with the increased number of physicians, they will have more time on their hands. As mentioned previously, office hours will be expanded. House calls are returning. Access will thus improve. With the increased time, physicians will be able to spend more time with patients. I quip that they will engage more both in the unusual practice of talking to patients and in the heretofore rare event of actually listening to one or two. Quality of care will thus improve. Countering this positive tendency will be the efforts of the payers to hold down costs, with potential threats to the health and welfare of the patients.[7] How we meet this challenge and the role of the physician executive in that challenge are the subject of the remainder of this chapter.

Where Do We Go from Here?--I: What Is the Nature of the Problem?

The problem facing American medicine is that, despite the excesses observed, the overprescribing of certain procedures, small area variation, the 37 million uninsured, and whatever other criticism one might appropriately address at American medicine, we have a success on our hands. Mortality rates for the bulk of our major killers are at historically low levels. The exception is cancer in the elderly, where longevity would appear to be contributing to the increased prevalence and death rates. Even our infant mortality rate is at a low--the recent cessation in its fall, notwithstanding.

Section I - The Context of Management

Not only are our mortality rates lower but a reasonable argument can be made for medicine's contributing to an enhanced quality of life for our society. We have developed an integral component of the late Twentieth Century American life-style, which is producing its desired outcomes and is highly desired by our citizens. The problem is it is, in and of itself, very expensive.

Where Do We Go from Here?--II: The Dual Challenge

There are two challenges that must be met for us as a society to be able to continue to provide health care at the level and to the extent found in America today. The first is that we in the health care industry must be able to say to the American people that we have done, and are doing, everything possible to reduce inefficiency in the delivery of health care in this country. The second is that we must be able to find the resources necessary to support the level of care people seem to demand. The first of these challenges entails institutional management; the second, social management. The first of these challenges is a necessary prerequisite for long-term success in the second, but they must be pursued simultaneously.

The Institutional Management Challenge. The challenge here is to increase the efficiency of the delivery of health care in the United States to the maximum extent possible. It is through aggressively pursuing this challenge that health care leaders can assure the American people that everything possible is being done to reduce the cost of medical care. The concept of efficiency in economics implies that quality is held constant. There is reason to believe, however, that in health care enhanced efficiency can bring enhanced quality.

In discussing this challenge, I am using the adjective "institutional" in the broadest possible sense, from the largest of our medical centers to the smallest of our physicians' offices. Preceding sections of this chapter have already addressed multiple aspects of this challenge and we have already made great strides in addressing it--far greater than many payers appear to appreciate or, in certain instances, appear willing to acknowledge. Good business sense alone would suggest that most in the health care industry pursue this goal aggressively. The competitiveness recently unleashed in health care has made the pursuit of this challenge mandatory for institutional survival.

Because of the special attention that must be paid to cost-quality trade-offs in the quest for efficiency, the physician executive has, as discussed above, a critical leadership role to play in addressing this challenge. What is at stake, however, is not simply enhanced efficiency. Rather, it is the credibility of health management/practitioner community and the potential for its enjoying the confidence of the American people. It is my bias that the unwillingness of citizens, as expressed in polls, to increase taxes to pay for care derives, at least in part, from lingering perceptions that the health care industry is wasteful, inefficient, etc. It is my belief that if a full-scale attack on inefficiency is waged and the fact of that attack is communicated effectively to the American people and they are educated effectively as to the risks to their own health from a failure to adequately finance our health care system in the future, they will tell their elected and workplace representatives to allow the dollars to flow to this sector of the economy. In so doing they will be acting to enable the requisite services and technology to be provided by the industry so that quality can survive. How to achieve this desired behavioral response is the social management challenge.

The Social Management Challenge. The dollars necessary for the continued excellence of our health care system are not under the control of the managers of that system. They belong to the American people--either in the form of taxes that will have to be raised or in the form of higher prices that will have to be paid for commercial products. The American people have been reluctant to part with these dollars for health care needs, in part because of the aforementioned perceptions that the health care industry is very inefficient and that they are not getting their money's worth at current levels of expenditures. They have also been reluctant to part with these dollars because the consequences of their failing to do so have never been effectively communicated to them. Health care leaders have not to date adequately addressed this challenge. What public education has taken place in the health care industry has, for the most part, and sadly so, entailed lobbying for increased (or at least stable) professional incomes and institutional revenues. Very little has been done to educate the American people as to what is at stake if our health care industry is not adequately funded and very little has been done in terms of lobbying for their health and welfare. The good news is that most arguments for enhanced insitutional and professional revenues are consistent with enhancing the health of the American people.

What is needed is a massive, honest, and straightforward public education campaign by the leaders of our health care industry as to what is at stake in terms of the health of the American people from a failure to allow the appropriate level of resources to flow into the industry.[7] What is at stake is the ability of future Americans to avail themselves of the latest in technical care provided in modern, well-equipped institutions by professionally fulfilled caregivers and timely and well-targeted ambulatory care. Americans place a high value on high-quality health care for themselves and their families. They are not aware of the risk to that quality.

In this campaign, basic issues such as efficacy of new technologies and their contribution to decreased mortality, decreased morbidity, and enhanced life-style need to be accentuated and, most critically, the threat posed to their availability by overly aggressive cost containment policies in both the public and the private sector. The need to continu-

Section I - The Context of Management

ally modernize facilities must be stressed, as does the need to have the resources to raise the salaries of nurses and other health professionals so our health system will have a labor force of the quality it merits.[14]

Once the issues are made clear, it is my belief the American people will vote for the dollars needed for high-quality health care--vote through the ballot box in the public sector and "vote" in their places of work by expressing their opinions and preferences to their vice presidents of human resources and union leaders. Central to the success of this strategy is the reorientation in the minds of citizens of health professionals and institutions as their "partners" in assisting them to achieve new, or sustain existing, levels of health, rather than as individuals and entities profiting from their illnesses.

There is a very special role for the physician executive in this educational process. Despite what one reads or hears, physicians are highly regarded by the American people. Physicians, however, have not traditionally perceived as among their roles that of the social or political advocate. Such a role, however, is part and parcel of the functioning of today's and tomorrow's physician executive. Central to it are some of the basic concepts of marketing, namely, ascertaining the basic needs and desires of one's "patients," and then effectively communicating those needs in the political arena and developing a national consensus so that those needs and desires can be met. Achieving, in the political arena, the goal of the American people's being able to continue to receive high-quality health care will guarantee that the resources necessary for our institutional and professional providers to function effectively will be available.

Where Will the Money Come From?

To achieve the above goal will require substantial resources on an ongoing basis. On the public side, there would appear to be two principal sources for these resources: general revenues and excise taxes. The raising of increased general revenue is difficult in that it calls for across-the-board income tax increases. My bias, however, is that if, in the context of the above campaign, the American people were convinced these new taxes would go explicitly toward health care, they would vote for them. A reasonable case can also be made that within currently raised general revenues, a greater proportion should go to health care as opposed to, say, defense. I find it fascinating that, to date, no effective campaign against increased defense spending has been initiated by the health care industry. The political problems of raising taxes are immense, however, and, once raised, the dollars are subject to diversion to other uses. It is for these reasons that I prefer starting with excise taxes.

Excise Taxes--A major source of revenue to support the future of our health care system is being overlooked in our lack of aggressive use of excise taxes on noxious substances to raise dollars explicitly for health care. Many of the diseases of senescence--for instance, cardiovascular disease, in its various manifestations, and cancer--are caused by, or are at least accelerated by, the consumption of noxious substances, including cigarettes, high cholesterol foods, and alcohol (despite its high-density lipoprotein effect). These items could be taxed heavily and the dollars thus raised added to the Medicare Trust Fund, and possibly even used create a Medicaid or long-term care trust fund. I would also place a tax on gasoline and automobiles because of the carnage they wreak and earmark those funds for health care.

Thus, individuals could make consumption decisions of their choice, but in full knowledge that some of the dollars being expended in those choices would be set aside in trust funds for the future medical care that their current behavior will require. Thus, those who choose to consume noxious substances would be paying, at least in part, for their future care. It would not be borne by society in general. This approach also has applicability to the handling of illegal drugs in our society. Though it is unlikely we, as a society, would be so bold as to avail ourselves of these potential sources of revenue.

How financially viable is this source of revenue? An increase in the tax on a pack of cigarettes from 16 cents to 32 cents would raise an additional $3.1 billion in 1990.[20] An increase to 64 cents would yield three times as much.[20] An increase in the tax on beer and wine to equal the rate on distilled spirits would yield $5.8 billion in 1990. Increases far greater than these could be voted, and they could be linked to the consumer price index to rise with inflation.

Such excise tax increases also have the salutary effect of diminishing the consumption of the noxious substances and therein enhancing health. The impact of these taxes on cigarettes and alcohol in reducing consumption is especially pronounced in the case of teenagers. An increase in the real tax on beer of $1.50 per case has been shown to reduce highway mortality by 27 percent in this group.[21]

Critics of excise taxes argue that they disproportionally affect the poor.[22] This allegation is correct. The effect would, however, be ameliorated through various income tax rebate approaches.

How politically viable is it? The intuitive logic of having individuals who through their own behavior would be fostering health care costs on others incur these costs would appear to lend this excise tax approach an element of political attractiveness. The immediate gain to health of young people is an added plus. Policy makers in Washington have spotted revenue-enhancing potential of the above excise taxes as a means of reducing the budget deficit. It would be unfortunate if they were used for these general purposes and not to support health care.

Conclusion

Despite all the efforts to date to reduce health care costs, they will only continue to rise. They will rise because the delivery of an ever-improving product, high-quality medical care, to an aging society is an expensive undertaking. Leaders in health care must leave no stone unturned in attempting to increase the efficiency of the delivery of health care while simultaneously educating the American people and their representatives of the need to continue to allow resources to flow to health care that a high-quality system requires. The resources exist in our society to enable our health care system to remain a very high-quality one. It is important that they be harnessed for health care. The physician executive has a very special role both in the management of our future health care system and in addressing each of the above challenges. If these challenges are effectively addressed, the "Search for a New Equilibrium" could have a very salutary outcome.

References

1. "Health Care Equals 11.2 Percent of GNP." *Medicine & Health* 42(4):2, Jan. 25, 1988.

2. The Future of Medicare. A conference sponsored jointly by the Congressional Budget Office and the Subcommittee on Health, Ways and Means Committee, U.S. House of Representatives, Nov. 1983.

3. Richards, B. "Many Hospitals Feel Financial Strain as More of Their Patients Need Public Aid." *Wall Street Journal*, May 3, 1988, p. 26.

4. Foulkes, F., and Paul, R. "Containing Retiree Health Care Expenses: Company Liabilities are Soaring." *New York Times*, Nov. 29, 1987, Section 3, p. 21.

5. Hsaio, W., and others. "The Resource-Based Relative Value Scale." *JAMA* 258(6):799-802, Aug. 14, 1987.

6. Division of National Cost Estimates, Office of the Actuary, Health Care Financing Administration. "National Health Expenditures, 1986-2000." *Health Care Financing Review* 8(4):1-21, Summer 1987.

7. Shortell, S., and Hughes, E. "The Effect of Regulation, Competition, and Ownership on Mortality Rates Among Hospital Inpatients." *New England Journal of Medicine* 318(17):1100-7, April 28, 1988.

8. Kramon, G. "Insurance Rates for Health Care Increase Sharply." *New York Times*, Jan. 12, 1988, p. 1.

9. Newhouse, J., and others. "Some Interim Results from a Controlled Trial of Cost-Sharing in Health Insurance." *New England Journal of Medicine* 305(25):1501-7, Dec. 17, 1981.

10. "Massachusetts Lawmakers Vote Dukakis's Health Insurance Bill." *New York Times*, April 14, 1988, p. 1.

11. Love, J. *McDonald's: Behind the Arches.* Toronto, Canada: Bantam Books, 1986.

12. Scully, J. *Odyssey.* New York City: Harper and Row, 1987.

13. Schwartz, W., and others. "Why There Will be Little or No Physician Surplus Between Now and The Year 2000." *New England Journal of Medicine* 318(14):892, April 7, 1988.

14. Tolchin, M. "Health Worker Shortage is Worsening." *New York Times*, April 18, 1988, p. 9.

15. Scitovsky, A., and Rice, D. "Estimates of the Direct and Indirect Costs of Acquired Immunodeficiency Syndrome in the United States, 1985, 1986, and 1991." *Public Health Reports* 102(1):5-17, Jan.-Feb. 1987.

16. Agins, T. "Chamberlain Resigns High Post at Avon Apparently Unhappy with Firm's Focus." *Wall Street Journal*, May 2, 1988.

17. Drucker, P. "The Coming of the New Organization." *Harvard Business Review* 66(1):45-55, Jan.-Feb. 1988.

18. Hughes, E. *Perspectives on Quality in American Medicine.* Washington, D.C.: McGraw-Hill, 1988 (in press).

19. Schwartz, W., and Aaron, H. "A Tough Choice on Health Care Costs." *New York Times*, April 6, 1988, p. 23.

20. "If Tax Rises Are Coming, Which Ones Will They Be?" *New York Times*, Feb. 21, 1988, p. E-4.

21. Saffer, H., and Grossman, M. "Drinking Age Laws and Highway Mortality Rates: Cause and Effect." *Economic Inquiry* 25(3):403-18, July 1987.

22. McIntyre, R., and others. *Nickels and Dimes--How Sales and Excise Taxes Add Up in the 50 States.* Washington, D.C.: Citizens for Tax Justice, 1988.

Edward F.X. Hughes, MD, MPH, is Director, Center for Health Services, Northwestern University, Evanston, Ill.

Section I - The Context of Management

CHAPTER 2

The Future of Medicine

by Eugene S. Schneller, PhD, Robert G. Hughes, PhD,
and Pamela Hood-Szivek

T he history of the medical profession in the United States is one of
an autonomous and predominantly self-regulating group of individuals. Through the sixties and seventies, physicians maintained a
virtual monopoly over the provision of services and defined, by themselves, the conditions and content of practice.[1-3] The position of dominance that had been established earlier in the century was rarely
contested by competing occupations, patients, payers, policy makers,
or the organizations in which clinical work took place. Indeed, the
substantial advances in clinical practice gave the American public great
confidence in the profession and in the abilities of its members to
intervene in the illness process. Professional autonomy and self-regula-
tion were further supported by the belief that medical work differed
from other forms of work. Each patient was believed to represent a
unique case, and the degree of uncertainty associated with the application of medicine to a particular person meant that accountability for
outcomes remained with the individual physician and, to a lesser extent,
the physician's peers.[3]

Major pressures, from both inside and outside the system, have contributed to substantial changes in American medicine. The autonomy of
physicians in their work and their influence in relationships with their
patients and with hospitals have been challenged. Although it is impossible to predict with confidence what medical practice will be like in the
future, it will certainly be different. Medical practice will be affected by
changes in the structure of the health care delivery system, especially by
changes in the hospital--its organization, mission, and relationship with
the human and nonhuman capital necessary to deliver health services.

Our intent in this chapter is to:

- Highlight the major factors in the historical development of the medical profession and hospitals.

- Specify the changes in the system that have led to the interrelatedness of the two entities.

- Detail the extent to which change may be viewed in the context of the introduction of organized patient agents, and the reconceptualization of medical work.

- Note how physicians may respond and develop new roles to cope with these challenges.

- Present an alternative view of hospitals and physicians that focuses on resources and their scarcity.

Physicians and Hospitals: Two Streams of Development

Traditionally, we have thought about physicians and hospitals separately. Physicians are viewed first and foremost as members of a profession. Physicians developed as solo entrepreneurs. Their organizational bases, at least through most of the nineteenth century, were their offices or clinics or simply the bags that carried their nostrums and rudimentary instruments. Much of their success or failure as healers and businessmen depended on their ability to attract and retain patients.

Hospitals, on the other hand, are viewed as organizations, with a sociological emphasis on their extensive division of labor and complexity and an economic emphasis on their behavior as firms and on the ways their behavior deviates from various normative expectations.[4] Historically, hospitals were primarily havens for the destitute and marginal members of society who had no alternative places to live and die. They were not viewed as advantageous, nor were they numerous. In 1873, the United States had only 149 hospitals (including mental institutions). The period between the 1870s and 1915 was a formative one for the American hospital.[5-7] The most important developments were in the area of science--most specifically the possibility of performing surgery with the likelihood of benefitting patients, rather than doing harm. By 1923 the U.S. had 6,763 hospitals (approximately today's number), mostly what have come to be known as community or general acute care facilities. By this time many physicians were using hospitals as their "workshops," but the profession was not in direct control. In general, the hospital was governed by nonphysician community leaders and managed by lay administrators and nurses.

This formative period in the development of American health care is important because the basic framework of hospital-physician relationships that persists today was established. The primary structural arrangement between hospitals and physicians is the medical staff, an organizational mechanism that developed to accommodate the interests of both hospitals and physicians. It allowed physicians to conduct their

Section I - The Context of Management

work in hospitals. They could make diagnostic and treatment decisions with the use of hospital resources, charge separately for those services, and work with few constraints imposed by the hospital. Most physicians practiced medicine as solo practitioners, in partnerships, or in small groups. With the exception of hospital-based specialists and the few who joined large groups, the medical staff mechanism allowed physicians to expand their entrepreneurial practice of fee-for-service medicine into the hospital.

For hospitals, the medical staff mechanism fostered the use of their facilities by physicians, who in turn strongly influenced where patients were admitted. The medical staff also developed out of a concern for quality by functioning as a means for a hospital to monitor the physicians who used its facilities. For both parties, the traditional, autonomous medical staff provided a flexible organizational structure that allowed many substantive issues to remain informal, and thus more resistant to outside influence.

What factors contributed to the establishment of this unique organizational arrangement between physicians and hospitals? An initial factor was the transfer of authority to admit patients from trustees to physicians.[7] Lay decisions to admit patients to a hospital, exercised by trustees, had been based on social, economic, and moral criteria as well as the health of the patient. Second, growth in the system led to excess bed capacity. Physician admission decisions, grounded in medical diagnoses, simultaneously reinforced their professional claim to define illness and to determine the illnesses that required hospital admission.

By the turn of the century, physicians were firmly in control of patient admission decisions. This constituted an important source of power in establishing favorable structural arrangements with hospitals. Hospitals and physicians were to become mutually dependent. As institutions were beginning to need financial support in addition to eleemosynary sources, hospitals needed the patients that physicians controlled. Physicians wanted access to hospitals, in part because it provided the means to practice a brand of medicine that would yield benefits for patients, and in part because such practice also was often more lucrative than office practice. Early on, some physicians exchanged charity care for the opportunity to learn new medical techniques by treating a hospital's indigent patients. As these physicians began to bring their paying patients to the hospital, hospitals began to augment their revenues, but also allowed physicians to charge separately for their services in the hospital.

Underlying the physician orientation to the hospital at the beginning of the century was a democratic, egalitarian ideology within the profession, as promulgated by the American Medical Association (AMA).[8] Substantial attention has been given to AMA exclusionary activities directed at delineating what constitutes a physician, clearly differentiating the profession from other health occupations and healers. But a complementary theme at this time was the preference for minimizing differences within the profession. This fostered a policy preference for the right of all physicians to admit patients and perform operations. The AMA, strongly influenced by general practitioners, who would be the "losers" in any system that recognized status differentials, did not want specialization within the profession along the lines of hospital and non-hospital physicians, as had occurred in England and other European countries.[8] Reinforcing this position was the argument that the doctor-patient relationship was sacrosanct, and thus quality and continuity of care were preserved when the physician could follow the patient into the hospital.

Throughout the century, the relative bargaining power of hospitals and physicians favored physicians. Most potent was their ability to use an alternative facility if one hospital instituted policies not to their liking. In extreme situations, doctors could open their own hospitals, since capital requirements at the time were not large. Hospitals, on the other hand, were dependent on physicians for patients and had no similar alternatives. In Hirschman's terms,[9] physicians could exercise both a voice and an exit option in their negotiations with hospitals, the potential of the latter strengthening the former.

The medical staff became an organizational affirmation of practices that were already in use: physicians who met a set of qualifications could admit patients to a hospital, use its equipment and staff, and charge for services separately. The structural relationships between hospitals and physicians thus avoided the organizational form that was transforming other sectors of society: bureaucracy.[10] Rather than being employed by a hospital and thus part of a single, formal authority structure, the physician could be, and often was, a member of more than one hospital medical staff. These patterns of activity have increased over the years. Now more than 90 percent of physicians have hospital admitting privileges, and the typical physician is a member of at least two medical staffs.[11] For all office-based physicians, over one third of patient time is spent in the hospital. The economic benefits derived from hospital practice are reflected in the higher earnings of hospital-based physicians when compared to their office-based colleagues.[12] Overall, it is clear that hospitals and physicians have been interdependent since the emergence of the modern hospital and that their interdependency has increased up through the present.

When hospitals and physicians have been considered together, the emphasis has been on the internal dynamics between them and not on the mutual dependence of both hospitals and physicians on external resources. Smith, in a classic article,[13] described the hospital as having two lines of authority: administrative and medical. Subsequent approaches have, in effect, built on this core observation and formulated models of the hospital as a physician's workshop[14] or as actually con-

Section I - The Context of Management

taining two firms (with the medical staff as the demand firm and the administration as the supply firm) in one organization.[15] Most recently, efforts to understand the factors contributing to high costs resulted in the conclusion that hospitals are characterized by a "power equilibrium" in which physicians dominate.[16] Overall these and other analyses have examined hospitals and physicians by looking at the internal organization in order to understand the outputs or consequences of their combined behavior along some dimension such as costs[16], quality[17], or profit-maximization.[14]

The history of physicians and hospitals demonstrates how a set of relationships evolved into two parallel lines of authority. The medical staff became a powerful group that successfully controlled the content and conditions of practice. The management system maintained the doctor's workshop by balancing the books and overseeing the day-to-day management of the plant. No third party shaped the work of physicians or the behavior of the hospital industry. Indeed, physicians, through their control of admission and discharge of patients, defined utilization patterns and accounted for the vast majority of health care expenditures. Interactions between the two decision systems centered on equipment purchases and space allocations during a time of continued growth. This expansion was supported by a cost-based reimbursement system.

Changes in the System

The system of relationships between hospitals and physicians was destined to change due to external forces. An important step in the change was the expansion and formalization of dependence on third parties.[1] The government's increased involvement in paying for health care services through Medicare and Medicaid was an infusion of dollars into the ongoing system of medical practice. These programs were intended to make services available to a wider range of the population.[18] Other problems addressed programmatically included a shortage of providers, the maldistribution of resources, and duplication of services in many areas of the nation. The initial approaches to correcting these problems included an expansion of the physician supply through established and new medical schools, the design and implementation of peer review processes to combat fraud, the development of alternative settings of care, and the development of new health practitioners to increase the flow of services to the medically disadvantaged. All of these initially reinforced the physician's claim to dominance in the system. The programs, which remained in place throughout the seventies and into the beginning of this decade, also laid the foundation for subsequent changes.

Perhaps the most important hint of what was to come was the passing of P.L. 93-641. This legislation established Health Systems Agencies (HSAs), which implemented certification-of-need legislation to encourage regionalization of health services and a more rational distribution of resources.[19] These agencies did not directly interfere with physicians' work nor advocate the growth of alternative services outside the hospital. Inherent in the mandate of the HSAs, however, was the belief that the health care system had inordinate duplication of services and often emphasized services that catered to the demands of the physician, who, after all, would fill available beds and use state-of-the-art (and thus the most expensive) technology.[20] The HSAs also assumed that hospitals, regardless of their ownership, would act out of self-interest rather than community interest. An important component of this self-interest was providing the "total workshop" for its physicians.[21] If rationality would not be achieved by collaboration between physicians and hospitals, the state would utilize its regulatory arm to achieve the systemwide balance necessary for an effective health care system. This legislation symbolized a shift in federal policies away from infusing more resources, with few constraints on their use, into a health care system organized to accommodate the historical interests of providers. The future would be one in which the government and other payers attempted to shape the system and influence how resources would be used.

The "crisis of cost," however, continued unabated as the driving force of change through the late seventies into the eighties. Regulatory responses were quickly joined, and then supplanted, by market-oriented approaches to controlling costs. Eliot Krause's "radical," and quickly dismissed statement[22] that health care would not substantially change until corporate America recognized the financial magnitude of the health care system and its influence on the economy, soon became conventional wisdom. The public and private sectors demanded greater accountability of providers and greater control over the distribution of health care dollars by directly influencing utilization patterns. At first the demand for cost containment was translated into the design and development of a variety of "cost effective" and "cost conscious" health care delivery organizations--especially the staff model HMO.[23] Acting on the belief that these settings would give attention to prevention, efficiency, and economy as they attempted to provide comprehensive care on a capitation basis, the federal government provided a variety of initiatives for the development of HMOs. At the same time, business coalitions attempted to influence health care policy on both the national and the local levels. And in some communities interactions between the business and health care sectors were characterized by substantial conflict.[24]

These actions, alone, did relatively little to change the power of physicians or hospitals. The hospital industry successfully acted, during the Carter administration, to head off cost containment efforts that would substantially restrict hospital spending, and physicians continued to control the majority of activity within the system. Increasingly it became clear that mechanisms that would directly affect the physician's behavior as well as more directly affect the hospital's incentives to constrain

Section I - The Context of Management

costs would be considered and, in some cases, adopted.

The eighties were entered with hopes of substantial reform in American medicine. The Reagan administration saw many of the regulatory mechanisms and government programs of the sixties and seventies as having precluded the principles of the marketplace from accomplishing their purported goal of balancing supply and demand and resulting in "natural" cost containment.[25] The new ideology of competition, deregulation, privatization, and monetarization[26-27] in Washington was supported by many hospital administrators who believed that the HSAs had stifled creativity, interfered with their ability to maintain a loyal medical staff, and indicated to physicians that administrators could not be trusted to make the truly important resource allocation decisions within the system. Not only were some physicians likely to shift their practices to hospitals where the latest technology was available; a growing number had moved their practices outside of the hospital. The sanctioning of competition would allow the hospital to become a player throughout the system.

Policies fostering competition dismantled the health systems agencies and encouraged the growth of a variety of forms of alternative health care delivery mechanisms. In very simple terms, it was believed that the rationality of the free marketplace would achieve systemic goals where regulatory efforts had apparently failed.

The marketplace that was to emerge in the eighties would be far from what many had envisioned as a classical "free market."[28] The aforementioned programs to constrain institutional behavior never really addressed the behavior of those who controlled the use of resources within the system--physicians. It was recognized that need for services was difficult to determine and the actual efficacy of medical procedures was increasingly difficult to define. By the late seventies, the cumulative evidence of studies conducted over the previous two decades cautioned policymakers that the rates of unnecessary hospitalization and surgery, as well as substantial variations in outcomes, average length of stay, and cost per case, were reason for concern.[29]

Such observations reinforced the belief that the traditional fee-for-service, retrospective reimbursement system offered few incentives for cost-effective behavior--on the part of physicians or hospitals. Suggested changes for controlling costs focused on the need to constrain the flow of patients and funds that fueled the growth of medical care. Two broad strategies designed to reshape the behavior of physicians and hospitals can be identified:

- The movement of large numbers of patients and physicians out of the traditional doctor/patient/hospital relationship into managed care systems such as HMOs and PPOs, thereby instituting patient agents to mediate, if not serve, the various interests involved.

▪ Reconceptualization of medical work and thus restructuring of the basis for reimbursing hospitals for the provision of care.

Both strategies lead to a redefinition of the traditional relationships between medical and administrative staffs.

Managed Care and Organized Patient Agents

The historical relationships between physicians, hospitals, and patients are logical if hospitals and physicians are the scarce resources around which the system is organized (i.e., the scarcity in the system is in the human and technological resources of the medical care system itself). It is our contention that a fundamental shift is occurring in the U.S. health care system. The predominant pattern of medical care organization, based on the aforementioned hospital-physician nexus of technology and expertise, is being replaced by the growing scarcity of paying patients. That is, the resources external to the medical care system that are the "inputs" essential for the medical care system to operate have become scarce relative to providers, and therefore constitute an important limiting factor in medical care organization.[30] The relative scarcity of paying patients strengthens the role of any organized patient agent that represents them in bargaining with providers for services.

Our health care system still needs the resources it has always needed to function. In the past, attention has been paid to the supply of physicians, facilities, and knowledge. These were the scarce resources around which the organization of medical care evolved. However, the relative abundance of these resources in the late 1980s, especially physicians and facilities, coupled with the increasing scarcity of paying patients, presages new dynamics in the ongoing transformation of the health care system. This suggests a fresh perspective may be useful in understanding these changes.

Physicians and hospitals have been the primary powers in determining the organization and financing of medical care. In the future, they will be joined by a third source of power, organized patient agents (or patient agent organizations). Organized patient agents may be any organizations that directly or indirectly control the flow of patients to providers.[31] This includes employers, insurers, unions, state and local governments, Medicare, and many others. The label "organized patient agents" signifies the important characteristics of these actors:

▪ They are organized in some form that is expected to endure, and they have a means of systematically influencing patient flows to providers (e.g., via payment mechanisms).

▪ They are the organizational analog to the physician role as "patient agent." They will act on behalf of individual patients (which will often coincide with their emerging institutional missions) in the organization and financing of medical care, just as physicians act on behalf of individual patients in the clinical realm.

It is important to distinguish between "organized patient agent" organizations and the structure of the delivery system. The delivery system includes those organizations that participate in the delivery of care, while patient agent organizations are those corporate actors that control the flow of patients into systems of care. Many HMOs and PPOs can be seen as the organizational mediating structures between the systematic interests of the providers on the one hand and the patient agent organizations on the other. The conflicting interests of physicians, hospitals, and organized patient agents will be balanced in the structural arrangements of the delivery system, e.g., through control of HMOs, PPOs, and other managed care systems. Emerging organizational arrangements may or may not benefit the interests of physicians anb/or hospitals, or both. Historically, physician and hospital interests coincided. The emergence of organized patient agents may bring latent divergent interests to light. Organized patient agents may even structure systems with opposing financial incentives for physicians and hospitals in an effort to maintain checks and balances in the system.

What resources do each of the three types of actors control? Hospitals control much of the advanced technological equipment that is too costly or complex for individual physicians to acquire. (An interesting trend is what may be a reversal in the decades long movement from office to hospital as a place to practice for physicians. This reversal is fostered by both the changing system of financial incentives and advancements in selected technologies that have reduced the financial and volume break-even thresholds for nonhospital acquisition of technology.) Hospitals also have a supply of human resources capable of caring continuously for very sick patients. Significantly, hospitals are often prominent community institutions. In smaller communities they may be a source of civic identity and one of the largest employers.

Physicians control the knowledge and expertise inherent in their training and experience. Collectively, they control the ability to make medical decisions through their legally enforced monopoly on medical practice. Physicians also have their patients and the loyalty and trust of established relationships developed, in some instances, over years of providing care. Thus their locus of control is in providing clinical care. The clinical mandate radiates out to others involved in providing that care (such as hospital staff) and to those receiving it (such as patients who follow doctors' recommendations for selecting hospitals).

Organized patient agents, as the label implies, influence patients or potential patients. Their focus is not, however, the direct clinical care of patients, but the organizational and financial arrangements surrounding clinical care. Their influence on patients is less directly tied to the discrete episode of illness than indirectly to the systematic organization

New Leadership in Health Care Management

of the medical care system in which that care will be provided. Influence is exercised via attempts to modify the behavior of hospitals and physicians (e.g., the imposition of reimbursement by DRGs, contracting for services on the basis of capitation, second opinion requirements, preadmission review, and concurrent utilization review).

The orientations of these three types of actors follow from their history, the resources they control, and the ideologies used to justify their control. Hospitals will continue to adapt to take advantage of their unique and complex community role and the ambiguity of their missions.[32] Indeed, some hospitals have attempted to short circuit the efforts of patient agents by forming HMOs and by purchasing physician practices. In these instances, hospitals serve the dual role of patient agent and delivery organization. Physicians will continue to use their clinical dominance to foster organizational and financial arrangements that protect their autonomy. Both physicians and hospitals will be confronted by organized patient agents that threaten to disrupt the symbiotic relations that have served them well for so long. Indeed, the key structural change in this perspective is the emergence of organized patient agents as actors who may have leverage similar to that of hospitals and physicians and who therefore have the potential to question established relationships.

A difference among the three types of actors may be the extent to which they have a national or local orientation. Medical care is, with minor exceptions, inherently local. Physicians, in keeping with their clinical mentality,[33] are most likely to have a local orientation. Hospitals share this orientation to some extent, although patterns of horizontal integration and systemization may introduce a tendency toward a regional or national orientation. Organized patient agents may be either local (a major employer) or national (the Health Care Financing Administration--HCFA). In any local area, the particular combination of the number of each type of actor and their orientations produces a different configuration and financing of services.

In order to understand the factors that influence hospital-physician relationships under conditions of "scarce patients," it is essential to recognize that they are mutually dependent on externally controlled flows of resources--patients and the funds to pay for their care. Again, this is not to suggest that health care is becoming a traditional consumer market and that the neoclassical economic models that are used to describe such markets will apply. Rather, we suggest that new, powerful corporate actors have and will exercise their power vis-a-vis both physicians and hospitals through their control of patient flows.

The Reconceptualization of Medical Work

Social scientists have provided important insight into the development of medicine as the model for our societal understanding of the concept

Section I - The Context of Management

of profession.[2,34,35] Under the professional model of medicine, each patient represented a unique set of circumstances. The clinical judgment of the physician required a substantial ability to apply "scientific" knowledge under a variety of conditions of uncertainty and indeterminacy. Given this "custom" view of medical work, few believed that medicine in the United States would lend itself to a form of social organization characterized by standard operating procedures, bureaucratic rules for the implementation of knowledge, and other features of the industrial sector. A professional principle, based upon the premises that medicine should itself formulate, control, and evaluate the strategic tasks of doctor's work, prevailed.[36]

As cost containment and competition have become important factors in the management of the health care system, the work of physicians has been subjected to both technical and bureaucratic control mechanisms formerly employed in industry only.[37] We are not yet prepared to argue that the professional model has been replaced by the bureaucratic model of work[36] or that physicians have been proletarianized.[38,39] DRGs, prior approval programs, second opinion programs, and PROs, however, all provide opportunities to question the physician's judgment and reorganize the physician's approach to work. Such systems mandate that cost, interpretation of test results in favor of less treatment, and other considerations not directly related to a particular patient become a part of clinical decision making. These mechanisms reconceptualize professional work as a series of steps "rationally" related to the production of what is believed to be a known product.

Since Taylor[40], the goal of standardization has been to ensure that the principles of successful and cost-effective outcomes are continuously applied to future work. This ideology about the nature of work poses a serious challenge to a profession that has long believed that its knowledge base is complex and esoteric. To serve the needs of the "unique" patient under conditions of uncertainty, work cannot be reduced to easily identifiable component parts. Today, the professional model is being challenged by a technical control model of work.

A more thorough understanding of technical control models allows us to understand the currents in the changing health care industry. The technical control model described by Edwards[37] is one in which management employs techniques not directly related to the product outcome for the purpose of circumscribing worker discretion. In industry, numeric-controlled machines and robots are applied in situations where work is easily routinized. These settings are characterized by repetitive tasks, predictable sequences of events, and little variation in the planned flow of work. This leads to the employment of assembly lines, piece rates, and automated systems to control labor. As work becomes repetitive and more predictable, workers become more interchangeable, and the labor force and jobs under technical control become more homogeneous.

Technical control in medicine is now related to computer and other modern technologies only indirectly. The important effect of these technologies is not tremendous increases in the predictability of outcomes so much as a "demystification" of professional knowledge and the trappings surrounding the profession.[41] A latent function of describing the physician's work in great detail and in standardized formats was the provision of information to third-party payers and planners who could unbundle medical work into component parts. The availability of this information fostered the application of cost accounting and industrial engineering techniques. Once the variation in parts was analyzed, the "repackaging" of medical work, as in DRGs, became possible. Employers may also engage in technical control by applying standards of time to be allotted to a given patient or procedure. The effect, in terms of scheduling patients, may be no different from the assembly line. In some instances, physicians are even rewarded for their collective efficiency (e.g., an HMO sharing surplus with employed physicians).

The full shift to a form of medical work organization not dominated by the physician could evolve only if the knowledge and skills associated with the occupation could be routinized, split down, or taken over by technicians or, as in conventional industry, by machines. This is not a likely scenario for modern medicine. To date, however, the application of industrial control mechanisms in medicine has been supported by a pool of physician/workers who are willing to collaborate and comply with those designing and implementing management control systems. Many physicians comply with bureaucratic mechanisms, supported by computer technology, to monitor the quality and quantity of outputs in the health care delivery system. This provides fuel for laymen to become involved in the reconceptualization of medical work and provides a set of ideas drawn upon by organized patient agents in their efforts to influence the organization and financing of medical care delivery systems. They rationalize increasing managerial control and challenge traditional professional autonomy, primarily through the development of a variety of managed care arrangements. These developments have stimulated strong responses from hospitals and physicians.

The Integration of Clinical and Managerial Cultures

It is noteworthy that the interfacing of clinical and managerial cultures takes place in the face of a wide variety of factors that traditionally distinguish the two groups. Managers and physicians often differ on the basis of occupational values, nature of education, nature of tasks, observability of work, career anchors, life-style, income, professional needs, stratification within the occupational group, and form of quality control.[42] To the extent that medical schools and academic health centers have been highly resistant to change and continue to be controlled by physicians with academic values, physicians will not have the opportunity to develop an appreciation and understanding of manage-

Section I - The Context of Management

ment until after they have left these institutional settings. And only a few graduate programs in health services administration have placed an increased focus on managing "with" physicians.

If we are correct that the United States is entering an era in which the profession of medicine as well as provider organizations will break down many of the traditional lines separating their organization and control, there is a need for the two groups to understand one another and be prepared to restructure and negotiate their activities on the basis of the multiple realities of work life. Simendinger and Pasmore surveyed administrative physicians and key hospital administrators to identify the most important factors inhibiting enhanced cooperation.[43] Both groups indicated cooperation was inhibited by perceptions of dishonesty, incompetence, and a lack of initiative or enthusiasm on the part of the other. Beyond this, physicians were criticized for refusal to listen, arbitrary decision making, manipulation, and a lack of followthrough, while administrators were criticized for lacking intelligence and/or education, wasting time, and having divided loyalties. In addition to differences in training and perspective, the very structure of the hospital has worked against collaboration between physicians and administrators. Ruelas and Leatt[44] list the following issues faced by physician executives as a result of hospital organizational structure: unclear accountability, unclear definition of tasks, lack of adequate information for decision making, and an inadequate reward system for managerial functions.

A number of analysts, including Glandon and Morrisey[45] and Shortell[46] describe a variety of organizational strategies with the potential to resolve the tensions between hospitals and physicians:

- *Promotion of "shared common interest."* In this strategy, outlined by Glandon and Morrisey, physicians maintain autonomy, but the hospital or patient agent educates physicians regarding cost-benefit issues. For example, the hospital or organized patient agent may provide performance feedback by DRG and by individual physician, with the expectation that physicians will compare themselves to the norm and thereby self-correct. This system typically utilizes committees, requires high physician involvement, and works best with high admitters, surgeons, and physicians in sole community hospitals, all of whom are highly dependent upon the hospital.

Given the release of performance of both hospitals and individual physicians by HCFA, the shared common interest will, we believe, become increasingly important. Not only will hospitals be able to evaluate physicians in terms of their practicing cost-effective medicine, but physicians, hospitals, patient agents, screening agencies, and the community will all be placed in a position to evaluate, accurately or not, the performance of individuals and institutions on a variety of gross outcome measures including mortality and morbidity. The assumptions in releasing data and encouraging a "shared common interest" is that a convergence of practice patterns will result in higher quality and more cost effective care. Yet state-of-the-art medicine remains highly discretionary. Empirical studies with large numbers of patients, adequately controlling for case mix, are often lacking to demonstrate the effectiveness of one approach over another. Cost data are easily interpreted, while data on effectiveness are neither plentiful nor conclusive. This makes it especially difficult to determine the cost-effectiveness of different practice styles. Yet organized patient agents will make decisions on the basis of such data--requiring that hospitals and physicians enter into collaborative arrangements and pay close attention to costs and the documentation of patient benefits derived from care provided.

- *Joint ventures.* Joint venture rela' ..ships, in the form of preferred provider arrangements, merge the financial interests of hospitals and participating physicians to shape desirable practice patterns. Increasingly, joint ventures involve services other than in-patient medical care, including shared or co-financed laboratories, diagnostic imaging centers, ambulatory surgery services, and medical office buildings.[47] Relman has argued that physicians should not participate in such plans because of the inherent conflict of interest the strategy creates for the physician.[48] A major ethical issue, for example, arises for physicians who are owners and providers in the same organization. These clinicians may experience conflicts of interest when what is best for the individual patient (or for the greater good of society) may not be in the best interests of the image or economic security/profitability of the organization. This issue of self-interest, of course, is not a new one. The solo physician in fee-for-service practice is subject to many of the same pressures.[49]

- *Redesigning the medical staff.* Although medical staffs have traditionally been informally structured, and lacking integration, the trend is toward formalizing the structure and providing opportunities for physicians to have greater participation in hospital governance.[50,51] Shortell[52] builds the case for the formalization strategy by demonstrating the effect of medical staff organization on quality of care: Highly structured organizations have higher quality of care, and greater physician involvement in hospital affairs appears to be related to higher quality of care.

Glandon and Morrisey also recognize the advantages of the strategy of redesigning the medical staff through a limited access model.[45] Under this method, the hospital board evaluates applicants to the medical staff and reviews reappointments on the basis of demonstrated cost-effective practice patterns (in addition to quality of care and other utilization review data). There are a number of inherent legal and ethical problems in the board reviewing these decisions by merging economic and quality issues.

Section I - The Context of Management

Shortell[47] depicts several models of medical staff relations, including an innovative model that may accomplish the goals of restructuring the relationship between the medical staff and hospital by removing the medical staff from the hospital and providing for negotiations between the hospital and an independent physician group for comprehensive physician services. In this "independent corporate model," the medical staff is a separate legal entity and "negotiates with the hospital for its services in return for receiving the hospital's functional patient care and administrative support services."

- *Physicians as corporate employees.* Although it has been suggested that the employment of physicians is a sound mechanism for managing hospital-physician relations,[45] it is not at all clear that employed physicians have less autonomy or are more likely to follow clinical protocols.[53-55] Certainly Glandon and Morrisey[45] are correct that direct employment gives hospitals more control over administrative decisions, allows for improved scheduling and coordination, and provides the resources for contracting for alternative delivery systems. At the same time, the peer review structures that accompany employment may provide the medical staff with even more power to establish its own standards and operating procedures to meet the profession's views of patient requirements. This is consistent with Freidson's notion of the importance of colleague control.[49] Hospitals that have invested heavily in purchasing physician practices should closely examine the pros and cons of their behavior, lest they find themselves with an even stronger and more organized group of professional employees.

Physician Responses

Because the initiatives of the sixties and seventies were compatible with the culture of medicine, they affirmed the dominance of the physician.[1] Physicians were made responsible for organizing PSROs and for designing the new primary care training programs. Government initiatives for financing and delivering more medical services offered the profession some relief from full accountability for the outcomes of the "underdeveloped" U.S. primary care system and of "underplanned" allocation of specialists in the U.S. At the same time, the centrality of physician manpower to the continued development of the health care delivery system was maintained.

In the eighties, physician reimbursement has not yet been drastically changed, and physicians' practice of medicine has been somewhat sheltered from changes in the health care system. Hospitals, in their transition to DRGs, have introduced changes that affected physicians' hospital practice. Although organized patient agents, in their cost containment efforts, have recently influenced patient volumes and reimbursement levels, physicians in different parts of the U.S. are unequally pressured and many have only just begun to feel the impact of and to respond to these changes. By early 1988, there were several new models for physician reimbursement under consideration. The implementation of such models has the potential to further change the relationship between the physician and the health care delivery system.

In recognition of the changing relationship between the physician and his "employer," Marcus[56] argues that physicians, to preserve their strengths as professionals, must embrace labor mechanisms, such as unionization and collective bargaining, that have worked well for other occupations. This, he believes, is the most effective way for physicians to maintain their workplace position as "de facto employees of the new multibillion-dollar corporate entities that have taken economic control of health care."

It is difficult to predict how physicians will react to continued changes in their world of work. Some analysts[57] have argued that physicians should maintain their mandate "to do all they can, within reason, for their patients." This may mean direct confrontation and defiance by physicians, with organized patient agents and the variety of control systems employed to monitor and shape clinical decision making. There are strong pressures upon physicians to conform and cooperate with the logic of a health care system based upon an industrial or corporate model. Yet the sounds of physician discontent with the day-to-day practice of medicine are mounting. Surely the physician, as a potentially alienated employee, is cause for concern. From what we know about other occupations, likely responses from physicians may include:

- *Manipulation of control systems.* Examples of this include the variety of "gaming" techniques emerging with DRGs and the use of physician capital to avoid rules aimed at the regulation of hospitals.

- *Job (setting) changes to maximize autonomy and minimize control by others.* The establishment of surgical and emergency clinics by individual physicians, for example, allows the physician to avoid some of the features found unsatisfactory in institutional practice.

- *Specialty changes.* As certain specialties are perceived as overpopulated and overregulated, physicians will seek to enter fields where there is a perceived need and a chance for autonomy.

- *Career (occupation) changes.* Physicians are increasingly expressing dissatisfaction with the practice of medicine and may search for careers that allow them to use their medical training outside of the clinical arena. The return of the physician to the administrative arena is one sign of this movement. Early retirement will become increasingly attractive to successful physicians.

- *The formation of central work values and attitudes around the*

Section I - The Context of Management

physician's working conditions–rather than around client-oriented issues. As a result of training that emphasizes cost containment and the values associated with an entrepreneurial system, physicians will overemphasize treatment of the patients in a customer-like manner. Although this may yield some of the desirable effects of improved consumer behavior, the latent function may be one of increased risk to the patient.

- *Collective action.* As suggested above, there is a movement among physicians to embrace collective labor mechanisms to deal with their dissatisfaction.[56] Unionization may not result in the physician repositioning himself as a "designer" of the workplace. Aronowitz has demonstrated that unions often become a tool for maintaining control and ensuring workforce participation of employees.[58] There is no reason to assume that physicians' unions will not succumb to the tendency to focus upon salary and benefits rather than changes in the actual conditions of work.

- *Increased stress and deviant behavior related to the workplace.* There is already a crisis in physician abuse of drugs and alcohol. The decreasing ability of the physician to control his or her own destiny in the workplace and achieve the social, emotional, and economic goals associated with a medical career may signal increased risk.[59]

- *Conflict between hospitals and physicians.* Hospital administrators have begun to assess the risk associated with institutional practice by a pool of attending physicians within the community. The result of this, as discussed above, may be restriction of access to a very select group of physicians. At the same time, "medical staff privileges may be granted on the basis of the physician's conformity" to the economic goals of the institution.[57]

Speculation about the future of medicine must recognize the changing demograpic pool of applicants to and graduates from medical schools. With one out of every three medical students being female, the increased feminization of the profession begs intensive study.[60] We have relatively little knowledge about the differential responses by male and female physicians to extra-professional control mechanisms and organized patient agents. As the public recognition of medicine as "the premiere career choice" changes, those who self-select into the profession may be less attached to the values and norms of the past and more willing to see their careers as legitimately affected by outside pressures from nonprofessional groups--including organized patient agents. Finally, as elites in academic health centers accept the mandates of cost control and are affected by organized patient agents, the professional socialization system may legitimize the imposition of values from outside upon the behavior of the physician.

The reconceptualization of medical work within technical control should not be seen as totally imposed by organized patient agents on unwilling physicians. The reorganization of medical work offers many advantages to some physicians. Predictability of work hours and freedom from the business aspects of establishing and running a practice are valued by many physicians. Substitutability of physicians may be decried by some practitioners who have labored to cultivate large patient groups that depend on them, but it does allow physicians more flexibility in vacations, scheduling, and even in changing jobs. The expansion of delivery organizations provides many opportunities for physicians who want administrative careers.

Discussion

Physicians, individually and as a group, have controlled the practice of medicine and have shaped the delivery system. That the truly important decisions about medical work would remain within the hands of the physician was affirmed throughout the sixties and seventies and into the eighties. We have indicated that a variety of environmental factors are pressing for greatly decreased clinical discretionary power for physicians. The practice of medicine has not historically included many formal mechanisms for coordinated decision making, but the need for these is growing. The widely different perspectives of physicians, hospital administrators, hospital boards, consumer interest groups, legislators, medical insurers, and others with a financial, professional, or personal interest in health care policy create conflicts as these groups all vie for greater control. Organized patient agents are setting policy that replaces much of the highly decentralized authority of individual physicians. The system emerging in the United States may well have many of the management components that have emerged in "totally" managed systems, such as in the United Kingdom.[61] It is possible that new health care delivery systems may result in more equitable, cooperative relationships between physicians, administrators, and payers, with clarification of the expectations and responsibilities of the parties concerned.

There is no doubt that many physicians recognize the erosion of their scope of influence. To these clinicians, the debate over moving from a model of health care based upon the "professional" principle to one based on the "industrial" principle may appear to be an academic exercise. When professional domain is challenged, any intrusion appears to be important. What is important to the clinician is the ability to deliver high-quality care at a level acceptable to peers. Should control mechanisms block this goal, forcing behaviors inconsistent with the range of normative behavior[33], the crisis of cost will be compounded by a crisis of quality.

In the face of the continuing crisis of cost, it is reasonable to assume that the physician may become active in national efforts to ensure an equitable system, one protected against collapse by unreasonable fiscal growth. There is reason to fear, however, that the physician will become just another commodity that hospitals or other delivery organizations and patient agents purchase, substantially removing the physician from deliberations within the system. To the extent that the physician is dropped as a real partner in the redesign of the system, the very foundations of the practice of medicine remain threatened.

The future roles of physicians in our health care organizations are uncertain. What does seem certain is that physicians will attempt to influence the evolution of how medical work is organized. This may take the form of physicians adopting new roles, many of them managerial, in the system. Rather than physicians' becoming bureaucratized, existing and emerging administrative structures may become professionalized in order for physicians to maintain their influence over the conditions of their work. There is emerging evidence that the professional model and the new forms of medical organization are compatible, allowing physicians to exercise autonomy. At the same time, there are doubts about the ability of these organizations to achieve the cost containment goals of organized patient agents.[62] If this ambiguity continues, the future of medicine will be even more dynamic and will offer more varied roles for physicians than in the past.

References

1. Starr, P. *The Social Transformation of American Medicine.* New York: Basic Books, Inc., 1982.

2. Freidson, E. *Profession of Medicine. A Study of the Sociology of Applied Knowledge.* New York: Dodd, Mead and Company, 1970.

3. Freidson, E. *Professional Dominance: The Social Structure of Medical Care.* New York: Atherton Press, Inc., 1973.

4. Ver Steeg, D., and Croog, S. "Hospitals and Related Health Care Delivery Settings," in *Handbook of Medical Sociology,* Third Edition. Englewood Cliffs: Prentice-Hall, Inc., 1979.

5. Rosner, D. *A Once Charitable Enterprise.* Cambridge: Cambridge University Press, 1982.

6. Vogel, M. *The Invention of the Modern Hospital: Boston, 1870-1930.* Chicago: University of Chicago Press, 1980.

7. Rosenberg, C. "Inward Vision and Outward Glance: The Shaping of the American Hospital, 1880-1914," in *Social History and Social Policy.* New York: Academic Press, 1981.

8. Stevens, R. *American Medicine and the Public Interest.* New Haven: Yale University Press, 1971.

9. Hirschman, A. *Exit, Voice, and Loyalty: Responses to Decline in Firms, Organizations, and States.* Cambridge, Mass.: Harvard University Press, 1970.

10. Weber, M. *Essays in Sociology.* New York: Oxford University Press, 1946.

11. Gaffney, J., and Glandon, G. "The Physician's Use of the Hospital." *Health Care Management Review* 7(3):49-58, Summer 1982.

12. Steinwald, B. "Hospital-Based Physicians: Current Issues and Descriptive Evidence." *Health Care Financing Review* 2(1):63-75, Summer 1980.

13. Smith, H. "Two Lines of Authority: The Hospital's Dilemma." *Modern Hospital* 84(3):59-64, March 1955.

14. Pauly, M., and Redish, M. "The Not-For-Profit Hospital as a Physicians' Cooperative." *American Economic Review* 63(1):87-99, March 1973.

15. Harris, J. "The Internal Organization of Hospitals: Some Economic Implications." *Bell Journal of Economics* 8(2):467-482, Fall 1977.

16. Saltman, R., and Young, D. "The Hospital Power Equilibrium: An Alternative View of the Cost Containment Dilemma." *Journal of Health Politics, Policy, and Law* 6(3):391-418, Fall 1981.

17. Roemer, M., and Friedman, J. "Doctors in Hospitals: Medical Staff Organization and Hospital Performance." Baltimore: Johns Hopkins Press, 1971.

18. Davis, K. *National Health Insurance: Benefits, Costs and Consequences.* Washington, D.C.: The Brookings Institution, 1975.

19. Bice, T. "Health Services Planning and Regulation," in *Introduction to Health Services,* Second Edition. New York: John Wiley and Sons, 1984.

20. Roemer, M. "Bed Supply and Hospital Utilization: A National Experiment." *Hospitals* 35(21):36, Nov. 1, 1961.

21. Pauly, M. *Doctors and Their Workshops: Economic Models of Physician Behavior.* Chicago: The University of Chicago Press, 1980.

22. Krause, E. *Power and Illness: The Political Sociology of Health and Medical Care.* New York: Elsevier North-Holland, Inc., 1977.

23. Brown, L. *Politics and Health Care Organization: HMOs as Federal Policy.* Washington, D.C.: The Brookings Institution, 1983.

24. Goldbeck, W. "Health Care Coalitions," in *Health Care Cost Management: Private Sector Initiatives.* Ann Arbor, Mich.: Health Administration Press, 1984.

25. Salkever, D., and Bice, T. "The Impact of Certification-of-Need Controls on Hospital Investment." *Millbank Memorial Fund Quarterly* 54(2):185-214, Spring 1976.

Section I - The Context of Management

26. Ginzberg, E. "The Monetarization of Medical Care." *New England Journal of Medicine* 310(18):1162-5, May 3, 1984.

27. Ginzberg, E. "The Restructuring of US Health Care." *Inquiry* 23(3):272-281, Fall 1986.

28. Enthoven, A. *Health Plan.* Reading, Mass.: Addison-Wesley, 1980.

29. Donabedian, A. "The Epidemiology of Quality." *Inquiry* 22(3):282-292, Fall 1985.

30. Pfeffer, J., and Salancik, G. *The External Control of Organizations: A Resource Dependence Perspective.* New York: Harper and Row, 1978.

31. Havighurst, C. "The Changing Locus of Decision Making in the Health Care Sector," in *Health Policy in Transition: A Decade of Health Politics, Policy and Law.* Durham, N.C.: Duke University Press, 1987.

32. Stevens, R. "A Poor Sort of Memory': Voluntary Hospitals and Government before the Depression." *Milbank Memorial Fund Quarterly/Health and Society* 60(4):551-84, Fall 1982.

33. Freidson, E. Professional Powers. *A Study of the Institutionalization of Formal Knowledge.* Chicago: University of Chicago Press, 1986.

34. Hughes, E. *Men and Their Work.* New York: The Free Press of Glencoe, 1958.

35. Wilensky, H. "The Professionalization of Everyone?" *American Journal of Sociology* 70(9):137-58, Sept. 1964.

36. Freidson, E. "Professions and the Occupational Principle," in *Medical Men and Their Work.* Chicago: Aldine-Atherton, 1972.

37. Edwards, R. *Contested Terrain. The Transformation of the Workplace in the Twentieth Century.* New York: Basic Books, Inc., 1979.

38. Haug, M. "Deprofessionalization: An Alternative Hypothesis for the Future." *The Sociological Review Monograph* 20(12)7:195-211, Dec. 1973.

39. McKinlay, J., and Arches, J. "Towards the Proletarianization of Physicians." *International Journal of Health Services* 15(2):161-95, Spring 1985.

40. Taylor, F. *The Principles of Scientific Management.* New York: Harper, 1947.

41. Haug, M. "Computer Technology and the Obsolescence of the Concept of Profession," in *Work and Technology.* Beverly Hills, Calif.: Sage Publications, 1977.

42. Friss, L., and others. Working paper, 1987.

43. Simendinger, E., and Pasmore, W. "Developing Partnerships Between Physicians and Healthcare Executives." *Hospital and Health Services Ad-*

ministration 29(6):21-35, Nov.-Dec. 1984.

44. Ruelas, E., and Leatt, P. "Roles of Physician Executives in Hospitals." *Journal of Health Administration Education* 3(2):151-169, Summer 1985.

45. Glandon, G., and Morrisey, M. "Redefining the Hospital-Physician Relationship under Prospective Payment." *Inquiry* 23(2):166-75, Summer 1986.

46. Shortell, S. "The Medical Staff of the Future: Replanting the Garden." *Frontiers of Health Services Management* 1(3):3-48, Feb. 1985.

47. Wolff, S. "Joint Ventures: the Trends and the Potential Pitfalls." *Trustee* 38(10):13-16, Oct. 1985.

48. Relman, A. "The New Medical-Industrial Complex." *New England Journal of Medicine* 303(17):963-70, Oct. 23, 1980.

49. Freidson, E. *Patients' Views of Medical Practice.* New York: Russell Sage, 1961.

50. Noie, N., and others. "A Survey of Hospital Medical Staffs-Part 1." *Hospitals* 57(23):80-84, Dec. 1, 1983.

51. Noie, N., and others. "A Survey of Hospital Medical Staffs-Part 2." *Hospitals* 57(24):91-94, Dec. 16, 1983.

52. Shortell, S. "Hospital Medical Staff Organization: Structure, Process, and Outcome." *Hospital Administration* 19:96-107, Spring 1974.

53. Sullivan, R. "Physician Extenders, Protocols, and Quality Medical Care." *Bulletin of the New York Academy of Medicine* 52(1):125-38, Jan. 1976.

54. Hall, R. "Professionalization and Bureaucratization." *American Sociological Review* 33(2):92-104, Feb. 1968.

55. Freidson, E. "Reorganization of the Medical Profession." *Medical Care Review* 42(1):11-36, Spring 1985.

56. Marcus, S. "Trade Unionism for Doctors: An Idea Whose Time Has Come." *New England Journal of Medicine* 310(23):1508-11, June 7, 1984.

57. Spivey, B. "The Relation Between Hospital Management and Medical Staff Under a Prospective-Payment System." *New England Journal of Medicine* 310(15):984-6, April 12, 1984.

58. Aronowitz, S. *False Promises.* New York: McGraw Hill, 1973.

59. Phillips, E. *Stress, Health, and Psychological Problems in the Major Professions.* Washington, D.C.: University Press of America, 1982.

60. Davis, K. "How Do Practice Styles of Women and Men Differ?" *Internist* 27(3):11-12, March 1986.

Section I - The Context of Management

61. Schneller, E., and Kirkman-Liff, B. "Health Services Management Change in the U.S. and the British N.H.S." Forthcoming in the *Journal of Health Administration Education*–Special edition on the Griffiths Report in the U.K.

62. Wolinsky, F., and Marder, W. *The Organization of Medical Practice and the Practice of Medicine.* Ann Arbor, Mich.: Health Administration Press, 1985.

Eugene S. Schneller, PhD, is Professor and Director, Robert G. Hughes, PhD, is Assistant Professor, and Pamela Hood Szivek is Research Assistant, School of Health Administration and Policy, College of Business, Arizona State University, Tempe, Arizona.

CHAPTER 3

Why Physicians Move Into Management

by Michael Guthrie, MD, MBA

Why would a successful physician choose to leave the rewards and satisfactions of practice to take on the uncertainties and unfamiliarity of a management position?

Many outsiders assume that the stresses of competition, relative incompetence, impending retirement, or neurotic impulses drive most physician executives from the noble practice of medicine into the bureaucracy of management. This chapter is designed to explore the real reasons physicians make this surprising, but increasingly common move. The reasons predicted by motivational theory are supported by a recent comprehensive self-report survey from physician executives themselves, compiled by the American Academy of Medical Directors.[1]

Understanding why physicians become managers is increasingly important, because surveys show that nearly two-thirds of all hospitals with 200 or more beds have medical directors or are considering medical director positions.[2] Data from this same survey show a steadily increasing number of hospitals interested in the medical director position. More physicians are also interested in medical management positions related to medical staff affairs, accreditation activities, quality assurance, medical education, and utilization review, or as directors or chairmen of clinical departments. Such positions are increasing in clinics and HMOs as well. With the rapid expansion of HMOs and PPOs over the past five years, and the predicted continuing growth of alternative delivery systems, the role of medical director in prepaid and other managed care programs is also rapidly increasing in importance.

The need for physician executives is increasing because there is pressure for more physician involvement in administrative decision-making in all of these medical environments--hospitals, clinics, group practices, HMOs, and PPOs. In addition, because businesses around the country are taking a more sophisticated approach to their dealings with the health care system, the physician executive plays an important role in negotiations and communication with industrial buyers and third-party payers. Finally, the political pressures on the health care system and increasing governmental control demand the response of a sure-footed clinical and business orientation provided by the physician executive.

Dissatisfaction or Motivation?

Why, then, does a physician make this remarkable transition into a managerial position? Both common sense and motivational theory[3] provide reasons that are confirmed by the self-report survey data. First, taking physicians as a select segment of the population, it is fairly obvious that physicians have to be bright and well-motivated to make it through the socialization and educational processes to finally become a medical professional. These individuals show a high need for achievement, recognition, and challenge, as well as an expectation for continuing rewards from their occupation beyond the pay and benefits provided. These rewards come in the form of personal appreciation for the significance of the tasks that they perform, the ability to operate with relative autonomy, the ability and opportunity to see their work completed from beginning to end, the chance to get some direct feedback from the work that they perform for others, and the continuing opportunity for challenge, advancement, social prestige, intellectual challenge, autonomy, and high levels of skill variety.

For many physicians, however, medical practice turns out to be something of a disappointment as the years advance. After a few years in clinical practice, a physician with a high need for growth and achievement may find that actual day-to-day practice offers little opportunity for continuing challenge and growth. Although individual patient care is still important and rewarding, many physicians look around for the opportunity to make a larger impact on the health care system or on society as a whole. Dissatisfaction is expressed in a variety of ways. Some physicians seek advanced certification or subspecialty training. Many physicians look to outside activities in their communities or in their subspecialty organizations, where leadership and challenge are a continuing part of the scene. Some physicians seek positions of leadership and authority in the organization with which they are associated professionally or in the political structure of a medical society or association. In recent years, many physicians have become active in organizing alternative delivery systems, entrepreneurial medical delivery alternatives, or political action groups that have a policy-making influence. Many of these same physicians have considered moving into part-time or full-time managerial positions in a health care organization.

Survey Data

In 1986 the American Academy of Medical Directors undertook a survey of physician executives, all members of the Academy, to ascertain their reasons for moving from practice into management and to analyze their satisfaction with the results of this move. From the approximately 1,100 responses to the survey, some trends and distinctions are apparent.

Though the reasons for the change from practice to management are multiple and individualistic, there are some common themes in the self-reports. Ninety-seven percent of the respondents said that a desire for leadership was somewhat or very important. One hundred percent of them cited the desire for challenge as important. These physicians were looking for more professional growth (99 percent somewhat or very important) and continued autonomy (92 percent).

The respondents wanted to have an impact on many people (89 percent) and to be involved in health policy decisions (73 percent very important).

The desire for income by itself was very important for only a limited number of the respondents (28 percent cited this as very important) and the desire for additional technical skills was important for only a third.

Given these desires, the physician executives who became managers frequently got what they were looking for in leadership opportunities, impact on people, authority, challenge, and opportunities for professional growth. Eight-four percent reported that they achieved opportunities for increased impact on people, 70 percent reported additional challenges, 89 percent reported opportunities for leadership, 80 percent reported increases in authority, and 61 percent felt they had achieved additional professional growth.

However, sometimes the physician executives did not get as much autonomy or control over working conditions as they expected. Income growth was less than they might have made in practice (53 percent reported less income than they expected). Thirty-five percent reported more autonomy, and 38 percent reported less. Thirty-seven percent reported more control over their everyday working lives, and 38 percent reported less.

Goals for Change

These same physician executives were asked to report on what their major goals were when they made the change from practice to management in a health care organization. The goals reported vary substantially, but several were mentioned by many respondents in similar words. Physicians wanted to improve health services and to be part of new directions in health care. They also wanted to influence health care policy decisions for health care as a whole. In addition, many physicians candidly reported that they wanted to improve their personal positions and to search out new sources of personal and professional satisfaction.

Section I - The Context of Management

Influences on the Decision

What do physician executives report as having been the major influences on their career changes? The attractions of management itself are reported by 58 percent of the sample as having been an important aspect of their willingness to make the change. The physician's family gave some or a great deal of encouragement for the transition 47 percent of the time and was discouraging only 13 percent of the time. Peers and colleagues in medical practice generally encouraged the physician to make the move (45 percent reported that they were somewhat or greatly encouraged by their peers), but there was more substantial encouragement from nonphysician colleagues in their organizations (65 percent reported that they were somewhat or greatly encouraged by nonphysicians in their peer groups).

Contradicting some speculation, competition from other physicians was reported by 81 percent of the respondent physician executives to have been of little or no influence in making the decision to move into management. Patient demands, however, were somewhat or very much of an influence for 43 percent. Physical demands, likewise, were somewhat or very influential for one-third of the respondents. Time and emotional demands played some part in the decision-making for about a third of respondents. Boredom with medical practice was reported to have been of significant influence by 24 percent of the respondents.

Given these influences and their goals for the change from practice to management, how do the physician executives look back on the personal success of this transition? For the most part, the outcomes reported by the respondents are very positive. Eighty-eight percent plan to remain in management, and 96 percent are somewhat or very satisfied with their managerial roles. Although burdened by the misconceptions of their medical colleagues (47 percent report that they are seen as "administrators" by other physicians), physician executives still report positively on the authority and prestige they have achieved in the move to managerial positions.

Conclusions

Physicians move into management positions for many positive reasons, most of them having to do with their personal need for growth, achievement, and challenge rather than their fear of the negative pressures of medical practice.

The positive reasons that are cited for interest in management include impact on people in a scope that is beyond that possible in private practice, influence on policy-making decisions, power in their organizations and in their communities, and authority for decision-making on a scale impossible for an individual physician.

Negative influences also exist that push physicians in the direction of management, including some dissatisfaction with the everyday aspects of medical practice, physical demands, the demands of patient care itself, and boredom.

Most physicians are encouraged by family and friends to make the change, even though nonphysicians seem more encouraging than peers. Most physician executives report that they are satisfied with the change, identify themselves now as managers, and plan to remain in their management positions. When asked if they ever miss medical practice, many physicians state clearly that, although they enjoyed patient care, they have found they can help more patients by being managers than they would ever have been able to help as solo physicians. Their roles are increasingly recognized as important for the future of the health care system, particularly in balancing the demands for high-quality patient care with the economic issues in our turbulent health care marketplace.

As these physician executives mature in their managerial roles and acquire greater self-definition and professional definition, they will function as role models for career decisions by many other physicians facing the same personal issues and seeking additional challenge and impact. More and more physicians can be expected to select a medical management option. As the profession grows, it is also likely that its interests will move, perhaps slowly but definitely, to a more general view of management. While physicians can be expected to continue to play major management roles in the medical areas of organizational management, they can also be expected to take on nonmedical management roles.

Why do physicans move into management? When physician executives themselves are asked, it is because of the challenges and opportunities that this new profession offers.

References

1. Montgomery, K. "Today's Physician Manager: A New Breed." *Physician Executive* 12(5):14-17, Sept.-Oct. 1986.

2. Lloyd, J. "Growth in Medical Director Numbers Continues." *Physician Executive* 12(3):10-13, May-June 1986.

3. Guthrie, M., and others. "Productivity: How Much Does This Job Mean?" *Nursing Management* 15(2):16-20, Feb. 1985.

Michael Guthrie, MD, MBA, is Vice President for Business Development, Penrose Health System, Colorado Springs, Colo.

Section I - The Context of Management

CHAPTER 4

The Unique Contribution of the Physician Executive to Health Care Management

or

"Does the MD Degree a Better Manager Make?"

by David J. Ottensmeyer, MD, FACPE, and M.K. Key, PhD

T his chapter assesses whether the physician executive is truly a management asset to the health care organization. What attributes make the physician more or less valuable in an executive capacity? One cannot simply assume that a good doctor will make a good manager or that preparation to practice medicine fosters the skills needed to manage organizations. In fact, some feel that physicians should only practice medicine and leave management to "professional managers." Through a review of historical precedents, physician involvement in health care organizations, the current context of medical practice, and the unique socialization of the physician, we will examine the tenet that physicians possess distinct qualities and experience suiting them for management in the health care field.

History of Physician Involvement in Medical Organization and Health Care Mangement

The health care industry of the past was not a management-intensive undertaking and provided few opportunities for physicians to develop management skills. The health care business itself was poorly organized and so required little management. Of greater importance, the commitment of the medical profession to "professionalism" created intense resistance to the management process.

The early health care system was fragmented and functioned with little structure, planning, or coordination. The "doctor" side of the business was an enterprise of small businessmen and women carried out in the style of a cottage industry. Starr describes medical practice as a profession derived from the European guild system of past centuries. It was caught up in the English class struggles of the 18th and 19th centuries and in the quest of the physician to gain some level of qualitative social recognition alongside the established aristocracy. This effort continued during the days of colonization of the North American continent, when the rootlets of the present medical profession were transplanted from England.[1]

The profession continued to evolve successfully into a "sovereign" profession--a term Starr uses to depict the social privilege, economic power, and political influence of the medical profession. Among the learned professions, it became the "profession among professions." It carefully and tightly controlled competition within its membership by control of the system of preparation (medical education), by restricting access with systems of licensure and credentialing, and by internally enforcing codes of ethics that upheld standards and controlled undesirable influences. These normative influences have all been incorporated into the doctrine of "professionalism," which has been strongly internalized by the rank and file membership. Professionalism focuses on concepts of self-governance and peer control by a collegial group, licensed and privileged because of its special body of knowledge.

Such professional sovereignty was ill-suited to management by non-peers (as kings cannot be ruled by lesser citizens)--indeed is averse to any management at all. Current manifestations of the historical resistance to management include the idealization of the solo practitioner, the notion of an independent self-governing medical staff, private practice of medicine, and physician scorn of the organized HMO. It is rationalized by the notion of "patient advocacy" and fortified by a fierce commitment to fee-for-service reimbursement, which ensures control of the economic exchange at a very basic level within the system. Thus the structure of the early health care system, the social positioning of the physician in society, and the professional structure of medicine did not lay a good foundation for development of management as a vocation concern of physicians.

In the first half of this century, the roles that did develop for physician executives were often token in nature or political in content. Characteristically, they were far removed from management policy or decision making. They usually derived from an organizational need for technical, not management, expertise. Initially the nature of physician involvement in organizations included the following:

- Bureaucrat

- Academic

- Technological supervisor or leader of a medical team

- Coordinator of a program

Section I - The Context of Management

- Advisor to management

- Interface between line management and the medical staff

- Elder statesman

- Public relation spokesperson

Physicians often filled the role of director in departments of public health, administering a *bureaucratic* subdivision of a jurisdiction's health operation. In this role, they depended upon their professional expertise for legitimacy. The *academic* is personified in the chairmanship of an academic department. The master/student pedagogical environment, as well as the Herr Professor/junior staff relationship, depicts the dynamic in that setting. In governmental organizations, such as the Centers for Disease Control, physicians similarly undertook the role of *technical supervisors* or *coordinators of programs*. The medical coordinator in a group practice is another example of a coordinator or facilitator of operations. *Advisors to management* are found in insurance companies and industrial organizations in a staff role. The military system frequently has a "staff surgeon" on the commander's staff. In the military, physicians assumed executive/command positions beginning in the early 20th century, when separate organizations (hospitals) were formed as identifiable entities in the troop list.

The need for an *interface agent between medical staff* and line management was the genesis of the "medical director" position, especially in hospitals. The medical director or director of professional affairs position was frequently filled by an *elder statesman*, who possessed the political savvy and wisdom to avoid "rocking the boat." Finally, the *public relations spokesperson* was seen in the public performances by Dr. Dennis O'Leary--who is now chief executive officer (CEO) of the Joint Commission on the Accreditation of Healthcare Organizations (JCAHO). His face became publicly known on evening television while President Reagan was hospitalized at George Washington University Hospital in Washington, D.C., subsequent to the attempt on the President's life in 1981. Dr. O'Leary was medical director at the hospital at that time.

These positions hold several things in common. Typically, physicians were hired for academic, professional, or scientific skills, not because they had management skills. Their promotion from mid- or entry-level positions to the ranks of manager/executive occurred from the need to oversee other physician-specialists/technicians and the professionally related operations of the organization. Their leadership was called upon to integrate other physicians into the organizational agenda. Some did then advance to broader areas of authority, moving into line management, policy-making, or executive roles within the organization. Thus, the physician was typically hired as a specialist within management. Over time, some were promoted to more management-intensive jobs. Entry into this career progression usually occurred after a significant number of years of medical practice. It characteristically involved little prior academic preparation to undertake management responsibilities.

The technical or staff positions held by physicians tended to have little or no institutionwide authority. As advisory positions, they did not constitute a threat to career management--nor did they offer substantial experience in organizational affairs. They were intrinsically narrow in scope. When leadership was desired, the selected physicians were often trusted elder statesmen within the medical staff, whose major qualifications were acceptance and trust by peers. They could be depended upon not to challenge management with their personal ambition within the management hierarchy. As a public relations person, the physician served as a diplomat, politician, figurehead, and "front man." This similarly did not challenge the authority of line management.

In the case of hospitals, custom and regulation tended to exclude physicians from management or governance. In practice, the medical staff of the hospital espoused the concept of the separate and independent, self-governing medical staff. In that mode, the medical staff itself was suspicious of any physician who joined the "Philistines" in administration. The '70s witnessed a greater schism between medical staff and administration, with the formation of physicians' unions and work slowdowns, complete to the 1975 doctor strike and the withholding of services. Moreover, as little as three decades ago, physicians were excluded from membership on hospital boards, in part due to the notion of conflict of interest.[2] In the 1940s and '50s, it was felt that doctors should keep their hands off administration, management, and governance.[3] The '60s brought change. The 1968 Report of the Secretary's Advisory Committee on Hospital Effectiveness,[4] known as the Barr Report, indicated that physicians should be involved in decision making and held accountable for decisions affecting costs of hospital care. Much of the writing of that era focused on strategies for physician involvement in decision making, to resolve conflicts between board, staff, and administration.[3,5] The position of medical director was the product of this strife. Physicians as a part of management took on the task of resolving hospital-medical staff conflicts, trying to replace conflict with cooperation.[5,6]

There were other factors that worked to reduce the number of physicians who devoted time to management of hospitals. While physicians had served as superintendents of hospitals in the late nineteenth and early twentieth centuries, this practice declined over time. An American College of Healthcare Executives survey found that, in 1972, there were 813 physician hospital administrators; by 1978, there were only 92.[7] In part, this was attributable to a shortage of physicians. But at the same

Section I - The Context of Management

time, a new "management professional"--e.g., one with a master's degree in hospital, business, or public health administration--began to populate the ranks of management in health care organizations, and peer attitudes ("real doctors practice medicine") drew more physicians into private practice and away from management endeavors. Only those who were "unable to compete" or had grown "old and tired" were pictured as suitable for organizational affairs. In sum, many disincentives existed for physicians to become managers. Those resulted from professional attitudes, prejudice, and historical constraints, real or imagined.

Emergence of the Physician Executive

Despite the barriers and problems previously described, the 1980s found physicians moving into management at an accelerated pace. This decade produced more opportunity and greater need for physician executives because of the changes in health care. Cost containment required physician involvement, because they traditionally controlled demand and price. In the face of increasing government regulation, successful financial management of hospitals became very complex, requiring cooperation and a more effective interface between doctors and administration. The advent of alternative health care organizations produced more need for management of the delivery process and more management opportunities.[8] The essence of managed health care is medical management: restructuring the delivery system itself by changing the behavior of physicians. This demands strong leadership and management effort that differs from the management of past health care systems.

The recent increase in the physician supply has also produced more physicians interested in management. Those who are insufficiently challenged by the routine of clinical medicine or who desire a career change are pursuing management opportunities. This is not limited to senior physicians. Recent graduates are now moving directly into management positions much earlier in their careers,[9] with more prior preparation and chance for on-the-job management education. The 13-year-old American Academy of Medical Directors (AAMD) has witnessed tremendous recent growth: the organization is now enrolling 100 new members a month, compared to 30 a month prior to 1987. Total membership by August 1987 was about 3,000 and steadily rising.[10] Kindig and Lastiri found that physicians in administration constituted 3 percent of all MDs, or 13,500 physicians, in 1985. In their survey of 878 of these physicians, they found 33 percent working in hospitals, 24 percent in schools, 23 percent in government agencies, 5 percent in health care corporations, 4 percent in group practices/clinics and in industry, one percent in HMOs, and 8 percent in others.[11] Thirteen percent of their sample belonged to AAMD--a figure they considered representative of the national distribution because of AAMD's concentration on medical groups and hospitals, with members having more

Table 1

Logical Niches for Physicians in Health Care Organizations

Organization	Niche
Group Practice	Executive Management [1] Line Management [2] Technical Management [3] Staff Support [4]
MeSH	Executive Management Staff Support
Independent Practice Association	Executive Management Staff Support
Managed Health Care Company	Executive Management Line or Technical Management of quality assurance, provider relations and contracting, utilization management Staff Support
Government/Military	Executive Management Technical Management Staff Support
Industrial	Technical Management Staff Support
Hospitals	Executive Management/Professional Interface --Management of Professionals --Management of Technology --Management of Interdisciplinary Teams

1. Executive Management refers to leadership/policy roles (CEO, Chief Medical Officer).
2. Line Management roles include medical director and department chairman (primary care, outpatient, and specialty departments), commissioners, and public health administrators.
3. Technical Management roles include department heads or specialties, such as radiology, pathology, and anesthesiology.
4. Staff Support includes occupational, industrial, and insurance medicine; medical coordinator; medical staff officer.

Section I - The Context of Management

extensive managerial involvement. These figures and trends suggest that the number of physician administrators or managers will increase in the future.

The present positions of the physician executive can be visualized in terms of organizations and the type of management positions they maintain. Table 1 illustrates the logical niches for physicians in health care organizations. Possible management positions vary on a spectrum of involvement from the practitioner team leader, through the departmental supervisor, the management staff support role, to line manager and at the other extreme, the executive manager. These can be arrayed with increasing percentage of management time and decreasing amounts of clinical time as the positions advance along the continuum. The positions are classified on the table as executive, line management, technical management, or staff support, with examples of each.

There is a characteristic difference between current roles for physicians and those bureaucratic or technical positions seen prior to 1970. New positions for physicians entail more management and executive responsibilities. Management has been defined as both a discipline and a culture--which, through the responsible exercise of authority, organizes people and resources to achieve organizational and societal goals.[12] Executives are responsible for planning, staffing, directing, and controlling entire organizations.[13] The AAMD recently estimated that 300 of its members are top executives--i.e., CEOs or board chairpersons.[10]

In conclusion, there are more opportunities now available for physicians with an interest in management, running the gamut from technical team leadership to top executive positions. The need for physician executives is increasing, and there are likely to be more candidates for these positions. Job descriptions are moving away from the administrative/technical/bureaucratic positions to genuinely executive-level roles. The question that remains to be answered is whether the physician is uniquely capable of filling these roles.

Does the MD Degree a Medical Manager Make?

We have seen that the physician executive is now assuming a more active role in health care management, especially with regard to other physicians. There are some circumscribing legal considerations in the management of physicians. The medical practice act varies from state to state, but usually places a prohibition on corporations employing or supervising physicians. In essence, only a physician is felt qualified to hire and supervise another physician (HMO legislation may serve as an exception). There are also the limits of licensure that prevent other professionals and lay persons from engaging in the practice of medicine. Therefore those individuals cannot supervise physicians. State quality assurance/utilization review legislation may have a mandate requiring that programs of this nature be directed by physicians. Regulatory requirements from JCAHO include a standard that licensed physicians hold the majority of positions on hospital medical staff committees.[6] Thus ready-made roles for the physician executive are "locked-in" by these stipulations.

The ability and acceptability of the physician as the manager of other physicians relates in no small way to identification with the medical culture. Physicians are more likely to follow the directives of their peers, particularly when their own values have been addressed. The status of the medical degree, common language, experience, and acculturation create a credibility that is not easily earned by a nonphysician executive. The mystique of the medical profession is reinforced by the politics of professionalism: "You can't be in the guild if you haven't served the apprenticeship"; "if you're not in, you can't lead"; and the preferred style of influence is "leadership," not supervision or management! That reality creates an incapacitating barrier to nonphysician, managers whose true claim to competency is training and experience in management affairs.

Professional networks are another asset that derives from cultural membership in the profession. The physician draws on a professional network that powers itself by professional referral. The leverage of the political relationship of one physician to another in that influential network is a key ingredient in the physician executive's effectiveness as a change agent. In hospitals, they are often leaders in the informal organization that controls most hospital medical staff decisions. These are all factors that derive from professional membership in the medical culture and enhance the ability of physicians to manage health systems.

One would expect to see the advancement of physicians to the management of professionals in the health care organization because of the primacy of the physician as leader of the medical team. Physicians are a logical choice, too, for supervision of the professionally related operations of the health care business. In competition with administrators or other health professionals (nurses, technicians, etc.), physicians' historical position of authority and scientific/legal role as licensed professionals affords them a strong advantage. Positions such as vice president of professional affairs are now filled by physicians, and they are beginning to extend their area of authority from medical staff-related operations to other professional services, such as nursing and ancillary services.

Presently physicians retain a large residual reservoir of respect in society, despite their having suffered some loss of status and control in the recent past. That credibility is a distinct advantage to the health care organization in the competitive marketplace. Physicians are particularly well positioned in ambulatory care, which is an expanding area of health care.

Section I - The Context of Management

In the strictly "doctor organization," such as a medical group, the imperative of the physician as the primary executive is most evident. Medical groups draw on an almost constant tradition of physician ownership, management, and control. Executive authority in most cases entails a favorable mix of professional competency, political savvy, strong leadership skills, competence in communication, and good networking within the medical group. The ownership of most doctor organizations by doctors makes this inevitable. However, the growing size and success of medical groups today is evidence of the accomplishment of physician executives in the operation of this successful and competitive type of health care institution.

A distinct asset for the physician executive is a wealth of knowledge about the health care system derived from patient care processes. Their technological knowledge of the business from a hands-on perspective creates an insight into the delivery process that is closely tied to the patient-consumer. Comprehension of the consumer's tastes and preferences has been acquired through daily contact with patients. Because physicians have played the provider role, they understand the resources (goods and services) required to effect medical treatment. Very important, Adams has pointed out that physicians are key personnel in connecting quality of output to quantity of resources (input) used in the delivery of medical care.[14] Where required to do so, they can gauge appropriate levels of productivity and thereby affect the cost-effectiveness of health care. Thus medical experience is a decided asset in the management of the health care delivery process.

While qualified in many respects, there is still a reluctance on the part of some physicians to get involved in management or to respect their peers' desire to do so. For physicians, autonomy remains an important value. Doctors resist being managed, as previously discussed, and look upon management with suspicion and distrust. One hears of the perceived ethical conflicts[14] between patient advocates and those who serve the interests of the organization. There is a suggested status differential, with administration appearing less prestigious and, sometimes, lower salaried. However, salaries are now becoming equivalent[15] or greater,[10] on the average. There is the contention that real doctors practice medicine--an item that draws frequent debate even within AAMD, i.e., "Does the medical director need to remain in practice to retain legitimacy in the eyes of other doctors?" Harking back to the original question, physicians may have the inclination to become executives, but they must be prepared to meet significant opposition within their own profession. Therefore, it is a hard choice for physicians to become managers.

By virtue of their medical training, physicians may have acquired less obvious assets for management. Medical education emphasizes problem solving, decision making, and interpersonal skills.[16] Physicians have been through a boot camp that drilled them in long hours, hard work, and high levels of stress, as noted by Doyne. The author states that by being thrown in over their heads, they develop creativity, innovation, thinking on their feet, and a mental toughness. They have learned to

---

Table 2

Traditional Characterizations of Differences Between Physicians and Managers[15,17-19]

A Physician	A Manager
Is autonomous; makes decisions alone	Uses teamwork; is probably involved in line reporting
Works one-to-one	Works primarily in groups
Is patient-oriented	Is organization-oriented
Is empathic	Is objective
Is crisis-oriented	Is a long-range planner
Is quality-oriented	Is cost-oriented
Enjoys immediate tangible results	Must often delay gratification and enjoy process
Accustomed to controlled chaos	Has a planned schedule, with more inherent flexibility
Sees people as material or objects	Sees people as resources to be managed
Is a doer	Is a delegator--gets things done through others
Reacts	Proacts
Is authoritarian in practice style; antiauthoritarian as it pertains to leadership	Delegates authority; deals with people as equals--participative style
Has a specialist orientation	Has a generalist orientation
Is a classical scientist	Is a social scientist
Is discipline-oriented	Is socially oriented

Section I - The Context of Management

examine the facts, analyze information, and arrive at a timely decision. They are taught to deal with crises and pressure-filled situations. Communication and people skills have been honed by the practice of medicine.[17] By completion of a medical education, they have demonstrated that they are intelligent, highly motivated, and educable and possess certain personality traits (perseverance, aggressiveness, competitiveness). The medical degree alone represents a substantial investment in human capital.

On the other hand, medical training produces results that are orthogonal to good management practice. Collegiality runs counter to the management notion of scalar authority in the organization. Several authors, including the present, have described distinct differences between the physician orientation and that of a manager.[15,17,18,19] For simplicity, Table 2 presents the major characterizations of these differences. While most are self-explanatory, a few require further elaboration.

Physicians have been trained to work in one-to-one situations, where the doctor is dominant. They are excellent short-term diagnosticians, trained to make decisions based on data. Physicians function within the classical medical model--a scientific model in which, to arrive at a conclusion, data are required. If left to wonder, they are inclined to perform the infinite experiment, always asking "where are the data?" By contrast, managers often tend to deal with problems using limited data, trusting their reason, intuition, and experience. The two camps clash when the manager desires to act and the physician holds back, striving to be objective. The two professions are also different in their orientation to people and organizations, leadership and behavioral styles, and constraints of their working environments.

Lack of academic preparation for management is a clear shortcoming of most physician executive candidates. By virtue of their medical education, physicians do not have adequate backgrounds or formal training in management disciplines. Fortunately, they have come to recognize this, and many are now working to compensate for this lack of preparation. While much of their past training has been experiential and on-the-job, physicians are now seeking postgraduate education. A large number of physician administrators surveyed by Kindig and Lastiri[11] feel that formal graduate course work or advanced degrees are advisable (62.1 percent) or should be required (21.5 percent). Physicians are seeking continuing education through AAMD, American College of Healthcare Executives, American Hospital Association, American Management Association, and American Group Practice Association seminars in management; through concentrated courses taught at universities such as Harvard Business School and Sloan School of Management at the Massachusetts Institute of Technology; and by returning to academia for graduate degrees in business or health administration. The Geisinger Foundation has presented a mini-MBA program in management, the University of Wisconsin has a master of science in administrative medicine, and New York University gives an MS in management, organized for physicians. Physicians are seeking to fill the deficit in their training-- an education that was formerly acquired only by mentorship or apprenticeship, self-teaching, and on-the-job experience.

Challenge of the Modern Health Care Organization

Today, many forces are working to challenge the authority of physicians. Pressures confronting the profession include:

- Corporatization of health care

- Paraprofessional and midlevel practitioners

- Managed health care

- Consumerism

- Demands for accountability in health care cost and quality

- Technology (data collection and management information systems, computer-based decision making)

The health care organization is becoming an increasingly dominant part of the health care business. Physicians have historically viewed the organization with some suspicion and even disdain. But the balance of power is shifting toward the organization because of the importance of capital, management skills, marketing expertise, entrepreneurism, etc. Power, influence, and authority in the organization generally reside within management. To have impact in organizations, a constituency (in this case, the medical profession) needs representation at the top in organizational management.

The historical position of the physician in the separate and independent medical staff now creates a problem for the new health care organization. There are problems with the traditional organization entailing two lines of authority, i.e., administrative and professional. The modern health care organization cannot tolerate the resulting struggle between administrative and medical staff thinking. That divided authority impairs the ability of the organization to act decisively in response to external change and challenge. Driven by the demand for efficiency and competitiveness, the effective organization must be capable of evaluating its environment, making decisions about indicated courses of action, and reorganizing and moving quickly to take the necessary action. With a high premium on decisiveness, the historical bipartite health care organization is inefficient. The independent, self-governing medical staff is a defective construct in that environment.

Today, the physician executive is beginning to offer a solution to the

Section I - The Context of Management

internal structural conflicts in health care organizations, as they serve to resolve these tensions. As physician executives compete within the ranks of management, some will logically rise into top executive positions. Some physicians have already done so or are in the process. This promises to serve the medical profession by ensuring that physicians (in the management role) sustain the profession's authority in the areas of clinical decision making and quality control of the health care product. The long-term implication is that the profession will tend to change in its relationship to the health care organization.

For the medical profession itself, one of the most compelling arguments favoring broader involvement of physicians in management is the profession's deteriorating control over patient care. As the medical profession moves into an era of surplus professional manpower and organized health care, the autonomous physician is becoming more and more circumscribed in authority and influence. If physicians desire to maintain control by their profession, they can do so by moving to the helm of the new health care organization. This is potentially a rallying point within the profession in support of the physician executive. There is evidence that this strategy is becoming a reality. The AMA has granted delegate status to the AAMD within its House of Delegates. The American College of Physician Executives is working to gain recognition of medical management as a legitimate specialty for physicians.

As the Dust Settles

Over the past decade, the critical place for physicians in the management of health care organizations has become much more evident. The success of the organization requires effective decision making in an environment of synergism between both the medical and the management components of the institution.[12] There is an evident need for an arbiter--an executive who can bridge the gap between the resource allocators and the deliverers of service.[14] Getting control over health care expenditures is not likely to be accomplished without physician involvement. The public good will be best served by a blending of practice and management concerns.

For the physician who is willing, who can work to acquire the management knowledge and skills, and who desires to be a manager, there is a place. As a manager, the physician has some unique attributes, skills, and experience to offer. Physician executives have demonstrated their ability to function in all types of positions and at all levels of organization.[15] Physician executives benefit from their practical knowledge of health care, certain legal realities, societal attitudes toward physicians, and the status of the profession. Physician executives can speak the language of patient care and of management, bringing a "legitimate authority to health care to which neither nonphysician executives nor physicians without management training can aspire."[20] As a specialist in management, the physician executive can serve the medical profession and the patient by sustaining the influence and authority of physicians within the increasingly complex health care organization.

References

1. Starr, P. *The Social Transformation of American Medicine.* New York: Basic Books, 1982.

2. Smith, R. "The Case for Physician Involvement in Governance and Management." *Hospital Medical Staff* 5(5):28-30, May 1976.

3. Schultz, R. "How to Get Doctors Involved in Governance, Management." *Hospital Medical Staff* 5(6): 1-7, June 1976.

4. U.S. Department of Health, Education and Welfare. *Report of the Secretary's Advisory Committee on Hospital Effectiveness.* Washington, D.C.: U.S. Government Printing Office, 1968.

5. Noie, N. "Doctors Move Beyond Medicine." *Hospitals* 50(7): 69-72, April 1, 1976.

6. Morrisey, M., and Brooks, D. "Physician Influence in Hospitals: An Update." *Hospitals* 59(17):86-7, 89, Sept. 1, 1985.

7. Friedman, E. "Physician-Administrator Making a Comeback." *Medical World News* 27(12):34-38, 40-43, June 23, 1986.

8. Smith, H., and Piland, N. *The Physician Executive: A Survival Plan for Medicine.* Unpublished manuscript, 1987.

9. Meller, G. "Management." *JAMA* 258(16):2301-03, Oct. 23, 1987.

10. Nelson, S. "The Rising Incomes--and Numbers--of MD Execs." *Hospitals* 61(18):63, September 20, 1987.

11. Kindig, D., and Lastiri, S. "Administrative Medicine: A New Medical Specialty." *Health Affairs* 5(4):146-56, Winter 1986.

12. Fink, D., and Goldhar, J. "Management for Physicians: An Annotated Bibliography of Recent Literature." *Annals of Internal Medicine* 92(part 1):269-75, Feb. 1980.

13. Drucker, P. *Management: Tasks, Responsibilities, Practices.* New York: Harper & Row, 1973.

14. Adams, O. "Getting Physicians Involved in Hospital Management, Trends." *Canadian Medical Association Journal* 134(2):157-9, Jan. 15, 1986.

15. Wallace, C. "Physicians Leaving Their Practices for Hospital Jobs." *Modern Healthcare* 17(10):40-41, 44, 48, 55, 57, May 8, 1987.

16. Myers, T., and others. "An Approach to the Assessment of Learning Needs

for Physician-Managers." *Journal of Health Administration Education* 4(4):629-43, Fall 1986.

17. Doyne, M. "Physicians as Managers." *Healthcare Forum Journal* 30(5):11-13, September/October 1987.

18. Forkosh, D. "Good Doctors Aren't Always Good Managers." *Hospital Medical Staff* 11(5):2-5, May 1982.

19. Stearns, N., and Roberts, E. "Why Do Occupational Physicians Need to Be Better Managers?" *Journal of Occupational Medicine* 24(3):219-24, March 1982.

20. Hillman, A., and others. "Sounding Board, Managing the Medical-Industrial Complex." *New England Journal of Medicine* 315(8):511-13, Aug. 21, 1986.

David J. Ottensmeyer, MD, FACPE, is Executive Vice President and Chief Medical Officer of EQUICOR, Nashville, Tennessee. Before this position, he served for 10 years as President and Chief Executive Officer of Lovelace Medical Center and Foundation, Albuquerque, New Mexico. M.K. Key is a clinical-community psychologist and Director of Research and Development of EQUICOR.

CHAPTER 5

The Dual Role Dilemma

by Michael E. Kurtz, MS

W hile physicians bring unique characteristics to the managerial role, they are also unique products of the culture of the medical profession. They have made major personal commitments to a profession and a career very early in life, and the professional culture they enter definitely shapes their values, beliefs, ideas, internal and external perceptions, behaviors, and personalities.

Physicians spend the most formative years of their professional lives almost exclusively in the company of other physicians (teachers, mentors, preceptors, etc.) and the professional values and norms of the world of medicine are strongly inculcated and reinforced on a daily basis. Also, for a physician to be successful in the clinical role and to achieve acceptance and recognition from the medical community, he or she must be willing to accept and demonstrate these values and norms; otherwise the physician will find him- or herself treated as an unacceptable member of the community and severely criticized. To be able to pass through the ranks, rites of passage, and hierarchy of the medical community, one must be willing to comply and behave in accordance with these norms and expectations.

This socialization process of the "becoming-physician" probably has more direct influence on behaviors exhibited later in practice than anything else. Upon examination, I have found that although most physicians share similar values, have experienced similar initial training, and identify as a distinct professional group, the individual specialties of medicine provide further socialization, demand specialty identification, and develop unique behavioral characteristics within their subgroups.

When analyzed through a series of behavior-oriented assessments, each specialty is found to use behaviors that are unique and specific to it; i.e., most surgeons act and behave as other surgeons, most pediatricians act and behave as other pediatricians, etc. These behaviors (whether successful or unsuccessful in achieving the individual's goals) are reinforced by other members of the physician's primary identification group

Section I.   The Context of Management

and are constantly rewarded and reinforced in the clinical setting.

In general, most physicians (i.e., all specialists) are oriented to certain behaviors and values in their clinical practices, and these behaviors are successful for them and most likely are needed if they are to achieve the desired outcomes and acceptance of colleagues and peers.

When the physician moves away from the clinical role and into the world of management, administration, and leadership, we find that he/she most often will continue to use these learned clinical behaviors, professional norms, and values. A negative result is seen when this occurs. While clinical behaviors are critical for success in the practitioner role, they tend to create conflict, resistance, and tension in the managerial role.

Through an ongoing study, a long list of differences between effective clinicians and effective managers has been defined. When factored to determine those that are most critical, a list of nine major differences emerges (see figure below).

Clinicians are *action oriented*. They are "doers" and hands-on oriented. They prefer to be directly involved in their work, and see themselves as the primary interacters in most situations (e.g., diagnostic workups, treatment, etc.). Managers, on the other hand, see their primary role as being in *planning and designing*. Managers work through a process that establishes goals and objectives, and then facilitate the planning and designing of activities that will accomplish these goals. They are not "doers"--that role is delegated to staff. Once you become a "doer," you are a worker, not a manager. When clinicians actively participate in the work itself, they are most often seen as interfering in organization operations.

Clinicians feel most effective, and report feeling most comfortable and

Major Differences Between Clinicians and Managers

CLINICIANS	MANAGERS
Doers	Planners, Designers
1:1 Interactions	1:N Interactions
Reactive Personalities	Proactive Personalities
Require Immediate Gratification	Accept Delayed Gratification
Deciders	Delegators
Value Autonomy	Value Collaboration
Independent	Participative
Patient Advocate	Organization Advocate
Identify with Profession	Identify with Organization

most successful, in *one-to-one* encounters and interactions. They prefer to deal with others on an individual basis, whether this be doctor/patient, doctor/nurse, doctor/family, doctor/doctor, etc. In a study of 800 physician-managers, I found that they tended to be very selective in the groups they join. They prefered to be left alone and were somewhat detached, independent, and self-sufficient. They demonstrated low interest in being included by others (especially in social activities) and had little concern about prestige or what others thought. (This may be a result of the medical training process, which traditionally prepares physicians for solo practice and for orientation to the private doctor/patient relationship.)

This low inclusion behavior may prove to be successful for the medical practitioner, but it lowers effectiveness for the physician-manager. The managerial role demands a high degree of *group interaction* in the organizational setting in order to accomplish effective decision-making and problem-solving and, where appropriate, to establish participative and collaborative team management. Approximately 73 percent of a manager's time is spent in meetings and group settings. Physicians find these situations (i.e., meetings) intolerable and perceive them as a waste of time.

Clinicians are trained as *reactive personalities*. They are inclined to wait for their clinical services to be needed and/or requested. The physician waits for the patient to present himself, or to be referred; the physician most often responds to a need already defined and/or in progress. To be effective in management, the individual must work from a *proactive stance*, which means that the manager must anticipate future needs and requirements and initiate and/or invent processes to address them.

Obtaining short-term and/or *immediate results/gratification* is reported as being extremely important to the physician, who desires to quickly see a result from taking an action or initiating an intervention and experiences frustration when this is not realized. Managers very seldom experience immediate results from their work. Because they most often work in planning and designing processes, anticipating future events, etc., they are forced to accept *delayed results/gratification* for the investment of their energies. A manager may not see the result of his or her work for months or even years (anyone who has been involved in a building project can easily understand this dynamic).

Physicians are trained to be independent problem-solvers and perceive themselves to be the *deciders* in almost all medical/clinical decision situations. They see themselves as having the ultimate authority and responsibility, and they will almost always assume this role and display this behavior. While managers have the "right" of decision-making and reserve the "right to veto," they will most often *delegate* decision-making to their subordinates. As stated above, organization leaders

Section I.   The Context of Management

manage the process of problem solving and decision-making. To always be the deciders would place them in a position of being perceived as autocratic, authoritarian, and mistrusting of their subordinates. Also, it is important to recognize that with the high degree of specialization and subspecialization that has evolved and developed in both the clinical and managerial fields, no one person can be expected to have all of the expertise and/or knowledge required for complex decision-making. Multiple resources will always be required.

The perception of being the "decider" held by the physician is further reinforced by the clincian's *value of autonomy*. Physicians tend to see themselves as autonomous professionals whose responsibility is to their patients and their profession. They are the ones to determine their level of involvement and interaction, and they don't perceive themselves to be subordinate or subservient to others. They prefer to perform their roles independently and autonomously, only involving others as *they* determine. While this value of autonomy protects the clinician from being politically influenced, it can significantly interfere with his or her effectiveness in a leadership/managerial role. Managers cannot function autonomously by the very nature of the definition of their role and function. Managers value *collaboration* and integration. They see their primary function as being one of facilitating and supporting the merging of ideas through the collaboration of organizational functions and related personnel. The actions of any one part of the organization affect every other part of the organization. Therefore, shared information, integration of ideas and resources, and collaboration of team members with other managers are absolutely requisite in maximizing the larger whole (i.e., reaching the goals and objectives of the organization). All decision-making and problem-solving must be entered into with the orientation of what will be best for the greater good (of the organization) rather than what will be best for the individual. The value of autonomy held by most phsycians results in a fairly high degree of self-centeredness and is often perceived as selfishness by nonclinical members of the organization.

Concomitant with the value of autonomy is the *value of independence* held by the clinician. Physicians are trained to work independently, to make independent decisions, and to take independent responsibility for outcomes. They don't want to feel that they are dependent on others for the successes or the failures they experience. Research data demonstrate a very low need for inclusion of and involvement by others, a low need to participate with others in situations that don't directly affect them, and a relatively high need to take charge. Physicians enjoy making decisions and influencing others and resist allowing others to influence them. They don't want others (especially nonphysicians) to tell them what to do, and they consume a great deal of physical and psychological energy protecting this autonomy and independence.

Concomitant with the value of collaboration, managers strongly value *participation* and avoid independent behaviors and actions. To ensure quality and commitment in decision-making and problem-solving, managers recognize the need to involve others in the process. They see their role as one of facilitating and supporting the involvement and participation of others in order to obtain maximum synergism. An effective manager is a person who designs and plans an organizational system that creates a culture and environment that encourages and supports participation by all members of the organization and one that discourages independence and ivory tower decision-making.

Another major difference between clinicians and managers is that the physician assumes the primary role of being an *advocate for the patient*. Physicians assume the responsibility of protecting the patients from undue outside influence and interference. In many cases, the outside influence is defined as the organization and the management and administrative system. Clinicians are oriented to the concept that "if the patient needs something, one gets it for him." To be asked to do a cost-benefit analysis, or to be told that certain interventions or services are inappropriate, is untenable to a clinician, and is seen as interfering with professional prerogatives and responsibilities.

While managers are not insensitive to patient needs and to an acceptable level of quality in patient care, they are required to primarily function as *advocates of the organization*. The manager's role, function, and responsibility require that he or she work to enhance and build the organization as a whole and to maximize its efficiency, productivity, and assets. When working with others, managers do not represent themselves; they function as representatives and advocates of the organization. The manager will constantly be striving to ensure viability of the organization, and, therefore, decisions will be made that will be in the best interest of the larger whole rather than in the interest of individuals. Clincians will often make decisions based on isolated, unique, and specific facts of a certain case that may appear (or be) inconsistent with decisions made in related cases. Managers, on the other hand, are expected to make decisions that are consistent with organization policy, values, and norms. This concept of consistency and predictability carries extreme weight in evaluating effective managerial behavior, otherwise the manager would be managing by exception to the rule, which would result in organizational chaos.

This difference in advocacy orientation is further exaggerated by the individual's identification with a professional group or organizational entity. Physicians identify with their *professional group* and, more specifically, with their specialization within the larger professional designation. When asked "who are you," a clinician will first respond that he or she is a physician and then further define this identity with his or her specialization. The next level of identification is most often as a member of a certain medical community or communities (e.g., XYZ Hospital medical staff, ABC Physicians, or as a recognized member of

Section I.   The Context of Management

several different hospital medical staffs within a community). The very last identification will be as a manager, administrator, or as a representative of a specific organization. The clinician identifies with the organization only insofar as it allows the practice of skill and demonstration of the clinician's expertise. Physicans do not relate to the concept of "employment" or "unemployment." They perceive themselves as being able to practice wherever and whenever they choose. Because of that orientation, the physician sees the organization as simply a place that provides the opportunity, facilities, and environment to "practice," and this place could actually be anywhere.

The manager is in quite a different situation; his or her identity is totally dependent on employment or unemployment by an organization. Therefore, the identification is with the organization and not the professional field. Without an organization to manage, the manager can no longer be identified as a manager. Managers derive satisfaction from the rewards given and by the value accorded by the organization, which, in turn, affords recognition and acceptance by the larger managerial community. When asked the same question, "Who are you?", the manager will respond that he or she is the chief executive officer or the manager/director of the computer sciences department of XYZ Health Center. The manager perceives him- or herself as "belonging" to the XYZ Health Center, and the organization provides, promotes, and dictates this identification. The manager's role and responsibility is to develop the organization and to protect its viability in the marketplace, which creates competitive behavior and further fosters the identification with "us." This feeling of "my country, right or wrong" is totally foreign to the clinician when translated to the organization context.

These diferences between clinicians and managers are but a few in a long list of practical and philosophical differences, but they are the major ones and they tend to create the greatest degree of role-conflict and dual-role dilemma for the physician-manager. It is important to recognize that each set of behaviors, practices, and skills is neccessary for satisfactory performance in the specific role demand (i.e. clinician or manager), but the physician who chooses to enter into management and administration will most often find him- or herself straddling the chasm between the two.

Most physician-managers feel that it is important to maintain a clinical involvement, and there is a strong argument for this. The clinician wishes to at least maintain, if not enhance, clinical skills and abilities, to learn and update knowledge and skills from participation and interaction with colleagues, and to continue identification with the medical community and specialty. The clinician has spent the major part of his or her adult life in this community and has developed almost an exclusive identity with it. To leave it and move into another "profession" and career path is a psychologically wrenching and threatening experience. It means turning one's back on the primary identification group, giving up membership in an exclusive and elite professional "club," and starting out on a new educational and professional road. This choice requires leaving an area of acquired personal and professional expertise and recognition that is very comfortable and highly rewarded and moving into a relatively uncomfortable area with little, if any, preparation. It demands leaving an area of recognized professional competence and moving into the role of neophyte, learner, and student. This shift, along with the basic negative attitudes and perceptions about managers held by most physicians, further feeds the role-conflict and dual-role dilemma for the clinician.

There is another identify issue that emerges for the physician-manager. Along with the personal identity dilemma is the question of identification that is raised for the medical community and the organization membership. The physician can never rid him- or herself of the title of "Doctor" and will always be perceived as a physician by the organization's membership. The clinician will always be one of "them" in the eyes of nonphysician executives and staff, and, historically and through training and experience, "them" has always been an adversarial group. Therefore, the physician executive's allegiances, commitment, and dedication will always be questioned.

At the same time, the medical staff and/or community will now perceive its colleague as a member of the management and administrative staff, which has always been a "them" to that group. This is especially true if the physician-manager is employed and paid by the organization and may lead to questioning and mistrust of communication and intent.

Some physicians and management experts will argue that it is impossible to maintain this dual role--that one cannot adequately and competently perform in one while also practicing the other. The concern of becoming a "Jack of all trades, master of none" is a very real one and must be addressed by the professional community as well as the organization. With the strong movement to "professionalize" the role of physician-manager/physician-executive taking place in the United States, it can be assumed that this role will require certification of competence and capability in the very near future and that this "certification" will require demonstration of education, training, skill-development, and experience in managerial roles and responsibilities. No longer can the physician simply assume an organizational leadership or management role because he or she is a good clinician; these successful clinical skills and behaviors are being recognized as creating problems in the practice of management and administration. A shift in thinking, philosophy, attitudes, and behavior must take place if the physician is to be seen as successful and as an asset to the organization.

I don't think that it must necessarily be an either/or question. Experience demonstrates that those physician executives who are recognized as the most competent, capable, and successful have, through their own

Section I.   The Context of Management

choices and the demands of their organizations, given up clinical involvement and have dedicated themselves to the professionalization of the physician-executive role. They have not lost credibility with their medical colleagues because they have developed competence and expertise as managers. They are perceived as being sensitive to the needs and values of the medical community while being accorded credibility through the quality and fairness of their decisions and human relations skills. Their organizations tend to be large and complex, which requires full-time commitment and dedication to the managerial role. They also tend to be organizations that are physician-owned and/or physician-run, so that the entire medical staff is in some way involved in the management of the organization.

It is probably not an either/or question; it is more a factor of the size and the complexity of the organization that will provide the answer. A 15-person medical group can't afford to have one of its physicians excluded from a clinical role, but a 60+-person group can't afford not to force the choice if it desires adequate and successful management.

I don't think that this dual role dilemma can be easily resolved for the physician-manager. It will require some soul-searching, self-analysis, and the development of self-awareness for each individual. For the physician to be successful in the dual role requires that he or she thoroughly understand which hat is being worn at which time, be adequately prepared for each in order to obtain and maintain credibility, and make sure that those people working for and with the physician executive understand which hat is being worn at any specific time.

It's also important for the physician-manager to use this unique position to develop and enhance collaboration and integration of the medical and administrative staffs in the daily management and operations of the organization. Through this mechanism, the chasm of the dual roles and its concomitant frustration and conflict can be bridged.

Health care organizations are struggling with a rapidly changing economic, political, and social environment. Many are developing successful new businesses and service strategies, while others are suffering failure. It is predicted that 20-25 percent of currently operating hospitals will close within the next two to three years, and 30-40 percent of health care providers other than hospitals (e.g., clinics, group practices, HMOs, etc.) will initiate major organizational restructuring, redesign, and redefinition, or be the targets of takeovers and mergers.

Upon reviewing more than 60 such situations, I found that, although various strategies are being tested, there has been one underlying theme that emerges: the activities of the most responsive and strongest health care organizations all, in some way, support the integration of their medical staffs into the operational management and leadership of the organization.

The traditional adversarial positioning of medicine vs. administration is being consciously challenged and new roles and activities are being invented and designed that foster collaboration and cooperation. This new "partnership" may be the key to future viability, and many professional resources are being focused on the development of methods to assist in accomplishing this goal. The active involvement of the physician-manager may be the single most critical element in this process.

The first step is to strengthen the formal medical staff organization. By-laws must be reviewed in light of current impacts from external sources, medical staff leadership must be enhanced and developed, and active participation in the organization by all members must be encouraged.

The next step is to provide training and education for the development of leadership and managerial skills of the medical staff, and then to provide structured opportunities for actual integration with management staff through team and group development activities. Each group expresses unique characteristics and cherishes certain values and self-images that are usually misperceived and misunderstood by the other. This results in negative and adversarial perceptions and attitudes.

Upon examination, the two groups actually share many values, expectations, and goals, but there are major differences in how they are communicated and what methods are developed for their achievement. The development of a common language, a clearer communication system, joint planning and problem-solving activities, and joint education and training must be given priority if an integration effort is to be successful.

My experience and data strongly suggest that all health care organizations, from single specialty groups to large comprehensive medical centers, need to first initiate an objective organizational assessment and analysis process to determine their current situation and state of integration. Second, a process of mutual goal setting and strategic planning must be established. Third, an integrated effort for planning and initiating activities that will lead to the desired change and/or objective must be developed.

An honest commitment to the development of collaboration and integration efforts by all parties may well be the key to future survival and viability. Assisting health care organizations in meeting this commitment is one of the primary roles and responsibilities of the physician executive and may be the most successful way to reduce the conflict and frustration of the dual role dilemma.

Michael Kurtz, MS, is an organizational psychologist and management consultant in Herndon, Virginia.

Section I.   The Context of Management

CHAPTER 6

The Credibility of the Physician Executive

by John M. Burns, MD

P hysicians are entering the field of health care management in growing numbers. In just three years, the American Academy of Medical Directors has seen its membership grow from only slightly more than 1,000 to more than 3,000. Just as important, official statistics of the American Medical Association indicate that approximately 14,000 U.S. physicians have some health care management role.

The challenge placed before those who aspire to the role of physician executive, in spite of that impressive growth, is to demonstrate that the position is indeed legitimate. While there may be little argument from within the membership of the American Academy of Medical Directors as to the appropriateness of and critical need for this emerging profession, the acceptance of the physician executive by peers and subordinates and by the huge external world of "management" requires the recognition of major barriers to that acceptance and the development of strategies to overcome them.

Credibility of Medical Profession

Current medical literature, legislative activities in health care financing, business's involvement in health care purchasing and management, and media attention all focus on a disturbing characteristic of the health care system in general and of physicians in particular. There exists tremendous variability in the costs and quality of medical care systems, in practice styles, in occupancy rates, and in outcomes. "Managed care" interventions, be they preadmission certification, second opinions for surgery, or mandated outpatient surgery, or any of a number of cost-reducing techniques installed at the insistence largely of third-party payers, all validate the perception of purchaser and consumer alike that the system has been and is being "worked" by providers.

Regulatory solutions abound. The protestations of physicians and of organized medicine in this regard fall on deaf ears. In the business world (and perhaps government), it is perceived that the medical/health care system is completely out of control. Does the medical profession itself have credibility? The physician executive must be prepared to answer this question and discuss the issue if credibility is to be ensured for the profession.

As for the profession of physician executive, demonstrated leadership in the medical community itself is critical. Physician executives must have credibility among their peers. Respect, followership, and judgment of competence by other physicians should be based on the physician executive's participation and demonstrated skills within the health care system. In addition, peer judgment of clinical or management competence should never be based on the practice affiliation or method of compensation of the physician being evaluated. Thus the first credibility characteristic of a physician executive:

■ Active participation and leadership within the medical community.

The Role of Health Management in Establishing Medical Standards

A basic role of the physician executive, regardless of position in the health care delivery system, is to participate in the process of establishing standards of health care. *Standards of care*, not *measurement of norms*, are needed. The medical profession must be held to these standards if credibility is to be regained or maintained. These standards will be based on defining care in terms of medical appropriateness and necessity. Diagnostic and therapeutic adventurism must be eliminated. The economic impact on providers of care, institutions and physicians alike, of a reimbursement system based on objective standards of medical appropriateness and necessity is formidable.

Any number of "stakeholders" in the health care delivery system will be threatened by the proposal that objective standards for intervention or reimbursement be established. Only those who are willing to take leadership positions and face obstacles placed in the way of their efforts to establish objective standards should pretend to management positions.

Credibility implies that a "gap" does not exist. It implies that there is no disparity between what is said and the actual facts. One's professed motives are accepted as the true ones. Health care has been accepted by patients, providers, and buyers without question as to need or appropriateness. There exists now a characteristic of the health care system that needs attention. I refer specifically to the subject of variations in practice styles.

The medical system employs a number of explanations to justify variations in practice. Regardless of the explanation, however, reimbursement is almost always an issue central to the argument.

Section I.   The Context of Management

"Doctor/patient relationship," "individual case," "usual and customary," "unique case," "protocol," "standard orders"--all these terms are used in the typically retrospective claims administration process where physician reimbursement is threatened or patient financial liability is an issue.

This same characteristic, variations in practice patterns for the medical profession, feeds the tort system and drives malpractice claims based on *post hoc' ergo propter hoc* outcome judgments. The same variability enablement that supports the reimbursement system absolutely encourages the malpractice claim.

The financial incentives attendant to the litigation process have encouraged the gathering of medical testimony (of course, in retrospect) to support the view that "something else *could* have been done" in cases where the medical care process has unintended results. The process has facilitated a new profession of expert witnesses. Prospectively established and communicated standards would reduce or eliminate the appropriateness of retrospectively based testimony as to what could have been done and require that malpractice be based on conformity to established standards.

Thus the second characteristic of the physician executive:

- The capability and willingness to participate in the establishment of standards of health care.

Management Credibility

A massive amount of management literature exists. Management seminars abound and academic programs proliferate.

Fueling the above is the phenomenon of emerging management specialties and subspecialties. A current challenge of some urgency is the need to specify the bank of knowledge that creates and defines the profession of physician executive. The monograph you are reading is one component of a process aimed at clearly defining this management specialty.

Basic training, skills, and experience in management are needed to construct the foundation of our profession. Certainly some basic management training should be a requirement.

In addition to experiencing and being exposed to the formal, didactic component of management training, the physician executive should broaden himself/herself through extensive reading of both general management and health care management literature. The classic efforts of Frederick Taylor, Alfred P. Sloan, Jr., and George Siemens and the works of Douglas McGregor and Peter Drucker but skim the surface of a wealth of knowledge and ideas available in the literature.

Management is a discipline. Thus the third characteristic of the physician executive:

■ Training and experience in the basics of management.

The Credibility of the Physician Executive

Credibility is established through a process over time. It is not an event attendant to completion of a course or attainment of certification. Credibility must be earned. The trained and experienced physician executive who is active in the medical community, engaged in the process of establishing objective standards of health care quality, and trained in management is positioned to earn credibility. That credibility will be established with superiors, peers, and subordinates; with the management profession; and throughout the health care industry.

More important, the physician executive will gain the support of business. This support will come with business's recognition of the management skills of the physician, exhibited through leadership and the willingness to set standards. Business needs and wants a partner in the management of health care. But that partnership requires credibility.

The credibility of the physician executive rests on three prime characteristics: participation and leadership in the medical community, a capability and willingness to participate in the establishment of standards of care, and possession of training and experience (and accomplishments) in management.

John M. Burns, MD, is Vice President, Health and Environmental Resources, Honeywell, Inc., Minneapolis, Minnesota.

CHAPTER 7

Key Management Skills for the Physician Executive

by Leland R. Kaiser, PhD

T his chapter is written for you, a physician executive employed in a modern health care organization. The chapter will help you re-conceptualize your job and identify some of the key management skills you must master to be successful. The skills I describe are drawn from the current management literature and from my experience in working with physician executives. A bibliography is attached for further study.

Role of the Physician Executive

You are an interface professional. You work on the interface between the disciplines of medicine and management. Most of the problems in our contemporary health care system fall on this interface. A good example of an interface problem is the trade-off between the cost and quality of medical care. This trade-off requires that both a medical and a management decision be made for each patient. You are qualified to make such decisions because you have expertise in both arenas and can simultaneously protect both the patient's and the organization's welfare.

Your role and function will vary with the needs and interests of your employing organization. As a result of the wide range of job functions that physician executives perform, there is no uniform job description. In each new position you must negotiate your role and function with your employer. You must match your interests and abilities to the job that needs to be done.

Advocating for both the patient and the organization places the physician executive in a value conflict situation. What is best for the patient is not always best for the organization. What is best for the organization is not always best for the community. What is best for the community is not always best for the federal government. A manager always faces conflicts of interest. The physician has the luxury of focusing only upon the needs of his patient. You must take into account the interests of all the parties involved. Learning to think like a manager as well as a physician is one of your greatest challenges. You have mixed accountability, and often what makes one party happy with you will make another party angry with you. Good managers try to plan "win-win" games, but it is not always possible to do this in the real world of the physician executive.

Any manager is expected to promote the institution's philosophy and uphold its goals. You must be a team player and accept your role as a co-creator of your organization. You must be concerned not only with medical/management problems, but with the general welfare of your organization. This requires that you identify with organizational interests and problems that transcend your day-to-day functioning as a medical care administrator.

An alert physician executive will keep his organization well informed concerning new developments in medicine and patient care. This requires careful monitoring of the literature and attendance at medical meetings. You are expected to be an expert source for medical management, and other organizational managers will depend upon your advice and direction.

The physician executive is expected to set the standard of excellence for physicians in the organization. You must play a leadership role in quality assurance and risk management. The medical staff should view you first as a doctor, then as a manager. The management team, by contrast, will view you first as a manager, then as a doctor. Because you live in both camps, from time to time you must engage in a little fancy footwork, convincing both doctors and managers that you are representing their respective interests.

Some physician executives continue to see patients; others do not. There is no simple rule to follow in this matter. The important thing is that you maintain clinical credibility with the other physicians in your organization. That is hard to do if you no longer see patients. Yet even if you continue to see patients, it will be difficult for you to maintain medical competence on a part-time practice basis and even harder to find enough hours in the day to also practice management. Most physician executives gradually move toward full-time management because of these twin pressures. Some physician executives want to keep a foot in both camps because they are not yet fully committed to the management role and want to keep their bases covered just in case they decide to return to full-time practice.

As a physician executive, you will be subjected to many organizational challenges and stresses. Being an interface professional is not easy work. Potential stresses include: (1) the time and effort it takes to stay current in two disciplines, (2) dual identity as both a physician and a manager (this can lead to an identity conflict or a feeling you are neither), (3) lack of role clarity in your organization, (4) less hands-on

Section I.   The Context of Management

satisfaction than you had as a pure clinician, (5) trying to quickly learn the required new management skills, (6) excessive work loads, (7) being in the middle between the medical staff and management (conflict), and (8) having few professional peers to relate to (loneliness). If you are successful in your organizational role, you will mediate, translate, integrate, and absorb shock. These situations are stress generating, and you must develop some good stress management skills if you hope to remain healthy in the job.

Of course, there are many benefits that go along with this exciting new profession: (1) exploration of a new career, (2) variety and change, (3) identification with an organization (security and protection), (4) exercise of power and control, and (5) the challenge of mastering a new body of knowledge. The pluses outweigh the minuses, but you must factor them both into the equation of overall job satisfaction.

Learning to think like a manager represents one of the biggest challenges you will face. Characteristics of the mindset of a manager include: (1) seeing the big picture, (2) adopting organizational values and standards, (3) engaging in objective analytical thinking, (4) acting in the face of uncertainty, (5) enjoying complexity, (6) developing goals and objectives, (7) translating goals and objectives into action plans, (8) measuring organizational effectiveness, (9) developing a distinctive style of leadership, and (10) assessing organizational effectiveness. Though these skills are not antithetical to those of a physician, they are not usually well developed as a result of medical school education or clinical practice. Some physicians have a natural bent for management and have picked up some of the necessary skills. For other physicians, thinking like a manager is something that must be learned and practiced before proficiency is developed.

A physician gets direct positive reinforcement from his patients. He is recognized and appreciated for what he does for them. A manager must depend upon vicarious reinforcement. He succeeds only through the efforts of others. Reward is second-hand at best. Often good management goes unnoticed and the only thing you will receive are a lot of complaints if something goes wrong. People are unconscious of good management and are therefore unlikely to notice it when it occurs. If you want to feel good about yourself, you may have to pat yourself on the back for a job well done. Some physician executives miss the "good old days" when they were really appreciated by their patients.

It is important for the physician executive to develop a strong working relationship with the nursing manager. Both are clinician executives, and working together can constitute a powerful force for change in the organization. After all, who can successfully oppose all the doctors and nurses in the organization? The nursing manager is working on the interface between nursing and management and must have many of the same skills and interests as the physician executive. They are major allies and should view one another as equals in the process of planning and delivering patient care.

Innovation is an important role for the physician executive. He should stimulate creative thinking in the organization and be a major force for new product development. Most physicians are trained to think conservatively, and innovation is often outside their interest and experience in providing patient care. An innovator is a risk taker and must be willing to make many mistakes in the process of developing successful business ventures. Although by temperament some physicians are entrepreneurs, few physicians have had experience stimulating innovation in organizational settings.

Managers spend more time communicating than engaging in any other management behavior. A primary role of the physician executive is to serve as a communication link between the medical staff and management. He must properly represent the perceptions of each to the other. Written and verbal communication, dyads, small groups, large groups, and public speaking all fall within his purview. The physician executive who is not an effective communicator might benefit from some further training in the communications department of a local college or university.

Ultimately, as the new kid on the block, you must make your own way in the organization. Your position as a physician executive will be what you make it. Your profession is new enough that health care organizations do not have a lot of preconceived notions about what you should do. You do not have to cut through a lot of history. You do have to become an architect of your future in the organization. If you are creative and quick to see how you can contribute, you will write your own ticket. If you wait to be asked, you may wait for a long time.

A major challenge may be resisting the avalanche of problems that beset you when you first arrive in the organization. We all have a tendency to react to whatever is demanding our attention. We have an inclination to do whatever we enjoy doing and are good at, whether it needs to be done or not. Discrimination is an important managerial skill. You must constantly ask yourself, "What most needs to be done in this organization at this time?" If you do not plan your work and your day, you will be swept away by trivia and will never have time to do the really important things that need to be done. Your time is your most precious resource--learn to guard it carefully. There are too many good things to do and too few that will make any long-term difference for either your organization or your patients. Stand back and get perspective. Ask yourself, "Why am I doing this?"

Becoming a Professional Manager

You will achieve success by doing what you do best. Where you are the weakest, you will fail. The effective manager concentrates on what he does well and hires other people to do what he does poorly. Be sure to hire associates that are unlike you and do not share your weaknesses. Much of your career success depends upon the match between who you are and where you are. Much also depends upon your skill in surrounding yourself with competent subordinates. How well do you fit your current organizational space? What do you need from your organization to really do the job? If you designed the ideal job space for yourself, how would it look? A manager that is a failure in one organizational setting is often a success in another organization. Everything depends upon fit. If the organization does not fit you--you are a misfit. You need a good fit between your personal profile and the map of your organizational environment. Here, self-knowledge is all important.

Where is your organization in its life cycle? Organizations, like people, have life cycles. Organizations are born, grow rapidly, reach maturity, and decline. It is more fun to manage an organization in its period of rapid growth than in its decline. Many physician executives are being hired by relatively new health care organizations. This adds an element of excitement and optimism to the position. The down side is that many of these organizations are unstable, economically risky, and subject to disappearance. You may be forced to trade the security of maturity for the excitement of youth. Managing an organization in decline is a no-win situation. Remember, as a manager, your destiny is tied into the destiny of your organization. It pays to be a little choosey and not necessarily pick the job with the highest salary and greatest fringe benefits. It may not be around long enough for you to collect either.

Are your organization's values consistent with your values? Values are the lowest common denominator of action both in people and in organizations. You cannot be an effective manager if you do not agree with what your organization is doing. The best management is management by value. What are the corporate values of your organization? What are your personal and professional values as a physician executive? Are both sets of values consistent? If not, what do you need to do? Some organizations do not have a very clear sense of their values and need to go through a value clarification process.

Are you overtrained for your job? A professional manager feels best when he is challenged but not overwhelmed by what he must do. Boredom is as difficult to live with as too much excitement. What is your optimal stimulus level as a manager? Do you feel a sense of accomplishment in your job and an opportunity to bring your full range of abilities into action?

Are you being adequately compensated for what you do? A physician executive should enjoy a high standard of living and a full return on the tremendous investment he has made in his career. You should compare your salary and benefits with other physician executives in comparable jobs. You may experience a decrease in income when you switch from fee-for-service, solo practice to an organizational salary. However, your expenses are less, you enjoy more free time, and the security is greater. As with everything in life, becoming a physician executive is a trade-off.

Did anyone precede you in your position? If so, you will inherit some organizational expectations created by the previous holder of your office. These may be good, bad, or, more likely, a mix. Talk to other people and try to recreate a picture of the world before you arrived. Decide what was right and wrong with that world and announce to the organization any needed changes you will be making. If you are going to make changes, the burden of proof is upon you. Organizations always resist change. You may experience some of this resistance as you try to cut a new groove for your position.

It also helps to know the history of your organization. Organizations are where they have been. Who were the founders? What were the major milestones in the development of the organization? By knowing the traditions and symbols of the organization, you enter its mythology and stand the best chance of helping in the transformation of the myth as the organization prepares to move into the future. The myth of the organization is its tap root and should always be taken seriously. Kill the tap root and the organization dies. Set yourself against the traditions of the organization and you will surely lose.

As a professional manager, you must build your knowledge base and remain open to new ideas. Every month you should peruse the leading management journals and read several of the best books on management. As we enter the turbulent information age in health care, new age managers will be practicing management by idea. Organizations that survive this "white water" period will be the "better idea" organizations. You will never be a better manager than your knowledge base permits. What you cannot think about, you cannot manage. There are few rules in management and little memory work. Management is primarily conceptual. A good manager is not a technician. He is a well-read thinker.

Because the role of physician executive is filled with ambiguity, it is important for you to project a strong self-concept. You must tell other people who you are and what you do. In some cases it is important to tell the organization what you do not do. It is tempting for an organization to load you up with things you should not be doing. You should be doing only what a person with your experience and dual training is qualified to do. If you are performing lower level tasks, the organization is wasting money and losing the unique contribution only you can make.

There are three big questions that any manager asks:

Section I.   The Context of Management

- What should I be doing (values)?

- How can I do that (knowledge)?

- Who can do it (power)?

This is the equilateral triangle of management. A physician executive must manage values, knowledge, and power. Unless you are willing to become a power broker, your values and knowledge will not come to fruition. Organizations are political creatures. Management decisions are often made on political grounds and fly in the face of both analysis and intellect. You must seek power in order to make a difference in your organization. You can only receive power from those who have power to bestow. For this reason your relationship to the CEO and the board is critical. Without the support of those higher up in the power structure, you will not be effective and you will end up frustrated--able to see but not able to do.

Any professional manager depends upon a network of colleagues to provide support and information. The physician executive needs such a reference group to avoid professional isolation. Begin cultivating professional contacts with other physician executives if you have not already done so. Stay in touch by phone and letter and arrange to meet together at the national and regional meetings of your professional societies.

Relationship with the Chief Executive Officer

Be certain the CEO supports you and your function in the organization. Work with the CEO to develop a clear job description and a location on the organizational chart that gives you a direct reporting line to the CEO. Obtain a commitment from the CEO for adequate budgetary and staff support. You should also request a three- to five-year employment contract after the first year or two of employment.

Work with the CEO to define your major goals and objectives for the fiscal year. Tie these goals to your budget and to your performance review. Make sure the CEO and you agree on organizational priorities and on your allocations of time and effort. Keep the CEO informed concerning your progress on goal achievement. If any unexpected events intrude on your projected work program, discuss them with the CEO and have him sign off on any changes in priorities.

Your value to the CEO will depend primarily upon the extent to which you keep your assigned organizational areas problem-free (do your job) and the degree to which you assist him with his own perplexities (help him with his job). It will pay you to spend some time every week worrying about the CEO's problems and suggesting possible solutions. Worry about what the boss is worried about, and you won't have to worry about the boss.

Request frequent feedback from the CEO and give the CEO frequent feedback. The most important part of your job is communication. If you want to enjoy a long and happy life in your organization, demonstrate consistent loyalty to the CEO and volunteer for some tough assignments. You want to become so central to the CEO that he depends upon your input every week.

Relationship to the Management Team

To be effective over the long haul, you must build a high level of trust with other members of the management team. Be certain team members understand your role and function. Be certain they are satisfied with your performance. Always be prepared for organizational meetings and perform well in them. Performance in meetings is a major criterion used to evaluate any manager. Most of the work of an organization is done in meetings. From time to time you will tire of meetings. Resist the temptation to bad mouth meetings. You will only lose ground with this or any other occasion of organizational criticism. Carry your share of the work load and always document your accomplishments with other team members. Encourage divergent options from the group, but avoid adversarial relationships with any team member. Aim for consensus decision-making.

It is important for you to be available and approachable. Display company manners. Give frequent praise. Be a good listener. You need to be highly visible in the organization and to practice management by walking around.

Become a student of the organization's written policies and procedures. Play by the rules. If a rule needs to be changed, volunteer to study the rule and suggest a new policy better adapted to the changing health care environment. You win points on any management team by being predictable, open, fair, and loyal in your dealings with all team members. The time may come when your job tenure is decided by your team members. Avoid making enemies at any level of the organization. Remember, it takes a lot more effort to fight a war than to maintain the peace.

Because many changes are taking place on the interface between medicine and management, you should conduct frequent briefing meetings for team members. Organizations do not like surprises, and it is your job to see that none occur in your assigned areas. If you have important fears or doubts about what is happening in patient care, share your feelings with the group.

Section I.   The Context of Management

Relationship with the Medical Staff

One of your most important functions is maintaining positive relationships with other physicians. In hospitals and clinics, this usually takes the form of your interactions with the organized medical staff. Some physician executives believe the medical staff cannot be organized, and that simple fact alone is the root of most of their problems. It is not easy to organize doctors, yet that is your job.

Your transactions with doctors can take many forms. You may be involved in recruiting doctors for your organization. You may call on physicians in their private offices, offer practice management consultation, and act as a liaison to the hospital. Office-based physicians often welcome help with marketing and sale of their services. If the doctors do well, the hospital should also prosper. It is a "win-win" game. Often physician executives develop orientation programs for new doctors joining the staff. The orientation program provides an excellent opportunity for you to explain the institution's culture and make organizational expectations clear to new physicians.

An important part of your role is to mobilize physician commitment to your organization's services. You may meet this challenge by initiating a medical staff development program that encourages physician input in organizational decision-making and makes doctors part of the family. If you can develop a core leadership group as a result of your medical staff development program, you will find your job as a change agent much easier.

By providing financial and clinical outcome data to physicians, you can improve their performance. Prompt feedback motivates doctors to do a better job. If possible, medical education should be geared to problems documented in the performance reviews. As a physician executive, you must monitor physician practice patterns and estimate their impact on quality and cost outcomes. Sometimes it is a simple matter of keeping physician skills up to date. It may, however, come to dealing with the impaired physician or the physician who must be given reduced privileges. You will have to discipline physicians who are bad actors and coach failing physicians. In matters of discipline, you will work closely with the hospital attorney to protect the rights of all parties involved.

As a physician executive, you must set up an accountability framework for physicians and enforce the ethical and legal standards of your organization and your profession. This is never a pleasant task for a manager, but it is one that must be done. In these matters the buck stops at your desk.

Part of your role as a physician executive is to teach other physicians to think like managers. You may need to hold some special educational sessions to explain all of the changes coming down the road that will affect doctors and hospitals. Physicians need help in learning to manage DRGs and admissions. Payer mix is an important variable in determining the hospital's economic survival. The physician is the major resource allocator in health care organizations. He needs to understand his economic impact on the organization.

An important future role for physician executives will be developing new corporate structures that bring doctors and hospitals together as financial partners. No longer can doctors and hospitals compete with one another or choose to go their separate ways. They will hang together or hang separately. Medical staff corporations, MeSH organizations, hospital/doctor-owned IPAs, and hospital-based group practices are new corporate forms that may or may not prove to be the answer. There is ample opportunity and incentive for creative experimentation in this area.

Future health care will be dominated by computers and robots. You need to view information systems as the new wave of medicine and management. How familiar are you with computers? Do you have hands-on skills? Now is a good time to begin experimenting with the new hardware and software being developed for medical diagnosis. Does your hospital provide computerized literature searches for your physicians? Do you have a special shelf in your medical library devoted to books on computers and medicine?

Product line management is a promising new way to plan and deliver health care in multispecialty group practices and hospitals. A production team composed of doctors, nurses, and other personnel plans the products for each specialty area in medicine. Market segments, packaging, distribution channels, volume, profit margins, and quality standards are determined for each specialty each year. Product performance is measured against production targets, and exceptions are noted and corrected. As a product manager, you can decide to position your products for cost, quality, service, or convenience. If you can position for all four, so much the better. Service is becoming an important emphasis in health care. As a physician executive, you should help develop a customer service strategy for your institution. You will need to develop your management skills in cost accounting, quality assurance, and productivity improvement.

The dispirited physician is a phenomenon of our times. Many doctors are discouraged and have decided to leave the clinical practice of medicine. Early retirements and career changes are common. Part of your job is to maintain physician esprit de corps and do what you can to add hope and help to disheartened doctors who feel they have been sold down the stream by society.

Competition among medical facilities will increase during the next few years until re-regulation of health care occurs in the United States. You must develop an effective plan for monitoring the competition and meeting it in the marketplace. What is your organization's distinctive competence? Can you develop centers of excellence? Where do you have the greatest depth in your medical and nursing staff? Can you protect and extend your primary care base? Can you install more effective cost controls? Can you improve channels of distribution? How will the growth of managed care affect your profit margins? Are you ready for new methods of physician reimbursement? Does your governing board recognize the changing medical market?

An important role you have with the medical staff is that of change agent. You are paid to help doctors change the way they think. Each year you should take a carefully selected group of doctors and managers on site visits to view innovative solutions to problems experienced in your institution. One site visit will change more physicians' minds than years of admonition and pleading. This means that you must maintain a list of innovation sites. This can be done by a careful search of the literature and by calling upon your professional network of physician executives.

A routine but important job of the physician executive is work with the designated medical staff committee to review and update medical by-laws. The physician executive should also work with all other medical staff committees in an attempt to improve functioning and reporting. If the hospital takes regular physician and nurse polls, the physician executive should be involved in the polling and in the interpretation of results.

Joint ventures represent an important new area for the physician executive. Many joint ventures fail, so you should approach this area with caution. A good business plan will avert many of the disasters. You should read about and practice drawing up a business plan for a hospital/physician joint venture. Consultants can help you in this area. Do not hesitate to use them. Joint ventures provide one method for minimizing competition between hospitals and physicians. In the future, physicians will be more involved in hospital resource allocation decisions. There will be pluralism on the medical staff. Some doctors will continue as solo practitioners. Other physicians will join groups and corporations that promise greater power and financial return.

Essential Professional Skills of the Physician Executive

As I indicated earlier, as a professional manager you will spend more time communicating than engaging in any other organizational behavior. Listening skills, personal observation skills, self-disclosure skills, and the ability to write and speak well are essential. You will communicate one-to-one, in small groups, in large groups, and on occasion before large audiences. Your ability to influence, motivate, and persuade others will determine much of your success in the organization.

If you are a high-energy person, you can communicate your zest and vitality. If you are a serious, thoughtful person, you can communicate your solid grasp of problem situations. If you are a good listener, other people will seek you out to help them clarify their own thinking.

To win the confidence of your organization, you must avoid extremism. You will always be looking for the common denominator that will bring conflicting parties to resolution. You cannot afford to alienate a large part of the organization by adopting extreme positions. You are an organizational diplomat and must be able to see the validity of many points of view. Your constituents will promote conflicting ideologies and hold limiting assumptions. You must lend a friendly ear to both. You are a listening post for the organization and a mirror for those who want to see themselves through your eyes. If both liberal and conservative physicians respect you and view you as a friend, you are projecting the right image. Of course you have your own opinions, but they should not get in the way of your managerial function as an interface professional--equally at home on either side of the fence.

A physician executive needs to be a high-energy person. On every hand you will be confronted by organizational inertia and physician passivity. Many of the battles you fight you will win because you can hold out longer than your opponents. View yourself as a spark plug. You are there to excite others to necessary action.

Your body/mind vehicle is the only tool you have as a manager. Physical and mental fitness are a precondition to organizational success. If you don't take care of yourself, you will be unable to care for the organization. Try to play a lead role in wellness programs and encourage others to conserve their health.

What theoretical perspective do you bring to your job? In my opinion, the systems perspective is the appropriate one for physician executives. You must be able to see connectedness and perceive interrelationships. Physician executives often work in complex health care organizations with multiple boards and overlapping jurisdictions. Vertical and horizontal integration, diversification, satellites, networking, joint ventures, and relationships with multis are management realities that escape any unidimensional approach to management. You will benefit from readings in general systems theory and systems analysis.

As a physician executive, you are a change agent and must stimulate both organizational stability and organizational change. If you are prepared, you can capitalize on organizational crisis. Often managers must wait until crisis occurs before they can motivate people to act. The good manager anticipates change and helps his organization manage it. The collective mindset of the organization is its ultimate limitation. An organization can change its future as quickly as it can change its mind. The effective physician executive is a mind changer.

Section I. The Context of Management

You need to develop your financial management skills. Everything in the organization reduces to economics. If you understand how the money flows in an organization, you understand most of the organization's dynamics. If you understand how physicians are reimbursed for their services, you can explain a lot of the variance in their practice patterns and professional behavior. You must be alert to the financial impact of all the decisions you make. Courses in cost accounting, pricing, taxes, financial management, budgeting, and investments will help you do a better job in your organization. As profit margins erode, you will become involved in downsizing, or resizing as it is often called. This may require taking beds out of service, dropping clinical services, letting employees go, and breaking relationships with managed care systems. In these instances, the required organizational decisions have both medical and managerial dimensions. Retrenchment management, as it is called, is not much fun, but may be a necessary part of your job for the next few years.

In a rapidly changing market, your organization must each year decide what business it wants to be in. You should help your organization assess its strengths and weaknesses and reposition itself in the medical marketplace. The position your organization chooses to occupy will be translated into the type of doctors and nurses you recruit and the array of services you provide.

Effective managers create positive organizational climates and cultures of excellence. It is part of your job to clarify institutional values and convert these values into organizational behaviors. You should view yourself as a designer of the organization's culture. What kind of a medical care setting is required to assure quality of care and cost containment? What type of organizational climate turns physicians on and encourages physician teamwork? What does your organization really believe in and what is it trying to accomplish. You must ask and help answer these questions.

As profit margins deteriorate in your organization, you should be looking around for new revenue sources. An effective manager generates resources. New medical care products, new market segments, more effective marketing and sales programs, trendy packaging, optimization of existing product lines--these and other strategies will generate additional revenue.

The health care field is moving toward integrated databases and data-based management. Hard facts will replace opinions as health organizations upgrade their management information systems. The physician executive needs data concerning the impact of physician practice patterns on the financial welfare of the organization. He can use these data to modify physician behavior. Without data, you must fly by the seat of your pants and outshout your opposition. You should update your knowledge about competing computer vendors and the information capability they provide. You should participate in the organization's decision to purchase a new computer system. Often the information needs of the medical director are not taken into account in the buy decision. You should own your own personal computer and use it as a personal productivity tool. For better or worse, you will have to learn to manage with numbers.

Managed care is creating a major financial problem for many hospitals. You should view yourself as a managed care consultant and help the hospital select the plan that best fits its needs and financial survival. If you work for a managed care organization, you can use the same skills to design a better package for hospitals. Managed care is here to stay and is something you must understand. Most of the rules you have learned in fee-for-service, solo practice do not apply in this new arena.

Each year you should review the unmet health care needs in your community and determine if these represent a desirable new market for your organization. Unmet needs may be documented and made available to the public in written reports published by other organizations in your community, such as the public health department or a local planning agency. You may have to determine the unmet needs yourself by conducting neighborhood interviews, leading consumer focus groups, or talking to the various gatekeepers in the community, such as pastors or social workers. Many communities do not offer adequate wellness programs, and there is a growing interest in such programs. Consumer interest is a key factor in your marketing effort. Who wants and is willing to pay for a product that your organization can produce? The aging population represents a growing market segment. Industrial health services is a growing niche for many health care providers. By forecasting changes in your service area, you can often spot new product opportunities.

Changes in reimbursement policy and procedure are a constant problem for all health provider organizations. The physician executive needs to examine the impact of such changes on physician behavior, organizational response, cost and quality outcomes, and organizational repositioning in the marketplace. Reimbursement is perhaps the most important dimension to understand in the business dynamics of any health care organization. Reduced reimbursement often requires cost reduction and may lead to organizational retrenchment.

As a manager, you should be alert to signs of organizational decline. This may take many forms including an eroding community economic base, new competitors that arrive on the scene, large industries that move out of the area, increasing obsolescence of your plant and equipment, growing ineffectiveness of your board of directors, deteriorating leadership of the CEO, aging medical staff, decreasing utilization of your services, declining market share, declining net worth, increasing morale problems, a talent exodus from the organization, increasing patient care

Section I.   The Context of Management

incidents, increasing litigation, renewed interest in collective bargaining, reduced quality and output, and increasing problems with third-party agencies. Organizations slowly slide into collapse if managers are not alert to the signs of decline and if they fail to engage in turnaround strategies. As a physician executive, you share responsibility for the welfare of your organization. You must alert the other managers of the team if you see signs of decline. Of course, the CEO and the board of trustees must also act. You cannot do it by yourself.

An important organizational skill for the physician executive is the ability to sell ideas and build people's enthusiasm for a better organization. You must be able to visualize a better organization and communicate that vision effectively to your fellow managers. The physician executive should be a visionary. Perhaps you should develop a think tank or futures group and get other people involved in your envisioning efforts. By creating images of possibility, the manager motivates others to excellence. Good management is high play and is fun. Imagination is the key to a more abundant future for your organization.

Performance Outcomes for the Physician Executive

How do you know if you are doing your job? How will the organization measure your managerial effectiveness? Of course, your performance objectives will vary depending upon the kind of organization you are working for and the specifics of your job assignment.

The most important indicator for continued job tenure is usually how you get along with the CEO. If the CEO views you as a valuable resource and frequently consults you before making important decisions, you know you have arrived.

How popular are you with other members of the management team? Organizational satisfaction with your services is a valid indicator of your value to the organization. You can't do your job if other managers do not like and respect you. You will be evaluated on your technical expertise, interpersonal ability, and organizational participation.

Patient satisfaction is another indicator of your value to the organization. Although this is a difficult dimension to measure, you should be concerned with it. How can you increase the satisfaction of your customers? Satisfied patients tell their doctors and their friends and become repeat customers. When you manage customer satisfaction, you are managing the bottom line.

In general, the physician executive is expected to help the organization survive in the rapidly changing health care marketplace. Do you make a major contribution to the bottom line of your organization? If your organization is in the growth mode, you help it grow. If the organization is in a period of retrenchment, you help it resize. Have you been effective in your efforts to reduce costs? Whatever you do, it must be essential to the survival of the organization. If you are viewed as a luxury, your organization may not be able to afford you in a period of economic decline.

A physician executive can often help the organization expand its patient base by reaching into unserved markets. Who are potential buyers of your products that are not yet customers? A good working relationship with marketing and planning is essential in your attempt to find new patients. If you can convince "splitters" (doctors who admit patients to other hospitals) to admit more of their patients in your facility, you can greatly expand the patient base with very little additional effort. Sometimes all that is needed is a word of encouragement or appreciation. It may be necessary, however, to buy new equipment, improve facilities, make changes in nursing, or fix production problems before you get more admissions from a splitter. It is usually easier to get more business from existing customers than to find new customers. You should carefully monitor the admitting behavior of each physician, note any changes, and act to improve the situation. Even if you are not hospital-based, you need to be actively involved in bringing more business into your organization. In a sense, you should view yourself as a professional sales person. You are selling your organization and its products to potential buyers. You may no longer be involved in manufacturing (the direct provision of patient care), but you should be involved in strategic planning, quality assurance, cost reduction, productivity improvement, marketing, sales, and advertising.

The physician executive knows he is doing his job if the quality of care in the organization is improving. You are a major control point for quality assurance, and if quality deteriorates, it is your fault. You should also be involved in determining quality standards and in setting specifications for computer systems that monitor quality of care. Have you made a major contribution to the risk management program?

Problem-solving and decision making are traditional management functions. What organizational problems have you solved in the past 12 months? Have you studied and improved the way your organization makes decisions? If you can streamline medical care decision making in your organization, you are accomplishing an important job function. This may require intensive work with the medical staff, redesign of staff committees, or the development of a new corporate structure for physicians.

Better management of patient care is also an outcome that should be traceable to you. Providing patient care is a production process, and you should view yourself as a production manager.

It is important that you periodically assess physician, nursing, and patient satisfaction with the production process. Are waiting times too

Section I.   The Context of Management

long? Is there confusion regarding referrals? Are procedures inefficient? Is documentation of patient care inadequate? Are the nursing units understaffed or overstaffed? Are admitting and discharge procedures quick and painless? You should diagram the flow of production in each patient care unit with the times, procedures, and costs carefully noted. You may have to buy a stopwatch and do a little management engineering to determine if you have optimal production efficiencies. In our current reimbursement environment, a dollar saved is a dollar earned. Productivity improvement can offset eroding profit margins.

Another index of your performance is the quality of relationships you maintain with third parties. Do outside companies like to do business with your organization? In addition to being a physician, you must fulfill the roles of diplomat, negotiator, and public relations representative for your organization. It is important to maintain the right image and to facilitate working relationships with outside parties.

Physician satisfaction with your role in the organization and an absence of problems in your assigned areas of medical responsibility are important indicators that you are doing your job well. You are hired to solve problems, not create them. A well-organized and well-functioning group of physicians is a tribute to your capacity as a physician executive.

Are you successful in your attempts to recruit and retain physicians? If this is part of your job description, it is an outcome that should be measured. The right age and mix of the medical staff is important to the survival of your organization.

Innovation is an important organizational outcome and should be part of your performance appraisal. Have you developed new medical services and products for your organization? Have you increased the organization's service area? Have you developed profitable joint ventures? Have you designed an innovative new organizational structure for physicians working with your organization?

Is the community experiencing an improved community health status as the result of your work? This is a difficult performance objective to measure, but it is the reason your organization exists. Your attention to wellness and prevention services is an important step in reducing morbidity indices in your community.

Career Development

A physician executive must learn to manage his career. Your destiny depends on how well you function and progress in organizations. You need to develop a career strategy and plan that is reviewed and updated each year. You must know three things to be a good career planner:

- Where you are presently in your career.

■ Your career destination.

■ A plan for getting from here to there.

It may pay you to get some help from a career planner or to attend a career workshop. There is a large body of literature in this field, and you will benefit from some directed reading.

Don't stay in a bad organizational space. If the organization or the job does not fit you, get out! You will lose time and confidence fighting a losing battle. Remember, a good manager in a bad organizational space is a failure. Even if you can get by, you are losing opportunities to make valuable contributions to the field. Many physicians have never had occasion to resign or have never been fired. They feel that if they are having trouble, it must mean that something is wrong with them. That is a possibility. Another answer is that the fit between the job space and the physician executive is wrong. The only way to know for sure is for the physician executive to leave and seek greener pastures elsewhere.

Develop a professional network. Each time you attend a professional meeting, make contacts and collect business cards. You should have a dozen or more peers with whom you regularly consult and share information. The best jobs come through professional networks. Often one of your peers has solved problems that stump you, and, if asked, will be happy to share the solution with you.

Maintain a high visibility in your profession. You should be a member of the American Academy of Medical Directors (AAMD) and/or the American College of Physician Executives. You should complete the Physician in Management Seminars offered by AAMD. You should attend the national meetings of AAMD. This builds a valuable network of contacts. If people do not know you, they can hardly help you.

Accept offices in national health organizations and serve on their committees. The practice is time-consuming, but it develops contacts and gives you valuable information not available to others in your profession. Remember, as a manager, you manage a knowledge base and you manage through the efforts of others. You have to stay in the mainstream to best serve your own interests and the interests of your organization.

Continue your formal and informal education. It may pay you to go for a MBA. The MD/MBA combination is a powerful vocational ticket. How much more education makes sense for you will depend upon how many more years you plan to work as a physician executive.

Redesign your job. You can enrich your job and increase your satisfaction by adding new job elements that represent your special interests and abilities. Think about your ideal job space. If you could have it all,

Section I.   The Context of Management

what would it be? Know what you need from your organization to be at your best.

Carefully analyze your successes and failures. Every manager learns from his intelligent mistakes. Debrief your actions. Why did I win? Why did I lose? What will I do differently next time? Good managers have a lot of experience and have made a lot of mistakes getting it. Unless you are willing to take risks and make mistakes, you will not learn. It is important that you work for an organization that will back you and take risks with you. No manager wants to be out on a limb.

Present papers at national meetings and contribute to the literature on physician management. As I indicated earlier, most management literature is not directed to your profession and is not easily adapted. If your writing skills are not up to par, work with a freelance writer. You will be the author and the freelancer will prepare your manuscript for publication. A test of any professional is the degree to which he contributes to the literature of his profession.

Do not be afraid to file your credentials with one of the many professional search firms. AAMD operates such a career center and placement agency, the Physician Executive Management Center. You are worth to your organization what you are worth to other organizations. Determine your current market value and talk with the search firm concerning what you can do to make yourself even more attractive to other employers. Maintain an up-to-date personal resume and be certain that it has some recent additions to it.

You may want to develop your consulting skills both inside and outside your organization. Consultation is an important organizational development skill as well as a profession in its own right. What is there after being a physician executive--perhaps a consultant in physician management?

In general, it is good to be active in your community and to develop power bases outside your organization. You may wish to serve on the board of other community agencies and become active in community development. The more power and influence you have outside your organization, the more you have inside it.

Summary

As a physician executive, you are a key player on the management team. You are an interface professional spanning the disciplines of medicine and management. Your effectiveness in the organization depends upon the appropriateness of your role definition and your possession of key management skills. This chapter has defined both of these. To further prepare yourself for success in your profession, consult the attached bibliography of current management literature. The bibliography is organized by topical area. Read in those areas where you will benefit most from further instruction. Although the selections are not written specifically for physician executives, you can easily adapt the material to your needs and interests. I have made no attempt to be exhaustive or necessarily representative of the vast literature available. I have instead included a few items in each topical area that I think will be of maximum benefit to you.

Bibliography

Career Planning

Bardwick, J. *The Plateauing Trap*. New York City: AMACOM, 1986.

Davidson, J. *Blow Your Own Horn*. New York City: AMACOM, 1987.

London, M., and Mone, E. *Career Management and Survival in the Workplace*. San Francisco: Jossey-Bass, 1987.

Rein, I., and others. *High Visibility*. New York City: Dodd, Mead & Company, 1987.

Change

Martel, L. *Mastering Change: The Key to Business Success*. New York City: Simon & Schuster, 1986.

Cognitive Style

de Bono, E. *Six Think Hats*. Boston: Little, Brown, 1985.

Sims, Jr., H., and others. *The Thinking Organization*. San Francisco: Jossey-Bass, 1986.

Competition

Kelly, J. *How to Check Out Your Competition*. New York City: John Wiley, 1987.

Kohn, A. *No Contest: The Case Against Competition*. Boston: Houghton Mifflin, 1986.

Porter, M. *Competitive Strategy*. New York City: Free Press, 1980.

Porter, M. *Competitive Advantage*. New York City: Free Press, 1985.

Sheldon, A., and Windham, S. *Competitive Strategy for Health Care Organizations*. Homewood, Illinois: Dow Jones-Irwin, 1984.

Creativity and Innovation

Albercht, K. *The Creative Corporation*. Homewood, Illinois: Dow Jones-Irwin, 1987.

Burgelman, R., and Sayles, L. *Inside Corporate Innovation*. New York City: Free Press, 1986.

Ray, M., and Myers, R. *Creativity in Business*. New York City: Doubleday, 1986.

Crisis Management

Fink, S. *Crisis Management*. New York City: AMACOM, 1986.

Customer Service

Albrecht, K., and Zemke, R. *Service in America*. Homewood, Illinois: Dow Jones-Irwin, 1985.

Desatnick, R. *Managing to Keep the Customer*. San Franscisco: Jossey-Bass, 1987.

Delegation

Jenks, J., and Kelley, J. *Don't Do. Delegate*. New York City: Ballantine, 1985.

Education of Managers

Johnson, J., and others. *Educating Managers*. San Francisco: Jossey-Bass, 1986.

Financial Management

Costales, S. *The Guide to Understanding Financial Statements*. New York City: McGraw-Hill, 1979.

Futurism

Foss, L., and Rothenberg, K. *The Second Medical Revolution*. Boston: New Science Library (Shambhala), 1987.

Leavitt, H. *Corporate Pathfinders*. New York City: Penguin Books, 1986.

Nash, D. *Future Practice Alternatives in Medicine*. New York City: Igaku-Shoin, 1987.

General Management

Badawy, M. *Developing Managerial Skills in Engineers & Scientists*. New York City: Van Nostrand, 1982.

Brown, W. *13 Fatal Errors Managers Make and How You Can Avoid Them*. New York City: Berkley Books, 1985.

Clifford, Jr, D., and Cavanagh, R. *The Winning Performance*. New York City: Bantam, 1985.

Harmon, F., and Jacobs, G. *The Vital Difference*. New York City: AMACOM, 1985.

Hornstein, H. *Managerial Courage*. New York City: John Wiley, 1986.

Giegold, W. *Practical Management Skills for Engineers and Scientists*. Belmont, California: Lifetime Learning Publications, 1982.

Ginsburg, S. *Ropes for Management Success*. Englewood Cliffs, New Jersey: Prentice-Hall, 1984.

Laureau, W. *Millennium Management*. Piscataway, New Jersey: New Century Publishers, 1978.

Mitroff, I. *Business Not as Usual*. San Francisco: Jossey-Bass, 1987.

Peters, T. *Thriving on Chaos*. New York City: Knopf, 1987.

Smith, M. *Maxims of Management*. Piscataway, New Jersey: New Century Publishers, 1986.

Van Fleet, J. *The 22 Biggest Mistakes Managers Make*. New York City: Parker Publishing, 1982.

Young, A. *The Manager's Handbook*. New York City: Crown, 1986.

Health Care Organizations

Charns, M., and Schaefer, M. *Health Care Organizations: A Model for Management*. New Jersey: Prentice-Hall, 1983.

Management Succession

Gabarro, J. *The Dynamics of Taking Charge*. Cambridge, Massachusetts: Harvard Business School Press, 1987.

Managing Professionals

Benveniste, G. *Professionalizing the Organization*. San Francisco: Jossey-Bass, 1987.

Shapero, A. *Managing Professional People*. New York City: Free Press, 1985.

Marketing

Coddington, D., and Moore, K. *Market-Driven Strategies in Health Care*. San Francisco: Jossey-Bass, 1987.

Negotiating

Fisher, R., and Ury, W. *Getting to Yes*. Boston: Houghton Mifflin, 1981.

Section I.   The Context of Management

Jandt, F. *Win-Win Negotiating*. New York City: John Wiley, 1985.

Organizational Politics

Block, P. The Empowered Manager. San Francisco: Jossey-Bass, 1987.

de Bono, E. Tactics. Boston: Little Brown, 1984.

Yates, Jr., D. The Politics of Management. San Francisco: Jossey-Bass, 1985.

Organizational Renewal

Waterman, Jr., R. *The Renewal Factor*. New York City: Bantam, 1987.

People Skills

Greene, Jr., R. *How to Win With People*. New York City: Hawthorn Books, 1969.

Stewart, D. *The Power of People Skills*. New York City: John Wiley, 1986.

Performance Appraisal

Rausch, E. *Win-Win: Performance Management Appraisal*. New York City: John Wiley, 1985.

Profit Making

Setterberg, F., and Schulman, K. *Beyond Profit*. New York City: Harper & Row, 1985.

Risk Taking

MacCrimmon, K., and Wehrung, D. *Taking Risks*. New York City: Free Press, 1986.

Strategic Planning and Policy

Aaker, D. *Developing Business Strategies*. New York City: John Wiley, 1984.

Below, P., and others. *An Executive Guide to Strategic Planning*. San Francisco: Jossey-Bass, 1987.

Cone, P., and others. *Strategic Resource Management*. Berrien Springs, Michigan: Andrews University Press, 1986.

Sawyer, G. *Designing Strategy*. New York City: John Wiley, 1986.

Yavitz, B., and Newman, W. *Strategy in Action*. New York City: Free Press, 1982.

Teamwork

Buchholz, S., and Roth, T. *Creating the High-Performance Team*. New York

City: John Wiley, 1987.

Garfield, C. *Peak Performers*. New York City: William Morrow, 1986.

Transformational Management

Adams, J. *Transforming Leadership*. Alexandria, Virginia: Miles River Press, 1986.

Adams, J. *Transforming Work*. Alexandria, Virginia: Miles River Press, 1984.

Kozmetsky, G. *Transformational Management*. Cambridge, Massachusetts: Ballinger, 1985.

Tichy, N., and Devanna, M. *The Transformational Leader*. New York City: John Wiley, 1986.

Leland R. Kaiser, PhD, is President of Kaiser and Associates, Brighton, Colo.

Section I.   The Context of Management

CHAPTER 8

Career Positioning

by Marilyn Moats Kennedy, MSJ

O nce you've decided to pursue a career in management, career planning--as opposed to job hunting--becomes very important. Career planning is the process for deciding three things: what skills you want to use (presumably you've chosen your management skills); where you want to work--in the service of what values and types of organizations and where geographically; and, finally, how you will find the right organization and get hired there. Getting a job is never unimportant, but the real issue is getting a series of right jobs and thinking about those jobs as parts of a whole career, not a series of unrelated steps. Career positioning is a key part of career planning because it's the framework within which individual job choices are made.

What is Positioning?

Positioning is the process of putting oneself in a particular relationship to a particular audience. For example, someone who positions himself or herself as a manager is signaling an audience to expect certain behavior. Someone who positions himself or herself as top management or potentially top management sends a different signal. The audience will make an independent evaluation but will be heavily influenced by your self-evaluation as expressed by the way you position yourself. Before you decide on your position, you need to examine your managerial goals.

Goal Setting

Why did you choose management? Do you have an agenda of things you want to accomplish? Are you trying to "straighten out" some part of health care? Is this a preemptive strike, because you don't see anyone else where you are who is capable of management? You need to clarify these questions in your own mind, because their answers are a prerequisite to positioning and career planning. They will influence your choice of organization. Understand that you may change your mind at any time, but saying, "I want to keep my options open," is drifting.

What timeframe have you set? Are you looking for the legendary fast track, a position to round out a career that began with clinical work, a way to maximize earnings now for a complete break in a few years? Each goal will require a different timeframe.

Finally, what are your plans for movement within management? Are you interested in top management, top medical management, or moving entirely out of medical management into the management of another function?

Targeting

Once you've answered these questions, you need to begin the process of targeting. Much has been written about organizational culture and its considerable impact on job and career success. Without repeating all of that, let's summarize and say that you will never be able to mold yourself to "fit" an organization. No surgical procedure known will accomplish that. Targeting is the task of finding an organization that will recognize your worth. In other words, if you have to sell yourself aggressively because there is no immediate recognition of mutual interest, you lose. Everyone must sell himself or herself in an interview, but a hard sell often foretells a bad fit.

The targeting process always begins with you. What are your values? In what environment do you manage best? Are you pro- or anti-meetings? Do you want a large or a small organization? Are you a workaholic or someone with outside interests? These questions must be answered before you can target organizations and position yourself in the right way.

As you mentally construct your ideal organization, there are four factors to keep in mind. An organization might be ideal for you culturally and might easily recognize your worth, but might be very bad for you because it has financial, structural, or marketing problems you could not solve. There are certain general guidelines for healthy, desirable organizations, and these are especially important to people who want to move up rapidly:

- Under $100 million in gross revenues.

- Fewer than 300 employees.

- Growth rate of at least 20 percent per year for the past 2-3 years.

- Not less than 5 and not more than 20 years old.

Of these factors, the growth rate is clearly most important. High growth creates jobs and bonuses. How does one subdivide nothing? In an organization growing at 20 percent a year, given normal turnover, virtually every employee below the CEO will have a chance to move up within two or three years. Contrast this with a shrinking organization. The work load will probably be greater in the latter, with little economic reward possible. Obviously, these criteria won't fit a hospital or group practice. However, growth of at least 10 percent per year, especially for a hospital, is important. A hospital that has a healthy census and expansionist designs (if realistic) is far more likely to provide opportunities for growth and advancement than one that has just announced its third layoff. The same is true of a growing multispecialty group versus one that is praying for several physicians to retire.

Deciding on Positioning Within the Organization

For top management. If the CEO position is your goal, you will need to look for organizations in which some, or all, of the following conditions exist:

A CEO who is at least 20 years older than you or one who is nearing retirement. If you are in your sixties, you're not out of luck. Most start-up organizations hire older managers simply because the younger the company, the older the top management team, excluding founders, tends to be. There is more risk in these organizations, but your contribution will be generously rewarded as the business grows--assuming that it does. If you're in your fifties, to become CEO you'll have to look for a fairly new or a troubled organization. In your forties, an organization with a 50-year-old CEO would be a poor choice. A 55- to 60-year-old CEO would be good. In your thirties, a 50-year-old CEO would be reasonable. A failing 45-year old CEO would not be good, because he or she will almost certainly be succeeded by someone in his or her fifties.

Besides the age of the present CEO, the ages of possible internal competitors need to be considered. If the rest of the top management team is much younger, the organization may already have done some succession planning, and one of those people may be in the process of being groomed to take over. A downturn in the organization's fortunes could eliminate this person, but that puts us in a turnaround situation again.

The ambitions of competitors must also be considered. It's not true that everyone who's a vice president wants to be CEO. Contented number twos are legion, although not one in 10 would own up to that.

A typical scenario for an MD/CEO of a hospital would be to be hired as medical director by the CEO who's planning to retire, voluntarily or not, within three years. There may even be whispers of a golden parachute. The board has decided to "play in" a new person. The candidate most likely to be considered would be in his or her forties, with at least a few years as a medical department chair of a similarly sized hospital in a similar community, or vice president of medical affairs in a smaller hospital who could show an agenda for whatever the board perceives as its institution's future. He or she would be expected to play on the CEO's team, never once so much as suggesting that he or she was "in waiting." The board would be most interested in establishing that the candidate had good relationships with his or her current CEO. Any hint of rebellion or disagreement with the current employer will squelch the deal.

The board of trustees/directors generally considers, although does not generally give the nod to, inside CEO candidates unless the organization is in trouble. In that case, an outsider will almost always be sought. If you're positioning yourself for CEO, no factor will be more important than being in a healthy organization, unless it's a turnaround situation and you literally are the physician applying the cure.

The worst strategy would be to go to an organization 20 years before you wanted to be CEO and attempt to bond yourself inextricably to the organization. This time frame is much too long for the current instability within the health care industry, indeed in U.S. industry in general. If you can't plot with some certainty a move into the top slot within five years, that organization probably isn't going to meet your needs. It's somewhat ghoulish to peg your upward climb to the probability that someone will die or leave in the interim.

Top Medical Management. If your goal is medical director or vice president of medical affairs, you'll have to target specifically the size and type of organization you want and whether you want to be a "first" or go in after someone has shaped the system. It's easier, with little management experience, to find an opportunity to be a "first." The organization doesn't really know what a medical director does, so you'll have time to develop the job. A job description that states "builds and maintains positive working realtionships with physicians" is not really a description, it's a hope. Chairing a medical department at a hospital would be good experience for becoming a medical director, because the chair will face many of the problems of a medical director, but on a smaller scale.

If you want the top medical management spot in a company, you'll need to network for companies just starting to take benefits planning and case management seriously. Then you and top management will have to agree on a set of tasks.

Going into an existing position means that the same rules apply as in any job hunt. It becomes a question of carefully matching your level of management experience--and the problems you're best at solving--with the organization's needs. Caution: what your predecessor did--and how he/she did it--will influence the organization's expectations. Be wary of a situation in which the job description is being "rewritten." It

Section I.   The Context of Management

means that your predecessor didn't do what was expected or did it badly. Organizations tend to react to mismanagement rather than act positively to encourage good management. They shop with a list of "never agains" rather than "must haves." You will need more leadership skills to follow a poor or disappointing performance. On the other hand, you will look much better with less effort, beause your predecessor depressed the CEO's expectations.

Outside of medicine. Should you wish to work in a nonmedical environment, your positioning will again be different.

You'll have to show the transferability of your management skills. That means you'll have to demonstrate the similarity between medical and nonmedical problems. We have watched many people make the transition in one jump by aggressively selling people skills and the concept of the generic manager, i.e., if you were good at managing people in one environment you'd be equally good in another. The argument was that serving as medical director of a 100-physician multispecialty clinic is necessarily a more difficult management task, with more personality problems involved, than managing any similar group.

Networking Nationally

Where do you find the right organization? You have to research this, and part of that will include networking. Nobody is likely to bare his or her organizational soul--warts and all--to a highly desirable manager--you. Without a national network, you might walk into any imaginable snake pit, moving your family thousands of miles only to find the situation untenable. Part of targeting is getting information on organizations that interest you long before any contact is initiated. If you don't keep ongoing files and regularly clip interesting stories from the business press about desirable organizations, you may find yourself wooed--and won--by a snake pit. This is true even if your strategy includes using search firms. It is not the recruiter's responsibility to reveal the client's problems. That's your homework.

It's not enough to be a star of the county or state medical society or well known in the specialty group. Management demands a network of managers, not practitioners. Certainly, for medical management, the American Academy of Medical Directors is an important group. A medical specialty group may provide second generation contacts, i.e., physicians who have access to the CEO, but is unlikely to have many CEO members, particularly of hospitals, HMOs, and companies.

Networking requires planning and organization. It means putting and keeping one's name and interests before key contacts in a positive way. More than for any other reason, people fail to reap the benefits of networking because they fail to follow up with contacts. No one can reasonably be expected to remember a person, regardless of competence or charisma, who is heard from once a year.

Job hunters need to be in touch with key contacts--e.g., those who hi
for positions similar to those the job hunter is seeking and people wl
are often tapped for names of potential stars--no less than once
month. No contact should languish for more than three months wit
out some contact. If you're using search firms, they need regul;
contact, too.

Pitfalls in the Career Planning Process

The saddest people we see are those who tried to short cut the care(
planning process, saying, "Forget goal setting. I will recognize the job
want when I see it." Wrong. The architecture underlying a job hunt :
critical. Here are some of the traps to beware of:

- Taking a job that does not represent a step forward toward your go;
  because you're "needed." This happens to physicians with depres:
  ing regularity, because by inclination and training, they respond to th
  needs of others. While medically sound, it's managerially bad prac
  tice. To be worth doing, the job must be the next step in a career, nc
  a detour.

- Kidding oneself about the importance of geography, the people envi
  ronment, or the kind/type of organization. Did you assume that
  because the organization has a strong religious affiliation, it would b(
  a less "political" environment? Then you didn't do your homework
  People feel free to do anything when they're doing it in the name o
  the Almighty. If you love New York City, you may find Butte a bit dul
  and the natives slow to warm up. Knowing yourself and your family':
  emotional and geographic needs is very important.

- Telling yourself that you're adaptable; you can stand anything for twc
  years. Wrong! You may not survive three months. Two years in a
  hostile or uncongenial environment might be two lifetimes. If there's
  pain going in, nothing positive will come of the experience. You didn't
  like the medical director, and the CEO was no prize. Still, you signed
  on as vice president, medical affairs. This has disaster written all over
  it. Those people were on their best behavior. That was as good as it
  gets! You're in for it now.

- Positioning yourself to work managerial miracles, because you were a
  medical miracle worker. "How bad can it be?" does not provide the
  frame, much less the picture. Never suggest that whatever problems
  they have would be nonproblems for you. Do you really have the
  managerial experience to assert that?

- Agreeing to take a turnaround job unless you are getting paid to turn
  the place around. Any turnaround situation is high risk. If it's not also

Section I. The Context of Management

high reward, it's not the monetary loss that worries us. It's the fact that the people won't believe a miracle not paid for has truly occurred. Someone else will get the credit and how will you trade that up to your next job?

- Positioning yourself on the fast track when you're actually there to ease burnout and into your retirement plan. They'll discover your real attitudes early on, as you unwittingly reveal your agenda--and you will. For example, maybe long-term planning is important to them, but you can't see the fine distinctions. That's because they don't affect your interests.

- Believing you're good at organizational politics because, as an attending, physicians and administrators like you. Being "good with people," especially when you're already in a power position, is not the same as being good at managerial politics.

- Positioning yourself as a manager and behaving as if you are still a clinician. This is a very common problem. Switching hats has to be a conscious effort. It's too easy to think like a physician when you ought to be thinking like a manager.

Finally, much of positioning is an ongoing process. It's not possible to decide now what you'll be doing in 20 years, even if you believe that's when you'll retire! Many people use retirement as a way to ease out of one career into another. It's important to reexamine your positioning at least every 18 months. That doesn't mean changing jobs at each career check point, but it does mean taking the time to reaffirm that what you are doing is a conscious choice, not something you've drifted into.

Marilyn Moats Kennedy, MSJ, is Managing Partner, Career Strategies, Inc., Wilmette, Illinois.

CHAPTER 9

Physicians in Management:
The Costs, Challenges, and Rewards

by James E. Hartfield, MD, FACPE

R arely does a blinding light from heaven suddenly surround the Chosen Physician as he trudges through evening rounds and a commanding voice proclaim, "I have created you to be CEO of St. Cedars General!" Although when such a promotion ultimately does occur, there is often more sublime serendipity than scholarly selection involved.

Until recent years, the designation of physicians as managers in medical complexes generally followed three criteria, professionally known as "SAG Factors"--Seniority, Accountability, and Gullibility. Within the scope of these salient features, little room for creative career design or targeting was possible. Given the unprogrammed and largely unprepared conscription of many physicians into early management roles, it is worth noting with pride the frequency with which these early, however "sagging," pioneers rose to the occasion. There is also competent support for the idea that good managers are born, not made, as the plethora of maximally degreed and minimally talented MBAs running loose in corporate ranks today attests.

This chapter seeks to summarize the preceding observations in this section and validate their accuracy with personal observations and experiences. While it is unlikely that any two physician executives would have duplicate management careers, some parallel insights may be useful for physicians entering this new specialty. The preceding introductory reviews of the current health care scene, with the evolving critical role of the physician executive as a major actor in this drama, provide an appropriate backdrop for the modern medical management stage. There is little tolerance of or excuse for relying on fate to plant a blooming medical executive in management's garden; today dedicated preparation and targeted matching of skills to job are expected. The professional conflicts that have been faced over full- or part-time management, credibility without some clinical practice residual, compensation, etc. remain as points for discussion to be sure, but they are now largely recognized for what they always actually were--smoke screens to cover the personal insecurity involved in making a major career change.

This accusation deserves amplification. Many of us who entered management did so in a part-time arrangement because our organizations needed our continued professional participation. This is particularly true in small group practices, in staff model HMOs or with hospital physicians. There is no magic number that automatically dictates full-time medical management commitment, whether that number indicates physicians, hospital beds, or health plan members. Clearly the appropriate time for a full-time physician executive is when those defining jobs and hiring personnel for the organization decide it has arrived. Throughout the country and within the wide scope of management opportunities, the range of those organizational decisions is highly variable. The physician executive who finds himself confronted with inappropriate part-time expectations by employers, credibility implications with his peers, or inadequate compensation for his labors has three basic choices: first, work to convince the organization of the necessity for acceptable changes; second, reluctantly but resolutely accept the status quo, or third, move to a more satisfying position. For some, that last alternative has meant retreating to full-time clinical practice and leaving management altogether. Many others convince themselves that they are pursuing reasonable change within their organization while in reality they are settling for the second, more secure, option.

From the viewpoint of one who has traveled the management road through all of these options, some observations regarding physician management behavior seem justified. The essential foundation for all of these activities and observations is my deep and abiding respect and admiration for the profession of medicine. There have been many exciting developments along with alarming alterations in American medicine that demand persistence of concerned physicians to preserve the integrity and heritage of this proud vocation. The physician executive has the critical opportunity of being a profession conservationist while also being a leader and catalyst in the current medical evolution.

Observations Regarding Physicians and Management

Most physicians entering management are inadequately prepared for standard managerial techniques.

If there is any justification for adding business degrees after the M.D., it would be to avoid the embarrassment many physician executives endure for having either basic ignorance of or deprecating attitudes toward those "basics" in management such as management by objectives, strategic planning, group dynamics, conflict resolution techniques, time management, etc. Even the most fundamental dynamic of how to utilize a good secretary or other support personnel effectively escapes many. It was not until I entered the corporate arena that I faced the stark nakedness of an empty appointment schedule. In clinical practice my patients clamored for every 15 minutes--how could a waiting corporate world find my presence so undemanded? The luxury was short lived fortunately, but it did provide a valuable lesson in time structuring for one whose schedule had always been regimented by rounds, conferences, nurses, and mothers. This cultural shock is equally severe in reverse for the academic physician whose private office and classroom regimen is suddenly confronted with demands for heavier clinical schedules by the faculty practice plan.

Physicians resist management practices that they consider sophomoric forays into busy work--as many regard job objectives, policy writing, employee evaluations, and such things as were overlooked in standard medical school curricula. Whether this resistance reflects unfamiliarity or a valid assessment of present situations, it is uniformly a reflection of the physician's discomfort with his job's management expectations.

The American Academy of Medical Directors was founded originally to address these educational deficits among physicians propelled into management. An honest appreciation of the essentials in management behavior is as needed as were the classes at Ft. Sam Houston in which those of us drafted into the medical corps were taught how to salute. We were at first extremely self-conscious; then we got the hang of it and even sort of enjoyed the activity, eventually accepting it as a tolerable part of military life and rank. Physician executives need to be cautious about having naive disregard for policies, traditions, buzz words, and personnel management. In the frequently alien world of management, MDs are the space invaders.

The skills required in good management often contradict the skills learned in good patient care.

Perhaps this observation explains much of the preceding paragraphs. Learning to move confidently and with dispatch through a crowded patient schedule or hospital rounds creates a self-assuredness and autonomy that is often foreign to business management. It is far safer to predict the results of treatment with penicillin or digitalis than to project the results of a marketing campaign or prosperity from a joint venture. Patient diseases are a piece of cake compared to corporate ailments.

Physicians are brainwashed from the first cadaver incision to the last residency prescription in the "scientific method" and the "proper" management of disease. With adequate clinical trials and experience, certain therapeutic regimens can be defined and results predicted, even expected. Organizational management is far less precise, and the effects of the most sincerely applied remedies are far less likely to be predestined. The confident demeanor and positive bedside manner that salvaged many despondent consumers of health care augur little more than false bravado in the board room. Conversely, the old reliable

Kildarian technique of "leveling with the patient" about your frustrations and perplexities is generally regarded as the theatrics of an incompetent or ill-prepared executive by corporate observers.

On the other hand, among the most distasteful exposures experienced in many management arenas are the "standard" techniques of Covering Your Flank and Blame Shifting, which are generally absent in medical circles. Rather than conspire jointly to solve a problem, there is cautious avoidance of any association with potential failure, and an endless line of memos documenting every glitch or glimmer when escape from association is impossible. That is probably understandable when one's bonus depends on how the boss perceives your performance.

As more physicians enter management, fewer will begin near the top of the organizational ladder. Even if those at the top are other physician executives, the culture is not, and will likely never be, the medical milieu of the examination room or operating suite. While the experiences may often contradict, they need not conflict, and the agile physician executive will eventually learn to enjoy hopping among frying pans.

Physician executives tend to overestimate their management capabilities but underestimate their management value.

In Chapter 8, on career positioning, one of the pitfalls cited for aspiring physician executives is assuming that saving lives adequately prepares the physician for saving organizations. Such near-omnipotence in the clinic is certainly commendable, but rarely does the opportunity arise to perform advanced CPR on the CEO. Although I occasionally suspected that my brilliant article published during medical school days on "Measuring Neurosecretory Material in the Pituitary of Sprague-Dawley Rats" could have had corporate application, I doubt that it was the highlight of my resume.

Frequently I am asked to review the curriculum vitae of physicians who are interested in management positions. Most are faced with a common problem: they have published little or nothing related to management and have limited management experience. The unfortunate reality is that both are important, although the latter is more desirable. In spite of these customary deficits, the general physician expectation is to enter management at a senior level with an associated executive salary and benefit plan.

Often the disappointing reality surfaces during these resume reviews that in the drive to assume some medical management role of significance, the "medical" credential is subjugated. Experience, however, indicates that the MD degree remains the most powerful force in the entire resume. Physicians still enjoy an enviable mystique and respect, even among corporation executives. The awesome responsibility and basic intelligence credited to most physicians command respect, and care should be exercised to avoid clumsily allowing these assets to fade. Physicians should be experts in dealing with other physicians, defining appropriate clinical practices, establishing quality controls, etc., which were usually among the reasons for seeking a "medical director" in the first place. No one expects financial genius, marketing savvy, or computer literacy in physicians. If any of these are part of the physician manager's talent bank, they are frosting on the cake, but they will not adequately ice over a basic inability to monitor professional behavior or deal with an impaired colleague.

Physician executives tend to avoid conflict rather than manage it.

An unusual paradox hampers the effectiveness of many physicians, and it spills over into their management careers. There is a tendency to flee from personal confrontation rather than attempt to focus the energy involved in such conflicts into positive action. This reality has been a major factor in the professional disdain for peer review organizations and has played a major role in the current malpractice epidemic. Although many colleagues would vigorously deny such a milquetoast malady, this is a major fault in physician executives and reflects an honest interprofessional empathy that is discussed later. Most physicians would rather be challenged or disciplined by peers regardless of the pain involved for both parties, and other nonphysician managers are delighted to relinquish this opportunity--they usually expect to be able to do just that. Physicians who are sincere and dedicated in clinical efforts simply do not want to believe otherwise of colleagues. Even the least productive and most aggravating associate is tolerated, and, in fact, the dances around confronting these individuals about commonly appreciated problems make Swan Lake pale by comparison. The business world, with its management hierarchy, titles, and status perks, excels in emphasizing the frailties of employees. It is no wonder that the recent runaway best sellers in management have been those that emphasize listening to employees, inclusion, praise, and other strange tactics taught in Psychology 101 at medical school. Perhaps we oversold the message to our students. Conflict usually means that people are alive and thinking, or at least reacting. Sure, it requires some digging to isolate a common framework of agreement for subsequent building or to displace emotional responses with constructive planning, but that is what should be expected when intelligent people address any issue. God spare us the robot mentality that prefers tranquil monotony over creative challenge.

Appropriate management requires as much concerted effort as direct medical care.

This observation is a corollary to the previous comments on overestimating management capabilities. After years of study, enduring the agonies of residency, mumbling through millions of phone conversations from patients, and surviving endless nights on call, it should certainly be a refreshing break to prop the old feet up on that huge desk and dictate to Miss Gorgeous. It's not that simple or pleasant. Begin with the realization that this is new turf, even if the new management responsibility is in an organization governed by physicians. Those who are being managed learn quickly to compartmentalize your efforts. The fact that you were an outstanding surgeon will only serve to reinforce those unspoken convictions that you should have stayed in the O.R. when the business begins to falter. Remember, those colleagues have likely not read this book and covertly believe that feet on desk and Miss Gorgeous routine. Medical management challenges are real. Addressing them appropriately will require intensive and extensive preparation. The "corporate culture" has a painfully real presence, whether in a major business, academic setting, the military, hospital, or group practice. Before it can be massaged and remolded, if needed, it must be defined, and that may mean developing a perspective of organizational history; knowing local, state, or federal ordinance impacts, appraising key personalities, and assessing existing organizational commitments or anticipated alliances. For a professional who either had personal mastery over health care problems or could find readily available consultants or referral sources, the shift to dealing with amorphous possibilities or responsibility isolation can be quite uncomfortable. Remember the security derived by dusting off Harrison's or Nelson's or even Current Therapy? The books do not exist, nor are they ever likely to be written, that neatly index the management problems that crop up with surprising regularity. Most require the application of principles and concepts rather than pills and cutting, and demand confident patience and thoughtful compromise.

The risks of failure for physicians entering management are greater than for their nonphysician counterparts.

In general, a conscientious physician who practices good medicine will be successful by almost any standard applied to success today. Even a sizable number of not-so-competent medical practitioners seem to enjoy considerable success. The same simply cannot be said for nonphysician managers throughout the broad spectrum of business endeavors. Endless possibilities exist in the corporate hierarchy to redefine the participation of marginal performers ranging from termination, demotion or lateral (dead-end) transfer to side-track (safeguard) promotions, or early retirement. To leave the security of a "sure thing" in medicine to opt for such management insecurity is undeniably risky, and on a much broader scale than for the nonphysician manager who never had it any better. The physician executive's risk is compounded by the extreme difficulty of reentry into full-time practice if the management golden opportunity begins to tarnish. A referral practice such as surgery or the medical sub-specialties is almost beyond recapture, and the rapid progression of medical technology and pharmaceuticals quickly escapes any physician who must focus on other priorities.

New Leadership in Health Care Management

In spite of the protests of "credibility maintenance" or "first love lost," the reluctance of many physicians to enter management on a full-time basis is rooted in the risk associated with leaving practice. While physicians are generally not regarded as being risk-averse, they are success-oriented (on behalf of their patients, they had better be). One should never underestimate the security concerns of the spouse as well.

I could almost set my watch by the regularity with which business colleagues ask, "Why did you decide to leave medicine?" Most of the time I am able to reply with some satisfyingly insipid remark. It is critically important that both we who are physicians entering management and those in the businesses we are joining recognize that physician executives are not "leaving medicine." We are merely changing specialties. My concern for the welfare of human beings has never abated. I have elected to transfer my efforts in support of those patients from the examining room to the board room, from prescribing therapy for specific diseases to developing pathways for fighting disease, from the practice of medicine to the preservation of medicine as an honorable profession for future colleagues and consumers.

Therein lies a further risk for the physician executive. To have significant influence in management, the physician executive must be capable. For the academic physician, it is understandably painful to fail an inadequately prepared medical student, yet the safeguarding of future patients is an overriding determinant. I have never been able to conjure comfort from any source when I had to terminate a physician executive. Of course, solid job performance must be expected from any manager, but can this colleague find a place of re-entry, either to practice or other management? This decision will have major impact on his family. The physician oversupply assumes new proportions when starting over at 55 years of age.

Perhaps this enhanced risk for physician executives is an argument for developing a management residency for the new specialty and forging a management career shortly following the academic years. I think not. While there are some attractive considerations, such as having an opportunity to gain experience, requiring lower starting salaries, and confronting less elaborate initial physician expectations, the time is not yet right for the physician community to afford leadership responsibilities to a colleague who has not "paid his dues." Roughly translated, for a physician executive that means "developed an appreciation for work in the trenches, demonstrated the ability to relate to patients and peers, and, in general, attained a position of credibility among a wide range of colleagues." This helps reduce the risks accepted by those being managed and currently goes a long way toward doing the same for the manager.

What Nonphysician Managers Think

Certainly these observations are not the only ones that could be or have been made regarding physicians as managers. They represent one physician's listing of impact assertions that need to be appreciated by those studying the field. A few years back, I was concerned about how nonphysician managers viewed the performances of physician executives under their direct supervision. Table 1, below, summarizes the responses from 31 nonphysician managers within the same company and with similar manager relationships. They were asked to identify the frequency with which some problems reported about physician executives were seen in the physician executive they directly supervised, and then to estimate by one to four checks the degree of job impact that problem produced for them. The replies are expressed as percentages of the choices given and the most commonly reported number of checks.

The most striking concern focused around time and task management, which is related in items A, E, F, and I and which had substantial job impact, as might be anticipated. The major shift from regimented appointment and O.R. schedules to personally directed time management seems difficult for many physicians.

For a profession in which talking to patients and families is a major time consumer, it is apparent that communication remains a problem (G). This charge is regularly leveled at physicians in general and has not been

---

PROBLEMS ENCOUNTERED WITH PHYSICIAN EXECUTIVES AS PERCEIVED BY THEIR NON-PHYSICIAN SUPERVISORS IN A LARGE CORPORATION

Manager Problems	Frequency Rare	Average	Often	Job Impact
A. Inadequate appreciation of job tasks.	30	40	30	!!!
B. Indecisiveness in dealing with staff physicians and other professionals	40	60		!
C. Inappropriate recognition of non-physician manager's job requirements	40	60		!!
D. Reluctance to confront service problems.	60	30	10	!
E. Inability to establish time and task priorities.	10	60	30	!!!!
F. Inertia in task completion.	30	40	30	!!
G. Failure to communicate effectively.	15	70	15	!!
H. Inappriate involvement in non-medical areas.	100			
I. Lack of relevant balance in addressing details.	30	40	30	!!!
J. Inability to accept or respond to constructive criticism.	70	15	15	!
K. Apparent insecurity or lack of personal confidence.	100			

New Leadership in Health Care Management

obviated by the transition into management. There is some reassurance in noting, however, that whatever and however the physician executive does, he does with conviction and confidence, regardless of how timely or well communicated (K).

Although this limited survey is far from definitive, a careful review of these responses is appropriate for all physicians in management. Given the high probability that no executive is perfect, the courage to expose imperfections is commendable. To discover them and then correct them is exemplary.

The Personal Bottom Line

She followed the rest of the preschoolers to the center of the stage and was immediately blinded by the harsh lights around the perimeter. Timidly glancing around, she noted one boy was screaming at the top of his lungs while another little girl was waving and smiling to the audience. One girl with long curls had wrapped her arms around a leg of the curtain puller--her face flushed with determination--and that little boy on the end had wet his pants. All of these seemed reasonable options at age three or four years when the time came for the first solo performance. Several decades later and after immeasurable trips to center stage, physicians who have been in some form of management need to appraise the health and stability of the only corporation over which they have ultimate control--themselves. This calculation of a "personal bottom line" should be done on a regular basis, not just when approaching retirement. It needs to begin with an honest realization of WHY. Why am I entering a new career phase? Why am I assuming the risks involved with such a move? Why do I presume to have the skills required? As indicated in Michael Guthrie's analysis reported earlier, most of us wanted leadership, challenge, influence, and involvement within the health care industry. So did you get what you want? Have you a prayer of ever fulfilling your ambitions?

It is unfortunately amusing that some of us are still on that preschool platform. Some are still clinging to security in the wings; others have moved bravely to center stage but are screaming about the injustices of our present situation (or are trying to be recognized by creating a disturbance), and others have soiled themselves so pitifully in public that they can neither advance nor retreat without pain or embarrassment. There will always be the upstagers who wave and smile at the crowd, but many of them keep doing only that long after the show has started, seemingly oblivious to the script or directors. Most of us will eventually start to sing or dance or recite, and while a few will be stars, most will be part of a chorus--performing as the essential, dependable, and indispensable backdrop for the panorama of modern medicine. Of course, that is all right, unless you wanted to be the star or unless you wanted to sing the aria or play the cadenza.

It is, in the final analysis, a matter of personal perspective--how the physician moving into management sees himself or herself. It is the standard of performance with which he can live, the degree of challenge he agrees to accept, and the end result with which he can be professionally proud and personally satisfied. There is a world of difference between cocky arrogance and quiet confidence. The world of medical management, just as the broad range of medical patients, is always looking for the latter and trying to avoid the former. While the chapters to follow are designed to provide the tools necessary to achieve management confidence, the appropriate and timely application of these techniques remains a personal challenge for physician executives. Your place on the stage is waiting.

James E. Hartfield, MD, FACPE, is Associate Vice President/Clinical Affairs, University of South Florida College of Medicine, Tampa.

Section II.

The Content of Management

CHAPTER 10

The Management of Professionals

by Irwin Rubin, PhD

As the profession of physician executive grows, an agreed-upon content, what it is that physician executives are expected to do, is being defined. That definition will change as physician executives move into a widening array of medical management positions in a variety of health care settings. No single definition can be expected to describe all physician executives in all environments, although a core description is sure to result. And physician executives will be judged on the basis of the degree to which they conform with the content of their jobs, regardless of the environment.

Mere job descriptions will not suffice, however. In order to adequately judge the performance of members of the medical management profession, however, it will be necessary to address process as well as content definitions. It will be necessary to define the behaviors that are expected in order for physicians to be granted membership in this new profession.

The survival and growth of any human organization rests upon a clear, agreed-upon sense of direction and purpose among its members. For a health care organization, this sense translates into the need for a mission statement, which provides a context within which fundamentally value-based choices must be made. Given an agreed-upon mission, the organization's members will be required to make decisions on how that mission can best be achieved. In the absence of a mission, a reactive, as opposed to proactive, stance toward the environment is inevitable.

Whereas an organization needs a *mission* statement, a group that would call itself professional needs an *identity* statement. To be in control of its own destiny, a professional group must exhibit a high degree of clarity and agreement around questions of direction and purpose. "Who are we?" "What is it that we uniquely stand for?" "How do our purposes and direction differ from those of other professions?"

Section II.   The Content of Management

The medical management profession has emerged from its "childhood" with a strength of numbers few would have ventured to predict at its birth some 13 years ago. To the profession's growing numerical strength must be added the strength of its resolve to grow in a particular direction with a particular purpose. The opportunity to begin the painful, difficult, and essential process of conscious identity formation for the profession flows directly from what has already been determined to be the primary concern of the profession. As a group, physician executives have as an overall concern, and purpose, the "management of professionals." The purpose of the physician executive, within that overall purpose, is to bridge the gap between the management of professionals and the management of physicians as a special subset of professionals.

Implicit in that purpose is a set of beliefs or assumptions that have carried the profession to its current stage of development. An examination of those beliefs and assumptions and of the historical foundation that they have allowed to be built is the first step in deciding the shape of the future that the profession plans to build.

The medical management profession has reached an important and very normal development threshold. As it moves into its "young adulthood," the profession should be prepared to take a proactive stance regarding its direction and purpose. It is time for the profession to consciously step up to the question, "What do we want to be when we grow up?"

A "Particular" Meaning?

Professionals are different. Too much can be made of those differences, but they exist. They have unique characteristics that differentiate them from others in terms of what is required of those who manage them. Whether for medical management or for any other kind of management, the characteristics and qualities of those being managed will play an important role in defining the content and context of the management function. Physicians, as a special subset of professionals, require even more differentiation. And, if the medical management definition is to be workable, the differences must be accounted for.

To understand the things that differentiate physicians from other professionals and from nonprofessionals, it is critical to look more deeply at what is involved in becoming and being a physician. By understanding what is involved in the process of producing a physician, one can understand what it is about becoming and being a physician that alters a person in ways that require that they be managed differently from nonprofessionals and from other professionals.

If you are a physician, you are experientially aware of what is involved in becoming a physician. A physician has "paid his professional dues" in ways that no outsider could ever fully understand. The best I can do is to articulate what I have heard physcians say in this regard.

To become a physician means making some very specific choices. A physician chooses to satisfactorily pass through a series of very intensive and extensive "hoops." Personal sacrifices have to be made to accommodate the time and energy demands of the education and training process for the profession. That process includes, for instance, the internalization of almost inhuman quantities of facts. Worse, after going through an initial exposure to such an accumulation of facts, when the physician is finally in practice, the information explosion makes it seem as if he or she is standing on shifting sands. The firm ground that science promised, in return for bleary, bloodshot eyes, loses some of its solidness.

Natural human emotions associated with the healing process are successfully desensitized during the physician's education and training. The purpose of this process is to lessen the pain of failure in individual cases, but the desensitization is complete. Emotional "programs" (the art of medicine) are successfully implanted alongside content "programs" (the science of medicine). The purpose of all this socialization is a successful physician, but it can make of the successful physician an emotionally handicapped individual.

So, the boot camps that medicine calls internships and residencies are powerful agents of socialization. The need to learn how to cope with "inhuman" expectations also has a powerful effect on the physician's professional development. The preponderance of jokes that equate physicians with "God" are not without significance. Nor are they without consequences. Many physicians may take these jokes, and their own "press clippings," too seriously.

Let me summarize what I believe it means to be a physician--a member of a particular subset of professionals. The physician has exercised intellectual muscles by pushing through a body of specialized knowledge. A personally acceptable level of truths from the science of medicine has been absorbed by the physician. In addition to the body of knowledge, an attitude has been instilled. The socialization process has yielded a bias. Physicians share a set of attitudinal, and therefore behavioral, *shoulds*. They exhibit a professionally consistent code of behavior. Physicians are independent, results-oriented, and impatient, for instance.

When the physician puts on a hat as a professional manager of physicians, two very familiar problems are encountered. The physician executive's clinical colleagues may resist managerial decision making. Success in passing through the education and training hoops carried the promise of autonomy--nobody would tell them what they had to do. This problem is compounded by the physician executive's need to shift his or her bias to that of a professional manager. The physician

Section II.   The Content of Management

executive's responsibility is to orchestrate the band, not to play the instruments. Managers make process decisions that dictate the what, who, and how of content decisions. For a physician, albeit a physician executive, this shift in approach can be wrenching. The initial socialization process does not fade easily.

A Contextual Conflict

The conflict in perspectives that the physician executive experiences daily is not personal or unique. Every profession imposes a set of behavioral expectations upon its members. It is the behavioral expectations that define what we mean by a professional in any field. The expectations result in a code of behavior that serves a crucial and positive function. The quality of the products and services associated with a profession is directly related to the degree to which professional expectations have been developed and enforced. The more professional a health care organization is, the better the care its patients can expect. The specific definitions of professionalism and high quality are, in the final analysis, personal. Most would agree, however, that they are, if not one and the same, very highly correlated.

The drive for high quality and a high level of professionalism puts enormous pressure on physician executives. It is the physician executive's responsibility to strive for the highest achievable levels of professionalism in the management of an organization's human assets. The challenge to a manager is to make a difference in the organization. Through the physician executive's own professional behavior, and through the manager's ability to influence the behavior of others, value is added to the organization's mission--the highest standards of professional care for its patients.

I need to reemphasize the fact that the existence of this conflict between the physician executive and physicians is not personal. It is a challenge faced by every organization in which professionals play key roles. Indeed, the science of management documents the universality of this contextual dilemma. Those who move from the ranks of "nonprofessional" producers to first-line supervisors encounter dilemmas that are qualitatively no different. Both the physician executive and the first-line supervisor experience this phenomenon, called "culture shock" and react in predictably human ways. While the first reaction may be nonproductive or counterproductive, the professional's concern with quality will eventually overcome socialization and produce the desired result.

A change in context also carries with it new meanings of rightness, new definitions of what constitutes the right behavior in a given situation. For the physician executive, a situation must now be viewed from a managerial perspective as well as from a provider perspective. If this were not true, there would be no difference in being a physician and in being the professional manager of that physician.

Professionals cannot, within the current context of health care, be left to manage themselves. This truth has ceased to be the subject of philosophical debate. It is a pragmatic reality thrust upon the profession by the marketplace. Health care has become an organizational activity that is governed by rules to a large extent imposed from outside the system itself. Even where physicians remain independent, that independence is tempered by the presence of a wide range of organizational entities--hospitals, health maintenance organizations, preferred provider organizations, and many more--with which they must deal on a dependent basis.

Implications for Management

If there is a profession of management and if it has any significance in the management of health care organizations, two requirements naturally follow. First, there needs to be a definable body of knowledge that must be internalized by those who would call themselves management professionals. Because of the work of the American Academy of Medical Directors, standards concerning requisite content knowledge for the physician executive are being forged. The "science" of this new profession is emerging, along with a willingness to enforce those standards. The creation of the American College of Physician Executives in 1980 was an important step in both recognition for the profession and in ensuring that the standards the Academy had established would have teeth.

It takes a great deal of courage for a profession to assume proactive control of its destiny in this way. The inevitable consequence is potential exclusion and disappointment for some aspiring members of the profession. The strength and maturity reflected by this step into professional adulthood is essential if the even more difficult second step is to be taken.

Another Requirement

The second requirement of any profession is, as mentioned earlier, a standard code of behavior. In medicine, this is referred to under the general rubric of "bedside manner." The science of medicine is ministered through the laying on of hands.

If there is a profession of management, it too must have its "artistic" side. The science of management (content) is ministered through day-to-day interpersonal behavior (process). It is in this domain that the next developmental challenge for the medical management profession lies.

Interpersonal skills are the tools through which managers shape the

Section II. The Content of Management

behavior of others. They are the tools with which managers make a difference. When the tools are skillfully applied, the result is higher levels of organizational professionalism and, consequently, higher quality of care.

The next step in the profession's control of its destiny is a definition of the "particulars" of a standard code of behavior for the medical manager. What does "rightness" mean in terms of how physician executives should behave toward their professional responsibilities?

It will come as no great surprise to those of you who know me that I believe:

- There is a uniform code of "good" managerial behavior.

- Human similarities far outweigh the impact of professional differences.

In other words, from a behavioral perspective, it is a myth to presume that there is any qualitiative difference between being a good healthy human being and being an effective manager of other human beings.

A good professional manager has mastered a body of knowledge. To utilize this or any other unique expertise requires the enactment of what is known (content) in a human manner (process). If a professional's code of behavior does not subsume a common code of human behavior, a paradox of awesome proportions has been created. It simply is not possible to be a good manager without enlisting some basic human behavior codes. Those who are to be managed will not respond well to a manager who is that alien.

Specialness of the Subset

To move this thesis ahead, I need to articulate another major quality that defines a physician. This quality is more elusive than those produced by the education and socialization experience. It has to do with how humans see and esteem themselves. For any person, this quality is central to the concept of identity.

Professionals feel a special kind of link with their colleagues. To have a strong reference group is to be part of a powerful culture, with all its attendant benefits and risks. So the management of professionals entails the management of a group of people who, for whatever reasons, feel and act special.

Professionals are expected to feel high levels of pride, self-respect, and commitment--higher levels for the most part than would be expected in nonprofessionals. Professionals are expected to approach their work, and consequently their organizations, with a "higher order" morality

New Leadership in Health Care Management

than do nonprofessionals. Physicians are therefore only a special subset of people who, for reasons unique in content but not form, feel special and expect to be treated accordingly.

When physician executives say that they must learn how to manage physicians as a special subset of professionals, they are saying they must learn to exhibit a special kind of caring--caring that acknowledges and reflects the specialness of those being managed. As managers, they feel a need to account in their managerial behavior for the investment others have made in internalizing a body of science, a body of knowledge. Physician executives feel a need to approach their role as managerial decision-makers within the context of the "prima donna" quality of their "troops." They strive to approach their managerial responsibilities with something labeled sensitivity and respect.

Ponder the following question. "What would happen if we approached the problem of managing all of our human resources with the same degree of care, concern, respect, and sensitivity as we do the management of professionals and of physicians as a special subset of professionals?"

It is to the benefit of a health care organization to acknowledge the special requirements of its professional employees. Professionalism and quality are virtually indistinguishable. But how can it not be of benefit to do the same thing for nonprofessional employees? Changing their perspective as professional managers is essential if physician executives are to find ways to have each and every employee feel and act and be treated as a professional.

Bridging the Gap

There is a gap that all managers need to bridge. It is a gap that transcends the boundaries of individual organizations. It is the gap between intentions, as driven by beliefs, and impact of managers on organizations, as driven by behavior. Douglas McGregor laid the challenge before all managers in his articulation of the correlation between managerial behaviors and X versus Y Theory belief systems.

The health care industry and physician executives are uniquely positioned to take the lead in creating a new, humanistic ethic of management. In a health care organization, the ability to care for patients is limited, in the long run, by the amount of human caring that managers create and nuture among those they manage. The question to ponder in this regard is virtually the same as the one raised earlier in this chapter. "What would happen if the management of all human resources was approached with the same degree of care, concern, regard, and sensitivity as would be accorded patients?"

The Next Step

If it is to continue to grow as a profession, medical management needs to articulate a uniform code of behavior. The profession's content standards are, as mentioned earlier, taking shape. It is time for the profession to shape to its process standards.

The question to be addressed can be stated as follows: "What categories of describable and observable day-to-day behaviors must a person learn to exhibit skillfully in order to be granted continuing membership in this new profession? The remaining chapters in this section will address some of the skills that physician executives will need to obtain and show how they can be applied successfully.

Irwin Rubin, PhD, is President, Temenos, Inc., Honolulu, Hawaii.

CHAPTER 11

Economics and U.S. Health Care

by Hugh W. Long, PhD

A bsent resource scarcity, there is no inherent tension between economics and medicine. But once we are confronted with scarcity of resources, medical decision-making must ultimately be tempered by economic reality.

By "resources," we mean anything directly consumed by human beings or used by human beings to produce something else directly consumed. General categories of resources are labor, energy, capital, raw materials, etc. The term "scarcity" does not mean that there is a shortage of any particular resource or even that we are running out of that resource. Rather, "scarcity" is a technical economic term used to refer to the following situation:

If we were to conduct a poll or census of all of the economic units in the society, both individual and organizational, asking the question, "How much of this resource would you like to have if it were free?" and we were to add up all of the responses to that question, the grand total would be a quantity of the resource larger than the known supply. Thus the concept of scarcity says every economic unit cannot have as much of a particular resource as it would like to have if it were free. Almost all resources used for medical care and health care are scarce.

The obvious decision that must then be made for each resource is which economic unit or units must "make do" with less of the resource than ideally desired. Deciding "who gets what" is also referred to as the "resource allocation decision." Allocating scarce resources is nothing more than the process, any process, that makes choices among competing alternative uses or users of the resource. From an economic perspective, the term "rationing" is simply a synonym for "allocating."[1]

Primitive societies dealt with the question of rationing or allocating scarce resources by reliance on tradition, custom, taboo, or caste. Society simply had an order that was passed down from generation to generation, and resource allocation occurred more or less automatically. Everybody knew who got what, and to what they were entitled, and anyone who challenged those traditions did so at great personal risk because of the threat that deviation posed to the continued orderly functioning of the society.

Modern industrialized society tends to abandon those original human traditions for alternative approaches. Two extremes among these new approaches are the "central planning model" and the so-called "free market or laissez-faire model."

In the central planning model, an individual or group of individuals with sufficient power and authority to impose and enforce their decisions on others simply decide by fiat who gets what. For instance, Industry A gets 100 million tons of steel, Industry B gets 50 million tons of steel, Industry C doesn't get any steel but does get aluminum. Those are the allocations, plain and simple, with no room for argument by any of the affected industries. This type of central planning is typically associated with Eastern Bloc countries, those that have communistic or socialistic systems. A historical example would be the Soviet Union's 5-year plans promulgated under Stalin.

In contrast to centrally planned allocation is the free market. For this method of allocating resources, we must invent something called money. Its function is that of a common denominator that we use to exchange all types of resources among ourselves. In physical form, money can be whatever we want it to be. It can be big round stones on the isle of Yap in the Pacific, or it can be funny little pieces of paper with green and black ink on them in the United States.[2] Whatever money's form, we all mutually agree by social covenant that we will hold money at least temporarily because all of us also agree to accept money in exchange for resources and resources in exchange for money.

Because we like to consume resources, and because money commands resources, it is a general proposition that we prefer more money to less money. This prompts us to always be looking at how much money equates to a particular quantity of each resource. We want to know how much money we must give up to get the desired quantity of each resource, or how much money we can get if we part with a given amount of a resource we hold. That ratio, the quantity of money to the quantity of resource, is called the "price" of the resource.

The notion is that if the price of a resource (the amount of money you have to give up to get it or that you receive for parting with the resource) is relatively high, people with money will tend to want less of that resource because they can use the money to command other resources. But people who already have the resource are willing to part with quite a lot of it, obtaining a good deal of money in exchange, increasing their capacity to command other resources. So the higher the price, the more people who do not have the resource do not want it, and the more people who do have the resource want to get rid of it. Conversely, the lower the price, the more willing are those who do not have the resource to obtain it, and the less willing are those who have it to part with it.

So all of the individual elements in the economy, individuals, organizations, money, and resources, interact in the laissez-faire, perfect-market world of Adam Smith in which large numbers of market participants, all on equal footing, exchange information, offer money for resources, offer resources for money, haggle, and negotiate in full "view" of all participants. After a while, says the theory, there will emerge for each resource a "market equilibrium" or "market clearing price" having the characteristic that at that particular price, and at no other price, the total amount of the resource that those who have the resource are willing to part with is exactly equal to the total quantity of the resource that those who do not have it are willing to buy. All transactions, purchases and sales, then occur at this unique price, and we have de facto determined "who gets what." We tend to associate this decision-making process with Western society, capitalistic countries like the United States, Canada, Western European nations, and Japan.

The reality, of course, is that neither of these economic models exists in pure form anywhere. One can find money and markets and prices and buy-and-sell transactions occurring in China and the Soviet Union. And in the U.S., one can go to almost any state in the Union and find a small group of people, empowered by statute and regulation, sitting around making decisions like Hospital A gets 100 beds, Hospital B gets 50 beds, and Hospital C doesn't get any but instead can convert square footage to outpatient care. In the public sector, this is called "budget-making." In the private sector, it's called "health planning."

These decisions generally are made with no consideration whatsoever given to the value of the services that might be provided in the presence or absence of beds, or to the cost to the public of providing services from those facilities, or to the alternative benefits of using the resources elsewhere. In other words, economic approaches are largely overwhelmed by fiat, by politics, by regulation.

Health Care: A Major Force in a Service Economy

At first glance, health care regulation in the United States over the past two or three decades is a curious phenomenon. The biggest private-sector service industry is health care.[3] Indeed, health care is exceeded in size only by government.

The service sector as a general class of economic activity has grown much more rapidly than the rest of the economy since World War II. Even in 1946, measured by employment, we were a service economy. Private sector services alone provide the vast majority of employment in the United States today. During the Reagan administration, total employment in manufacturing held stable at about 20 million people. Nongovernment services during the same period grew at about 4 percent per year to reach the 62 million level, more than three times the level of employment in manufacturing.[4]

Within the service sector, the major economic change besides growth has been its deregulation. We have deregulated the airlines, deregulated trucking, deregulated communications (e.g., the AT&T break-up), and deregulated financial institutions. There is competition with the postal service (e.g., Federal Express) and choice among many long-distance communications competitors, and we now have discount brokerage firms. It is even increasingly difficult to tell the difference between a bank and a savings and loan. The basic thrust of the economy under all administrations since Lyndon Johnson's, whether Democrat or Republican, liberal or conservative, has been to deregulate the service industry.

The single exception has been health care. There is, in fact, more regulatory control of the health care industry today than at any previous time in this century. Health care has been treated differently from all other services primarily because of who pays for health care and how health care is paid for. The lion's share for health services are funded directly or indirectly by government, and historically, government has not been a prudent buyer. Government, in turn, has looked at the skyrocketing costs, and rather than accept responsibility, complains that providers of care are "ripping us off." Government concludes that the only way to control costs is to regulate, to control, to punish the industry.

The Medicare End Stage Renal Disease (ESRD) program is a good example of why government views regulation as necessary. (Medicare administers the program, but it is really a program for all citizens of the United States, regardless of age.) The program provides payment for maintenance dialysis of patients with kidney failure. Since it began in 1974, the program has paid 80 percent of the cost of maintenance dialysis after the first 90 days of that treatment. In 1973, when the ESRD program was being considered by the Congress, the Congressional Budget Office estimated that the 1974 cost would be $75 million, and that by 1977, the cost would rise to $250 million. In actuality, the cost has grown to over $2.5 billion, which represents an annual compound growth rate of exceeding 25 percent.[5]

This rate of growth has often been cited in the media and by politicians as simply one more example of out-of-control health care costs and of irresponsible economic behavior on the part of health providers. What is omitted from this story is the fact that the number of persons receiving maintenance dialysis has grown by nearly 20 percent per year compounded during the same period, and that once one adjusts for inflation in the input resources used in dialyzing patients, the real resources actually consumed per program enrollee have absolutely declined at a rate of 3 percent per year since the inception of the program. These gains in efficiency reflect primarily the spreading of capacity costs over an increased quantity of service (economies of scale) and, to a lesser degree, learning curve phenomena and technological progress in dialysis.

But what accounts for this rapid growth in program enrollment, inasmuch as the U.S. population grows at only about 1 1/2 or 2 percent per year? It is not just an aging population that is a factor here. The average number of enrollees began at 15,000 and is now in excess of 90,000, more than 70,000 of whom would have died in previous years in the absence of the program.[5] This is simply one example of supply creating its own demand, one of the classic problems of the health care industry. Health care in general, and medical care in particular, is a victim of its own success.

The average Medicare beneficiary is now around 75 years of age, has one or two chronic conditions that are eminently treatable and certainly not life-threatening, and a remaining actuarial life expectancy of about nine years.[6] Nine years hence, about one-third of this cohort is expected to be alive, now with three or four treatable chronic conditions, and a then-remaining life expectancy of five years. However, because of the growing efficacy and quality of care, the actuaries are likely to be wrong, and it may be that 40 percent will be alive and have a remaining life expectancy of six years. And so it goes.

The economic reality is that generally, and regarding renal failure patients particularly, we're keeping more people alive on many fewer resources per person today than ever before. As a result, total expenditures continue to balloon each year.

But it is impossible to give serious consideration to economics without also considering the other dimensions of the medical care process. The vast majority of the 90,000 + U.S. dialysis patients have as their major economic activity being dialyzed two or three times a week. Fewer than half of them are employed or employable. They are net consumers. Mental health problems are also prevalent in this group. And a number of employees have voluntarily withdrawn from the program after 10 or more years of enduring this unpleasant regimen.[7-9] Most of the people in the program, and certainly most of their families, are happy that they are still alive. From a purely economic perspective, however, they are not paying their way economically. An economist will look at the total bill of nearly $3 billion (combining Medicare, Medicaid, and self-pay deductibles and copayments) and wonder what would be the next best use of all that money, such as dedicated nutritional programs and prenatal care for black, pregnant inner-city teenagers? How much neonatal intensive care expense could be avoided if we focused $3

Section II.   The Content of Management

billion on that social problem. Even politicians such as former Governor Lamm of Colorado are asking such questions.

If you were a 60-year-old citizen of the United Kingdom with kidney failure, and you went to the National Health Service (NHS), what would happen to you? You would die. The NHS will not provide maintenance dialysis to anyone over the age of 55 whose kidneys fail.[10] The therapy won't be initiated, and the patient won't even be told it exists. If you can afford to do so, you can buy dialysis today in England's private sector, just as you could have in the U.S. prior to 1974. But capacity was very limited in 1974, prices were high, and geographic access difficult. Those few hospitals offering the service had death committees to decide who would receive treatment and who would be allowed to die. Such decisions were relatively easy when the choice was between a 65-year-old wino and a high school valedictorian. The decision would not have been so easy between the valedictorian and a 24-year-old mother of three.

This is a dramatic example of the philosophical questions that surround decisions for allocating scarce economic resources. Those decisions may be made explicitly or implicitly, but they will be made, and, as a result, some people will live and some will die. Traditionally, physicians have avoided being part of the resource allocation decision-making process at the system level, focusing only on applying all indicated resources on individual patients, case by case. To avoid being led toward bad system results, however, it would be better to involve physicians in resource allocation decisions.[11]

Overview of the U.S. Health Care System

Table 1, below, shows the growth in U.S. GNP and in the U.S. health care sector from 1955 to 1985, with projections by the U.S. Department of Health and Human Services through the year 2000.[12] U.S. health care

Table 1. MACROECONOMICS OF U.S. HEALTH CARE
Billions of Current Dollars

Year	U.S. GNP	U.S. Health Sector	Health as a % of GNP	$ Ratio for Health	Current Health $ per Capita	1987 Health $ per Capita
1955	405.9	17.7	4.4	1 of 23	102	845
1965	705.1	41.9	5.9	1 of 17	206	1,181
1975	1,598.4	132.7	8.3	1 of 12	590	1,648
1985	3,998.1	425.0	10.6	1 of 9.4	1,721	1,979
1990(E)	5,414.0	647.3	12.0	1 of 8.4	2,511	-------
1995(E)	7,467.0	999.1	13.4	1 of 7.5	3,739	-------
2000(E)	10,164.0	1,529.3	15.0	1 of 6.6	5,551	-------

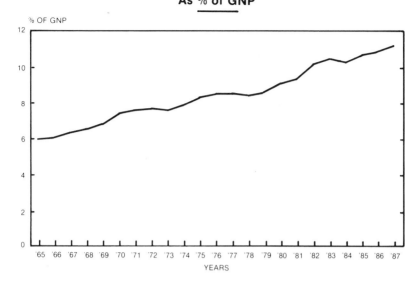

Figure 1(a). THE COST OF HEALTH CARE
As % of GNP

% OF GNP

YEARS

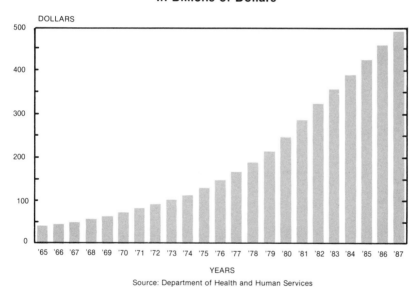

Figure 1(b). THE COST OF HEALTH CARE
In Billions of Dollars

DOLLARS

YEARS

Source: Department of Health and Human Services

expenditures of nearly $500 billion in 1987 represented 11.1 percent of GNP; one out of every nine dollars was spent for health, or about $2,050 per capita.[13] The United Kingdom, in comparison, spends less than one-third this amount per capita, 70 percent of which is covered by the state. Health status indicators in the U.K. are somewhat below those of the

Section II.   The Content of Management

United States in most categories, while those of Japan exceed the U.S. statistics. Japan spends only one-quarter the U.S. level per capita.[14]

You will note in figure 1(a), previous page, that there have been three years since 1965 (1973, 1978, and 1984) when health care went down as a proportion of the total economy. But from figure 1(b), previous page, it is clear that health care has, during this period, never had a bad year. Thus, the percentage declines can only be attributed to the fact that the rest of the economy had particularly good years (i.e., years in which growth was even better than the growth in the health sector, three times in the past quarter century).

An examination of the details of 1987's health care sector reflecting broad sources and uses of funds is instructive. (See table 2, below.) As to sources, in 1987, roughly 2/5 of the nearly $500 billion total came from government at all levels (federal, state, and local). Of government's $202 billion, the federal government accounted for about $140 billion, of which almost $80 billion was for Medicare. Of that $80 billion, nearly $50 billion was spent on services delivered to beneficiaries who died by December 1988. In short, almost two-thirds of all Medicare payments, or slightly more than 10 percent of total national health care expenditures, were spent on services for Medicare beneficiaries in their last year of life.[15]

The second largest source of funding for health care came from private health insurance, which provided about 1/3 of the total funding. Of that, about 85-90 percent is health insurance paid for by employers on behalf of their employees.[16] Payment by patients for medical expenses out of their own pockets accounted for 25 percent of the total. This

Table 2. U.S. HEALTH CARE EXPENDITURES 1987E
$497 Billions

SOURCE	From Whom $	%	USE	To Whom $	%
Gov't	202	41	Hosps.	193	39
HI	155	31	Phys.	101	20
SP	128	26	LT Care	42	8
Other	12	2	Medication	33	7
			Dental	32	6
			HI Cost	26	5
			Other Prof.	16	3
			Const.	8	2
			Equip.	9	2
			Gov't R & D	9	2
			Other	28	6

New Leadership in Health Care Management

includes payments for insurance deductibles, copayments, and non-covered expenses, as well as over-the-counter medications etc. The "other" category, accounting for 3 percent of the total, is largely international transfer payments from other governments and domestic philanthropy.[12]

The 1987 uses of funds in the health care system were as follows. Hospitals commanded 39 percent of the total. Their proportion has been declining over the past several years, from 42 percent of the total five years ago to the current 39 percent. Physicians received 1/5 of the total, a percentage that has increased from 17 percent five years ago. Long-term care is the next largest category, followed by medication, dental expenses, and health insurance cost, which is the difference between the premiums paid to private-sector insurance companies and the benefits disbursed. The next lower tier includes nonphysician professions, such as podiatrists, midwives, and chiropractors. At the end of the list are construction, equipment, and government research and development (private-sector R & D is imbedded in the other categories). Other items, including various public health programs, are included in the remaining 6 percent.[12]

In a very real sense, this itemization of sources and uses is a political road map. Major sources of funds will also be the sources of attempts to control expenditures. Government is clearly the number one controller or regulator, followed by private business through business coalitions, preferred-provider arrangements, managed care programs, and "by-right" initiatives. Everyone's number one target has been hospitals, and as hospital costs begin to increase less rapidly, physicians become the next most significant target.

When one compares the economy in general with the health care sector, differences in performance are evident. As a general proposition, health care has grown over the past 30-35 years much more rapidly than the rest of the economy, both in real output (a 50 percent greater growth rate) and in inflation (a one-third higher long-term rate). (See table 3, next page.[17]) Only during the Carter years of 1978-1980 was the rate of inflation for the rest of the economy higher than for health care. The Reagan years brought a major reversal in inflation generally, but the "victory" largely reflected declining oil prices and certainly not the medical care sector. While health inflation did decline, it dropped much less than in other sectors, so that, by 1986, the rate of inflation in health care (Medicare Care Service Component, MCSC, of the Consumer Price Index, CPI) was seven times the rate of inflation for the rest of the economy. (See table 4, next page.) Nineteen eighty-seven was not much better, with the MCSC rate around three times that of the overall CPI. And federal Medicare payments have gone up even faster than the rate of inflation because of an increasing number of beneficiaries.[18]

Section II.   The Content of Management

Table 3. AVERAGE ANNUAL COMPOUND RATES OF GROWTH 1955 - 1987

	Entire U.S. Economy	Health Care Sector
Nominal	7.8%	11.0%
Inflation	4.8%	6.2%
Real	2.9%	4.5%

Table 4. RATES OF INCREASE OVER PREVIOUS YEAR

Year	CPI	MCSC of CPI	Federal Medicare Payments
1955	0.3	1.4	--
1960	1.4	2.7	--
1965	1.6	2.2	--
1970	5.9	7.1	8%
1975	9.1	12.6	26%
1980	13.5	11.3	22%
1985	3.6	6.0	12%

Every administration subsequent to Lyndon Johnson's has considered health care costs (at least as embodied in the entitlement programs) as being out of control and requiring draconian measures to regain control. The post-Johnson Presidents have viewed these costs as a major obstacle to their pursuing primary political agendas, liberal or conservative. Health care continues to take for itself a disproportionate share of the incremental dollar of tax revenue, in spite of the Nixon and Ford Economic Stabilization Program, Carter's pleas for cost control legislation, or Reagan's TEFRA, PPS, and freezing of physicians' fees. Presidents are continually prevented from getting on with their favorite political agendas because every new tax dollar is largely precommitted to the entitlement programs. It is little wonder that health care and its providers are viewed as the "bad guys." The more health competes for system resources, the more the system will push back against health care. As health care has grown from 4 percent of GNP 30 years ago to 11 percent now, so too has the political pressure to stop the growth. With projections for health care to grow to at least 15 percent and perhaps 20 percent of GNP by the year 2000, political pressure will mount alongside that growth. Part of the major restructuring we shall see in health care will be the result of the industry struggling to meet the increasing

New Leadership in Health Care Management

expectations of the populace, to cope with the attendant growth in volume, and to defend itself from government and other third parties, particularly major private-sector employers and business coalitions.

Over the past few decades, the United States stimulated both the supply of and the demand for health care, increasing both physical and fiscal access, respectively. On the supply side, the Hill-Burton program provided incentives to build and expand hospitals. Other federal subsidies encouraged medical schools to double the size of their facilities and, hence, their entering classes. Similar programs produced corresponding increases in allied health personnel, and the space program as well as private research and development produced an open-ended flow of new knowledge and technology that expanded what could be performed medically.

Public-sector stimulation of the demand side began with the 1954 tax act, the last significant reform of the tax system prior to that enacted in 1986. The 1954 legislation provided, for the first time, that specified employer-paid fringe benefits would not be taxable to the employee receiving them but would remain tax-deductible as an ordinary cost of doing business for the employer.[19] Particular among these benefits was employer-provided health insurance. Thus, while an employer would be indifferent from the viewpoint of after-tax cost between spending a dollar on wages and spending a dollar on a health insurance policy for an employee, employees were no longer indifferent. Between the end of World War II and 1954, labor unions had fought exceptionally hard in the courts and at the bargaining table to expand health benefits from covering only 600,000 workers in 1945 to 7 million prior to the 1954 tax legislation.[20] Then it became easy. Within a few years, virtually all labor union contracts in the United States contained significant health insurance provisions as the result of the statute, collective bargaining, and their spillover effects in a competitive labor market.

Today, more than 150 million Americans have private health insurance, the vast majority of them as a result of policies purchased by their employers.[21] The importance of this mechanism for putting health insurance in place is shown in a study by the Employee Benefit Research Institute. Nationwide, nearly 20 percent of all workers having employer-provided coverage would choose not to have any health insurance at all were it not a part of their fringe benefit packages. Even more dramatic is the finding that over 60 percent of those workers earning $15,000 or less would not retain coverage.[22]

The second stage in the evolution of the U.S. national health insurance policy came in 1965, 11 years after the action on the income tax front. This second stage was the adoption of the Medicare and Medicaid programs. In concept, the 1954 tax subsidy had taken care of employed citizens and their dependents. The Medicare and Medicaid entitlement programs would now close the coverage gap for those not working,

Section II.   The Content of Management

specifically the unemployed poor (Medicaid), and those who had stopped working because of retirement (Medicare). Today these programs cover approximately 45 million citizens.[23]

Several years ago, the combination of the entitlement programs and private insurance along with other public-sector programs, including the VA, USPHS, CHAMPUS, and the active-duty military, accounted for coverage of over 90 percent of all Americans. In recent years, however, that percentage has declined to its current level of about 84 percent. That leaves approximately 37 million citizens of the United States without health insurance (Figure 2, below). A highly significant fact is that 55 percent, or about 20 million of those 37 million uninsured individuals, are part- or full-time employees, and nearly two thirds of the remaining uninsured individuals are their dependents (figure 3, next page.[24])

What has happened reflects the fact that the most significant employment growth in the United States in recent years has been in the service sector. Service industries, unlike manufacturing and construction, do not have a tradition of trade unionism, collective bargaining, and rela-

Figure 2. AMERICANS COVERED BY HEALTH INSURANCE

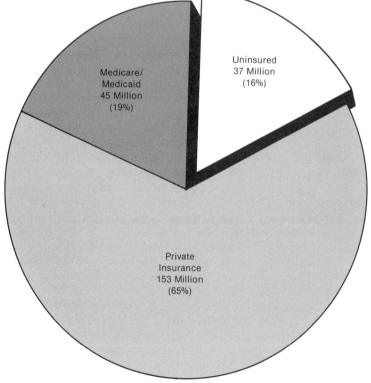

Uninsured
37 Million
(16%)

Medicare/
Medicaid
45 Million
(19%)

Private
Insurance
153 Million
(65%)

tively generous fringe benefit packages, and this sector tends to employ less skilled labor working at or near the minimum wage. Consequently, a fringe benefit package that is a relatively manageable percentage of a $12 to $16 per hour average labor cost in manufacturing and construction tends to be viewed as prohibitively expensive relative to a $4.50 to $7.50 per hour average labor cost in the service sector.[25]

Thus it is that more than three-quarters of the health insurance gap is filled with minimum-wage or near minimum-wage clerks, custodians, hamburger flippers, order takers, etc. and their dependents.[26] These persons tend to be younger and in poorer health than the population at large.

Proposed federal legislation would require all employers subject to minimum wage legislation to provide minimum health insurance to all their employees and their dependents. Passage of such legislation

Figure 3. NONELDERLY POPULATION WITHOUT HEALTH INSURANCE COVERAGE BY OWN WORK STATUS, 1985

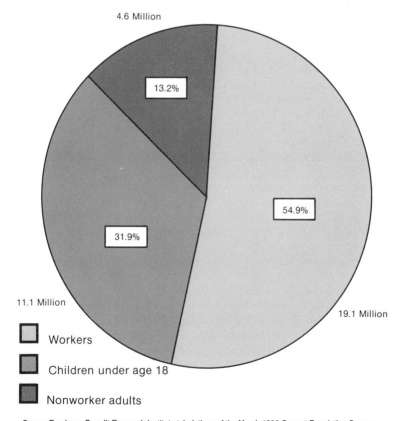

Source Employee Benefit Research Institute tabulations of the March 1986 Current Population Survey

Section II.   The Content of Management

would be a third major step of U.S. national health insurance policy. It would probably result in 96 percent of the U.S. population having health insurance and would almost certainly lead to 100 percent of fast-food hamburgers being more expensive. Keeping hamburger prices at levels consistent with employers not providing employees with health coverage significantly raises the likelihood of tax increases to finance a public-sector health insurance mechanism. Such a program, while motivated by the 37 million uninsured, would quite likely be enacted in a much more universal (and expensive) form than required to meet the basic need. (The Canadian system is most frequently cited by national health insurance proponents as a model to be emulated.[27-29])

In contrast, more expensive hamburgers would remove the primary argument for a national health insurance program and would have the salutary effect of causing the service sector/manufacturing playing field to become more level. Prices of the service sector's output would, for the first time, broadly bear their fair share of private-sector health services. Spreading the cost of health services more equitably through the private sector would cause consumers to view hamburgers and many other nonhealth services as relatively more expensive compared to goods. Consumers' responses to such price relationships would tend to move the economy toward a more efficient goods/services balance. Most important, however, would be the genuine closing of the existing health insurance gap, and the simultaneous strengthening of the private practice of medicine.

While increased physical and fiscal access have accounted for much of the real growth in the U.S. health sector, a second contributor to real growth has been increasing intensity of care. Factors identified with increased intensity include an aging population, new technology and growing medical knowledge, economic incentives (especially in fee-for-service and cost-based payment environments), "defensive" medicine, and regulation. Regulation represents intensity because compliance consumes real resources. There are forms to fill out, new computers, additional office employees, etc. Patients may never see the resources being consumed, but that alters neither their reality nor their cost.

The American Medical Association (AMA) estimates that between 5 percent and 10 percent of all health care expenditures are unnecessary, i.e., probably do no harm, but also don't improve outcomes, even though they are the result of physicians' orders.[30] Estimates by consumer activists are twice those of the AMA. Some of this excess comes from public demand; people hear about new treatments in the lay press and run to their physicians saying, "I know you can fix it; I heard about it on TV or read about it in the newspaper." But, of course, should there be an adverse outcome, those same people will find a trial lawyer and initiate a tort action. Hence, defensive medicine.

Beyond the factors that actually cause real growth, the consumption of

New Leadership in Health Care Management

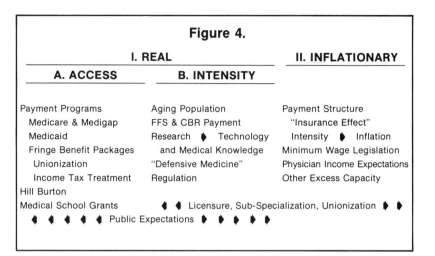

Figure 4.

I. REAL		II. INFLATIONARY
A. ACCESS	**B. INTENSITY**	

Payment Programs	Aging Population	Payment Structure
Medicare & Medigap	FFS & CBR Payment	"Insurance Effect"
Medicaid	Research ◆ Technology	Intensity ◆ Inflation
Fringe Benefit Packages	and Medical Knowledge	Minimum Wage Legislation
Unionization	"Defensive Medicine"	Physician Income Expectations
Income Tax Treatment	Regulation	Other Excess Capacity
Hill Burton		
Medical School Grants	◆ ◆ Licensure, Sub-Specialization, Unionization ◆ ◆	
◆ ◆ ◆ ◆ ◆ Public Expectations ◆ ◆ ◆ ◆ ◆		

more real resources, there are some things that are inflationary. By inflation we simply mean increases in prices without a corresponding change in the actual quantity of resources being consumed. The very nature of the payment structure not only increases intensity, but intensity itself begets inflation. Licensure and subspecialization also contribute through distortions of the labor market. Figure 4, above, summarizes various factors that influence both real growth and inflation.

In economic terms, licensure restricts supply and is a "barrier to entry." The limiting of competition allows everyone with the credentials to receive higher compensation than available in a price-competitive market to get wealthier. "Quality" is but one reason there is resistance to allowing foreign medical graduates to practice medicine domestically.

The fact that intensity begets inflation can be described graphically (figure 5, next page). The horizontal axis measures the dollar cost of resources that are consumed in producing health care. Along the vertical axis we measure value, the market value of those same inputs to health care, and the value of outputs from health care. The value of the inputs is a nice, straight 45 degree line. This implicitly assumes that we have an efficient market for input resources, which is generally true in the United States. In the case of input resources, value would be the market price. Presumably, if one buys resources (say, to build a hospital) and then changes one's mind, those resources can be sold back into the marketplace for about the same price (net of transactions costs) and used for something else (say, to build an apartment building). Fundamentally, value is retained by the input resources. The output value is different. It reflects what society would be willing to pay for health care, not what it does pay. The difference between what you would be willing to pay and what you actually have to pay is what economists refer to as "consumers' surplus." For instance, you might be willing to pay

Section II. The Content of Management

$20,000 for a car that you can get for $16,000. The curved line represents the value of the output. Its shape reflects the potential for consumer satiation. The more there is of a given output, the less valuable additional quantities become.

The four points A, B, C, and D depict value at various scales of activity. Point A is the maximum value of aggregate output occurring at a fairly large level of input and output. Point B is where the value of the output exceeds the value of the input by the largest margin and reflects a somewhat smaller health care industry. Point C, a small industry, is

Figure 5. ECONOMIC CHARACTERISTICS OF VARIOUS LEVELS OF INDUSTRY OPERATION

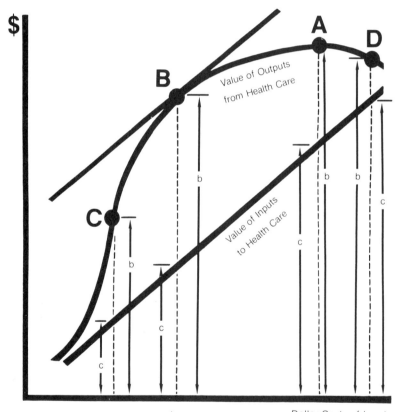

A - maximizes b
B - maximizes the amount by which b exceeds c
C - maximizes the ratio of b to c
D - maximizes c

where there is a maximum ratio between value and output value is attained. Point D is where costs are maximized, that is, where the health care industry as a whole is at its largest.

Different constituencies or interest groups have very different preferences as to where they would *like* to see the health care industry function. Generally, physicians and most patients with insurance like Point A. Point A is consistent with the Hippocratic Oath; you do everything possible for each patient.

Point D reminds us that in the desire to do all that is humanly possible, a physician needs to add an element of pragmatism. There *is* such a thing as doing a test too many times "just to be sure," in terms of patient discomfort and adverse side effects (e.g., increased risk of cancer caused by exposure to too many x-rays). Nonetheless, major economic forces continually press physicians and other providers outward toward Point D: Anyone supplying any input resource to the health care industry would prefer to sell the industry more rather than less of that resource. Whether it is medical supplies, I.V. solutions, labor, pharmaceuticals, high-tech diagnostic/therapeutic equipment, or office supplies, the more you buy, the happier the seller. Free samples of prescription drugs are simply one form of an invitation to move toward Point D.

Government has a bias toward Point C, not only because it lowers the scale of outlays, but also because, as the point having the maximum rate of return, politicians can fill their speeches with "efficiency in government" rhetoric, pointing with pride to each hard-earned tax dollar yielding the most health care bang for the buck.

Unlike everyone else, economists like Point B, where total net value-added is maximized. Beginning at the left side of Figure 5 and moving past Point C, each time the health care industry buys $1 worth of resources, it produces an output that society would value at more than $1. Unfortunately, each time the investment is repeated, the amount of additional output value generated exceeds $1 by less and less. Eventually, a dollar's worth of additional input yields just a dollar's worth of output. We have arrived at Point B. This is the point at which marginal or incremental cost equals the marginal or incremental benefit of the output. (Note the line tangent to the curve at Point B is parallel to the value-of-input line.) An economist would say this is the point at which to stop. If investment continues, each additional dollar's worth of resources will yield less than a dollar's worth of output.

Indeed, moving to the right of Point B is even worse than simply making an intrinsically bad investment. Because any additional input units must be bought in the market from their current owners who are at their own Point B, the potential health industry buyer must convince the current owner to part with such resources. The convincing is done with money.

Section II.   The Content of Management

Health care must bid $1.01 for the additional unit of input resource, raising the marketing-clearing price from $1.00. Somewhere else in the economy will be some other industry that will give up one unit of the resource, foregoing the production of some nonhealth output valued by society at $1.01--an output that would have been produced had the input cost only $1.00. Health care indeed competes with everyone else for the same input resources.

By offering $1.01 for a unit of resource, health care is implying to the market that the resource will yield at least $1.01 in output value, as would be the case at Point B. However, the additional value of health care realized is only $0.99. Thus, health care is lying to the market. Bidding the price to $1.01 from $1.00 is, by definition, inflation. This is why inflation is a lie. Because the health care industry has generally operated somewhere between Point A and Point B, where incremental value produced is less than incremental value consumed, the industry has had to lie to the market for the past 30 years, creating much of its own differential inflation. The resource market is told that something is worth more than it actually is, and an inefficient allocation of resources results. Because moving to the right on figure 5 is associated with greater intensity of service, the phrase "intensity breeds inflation" clearly describes a major health sector phenomenon.

The Health Insurance Phenomenon

For economists, the policy issue is how to move the health care industry back toward Point B. First, we must understand why any rational human being would be willing to spend one dollar on resources for only, say, 10 cents worth of additional benefit. There are two circumstances under which this could happen. The first is a life and death situation. When resources are required to save a life within the next 24 to 48 hours, the health care system just spends. But such situations represent a very small proportion of total health care expenditures, and such resource use is generally accepted.

The second circumstance under which it is rational to spend a dollar to get back 10 cents is when it is someone else's dollar. That is how health insurance has worked. Both the decision-maker, historically the physician, and the patient have been insulated from the cost of the resources consumed to produce the benefit.

In one sense, insurance resembles a gambling game. Imagine that you and nine other people get together to play a game. Each antes $125 a month, for a total of $15,000 a year for the 10 players. The house takes a 10 percent cut to pay for administrative costs such as writing and enforcing the rules of the game, making actuarial predictions (calculating the odds of winning), and managing the game's payouts of winnings. A $13,500 grand prize is thus available. Now suppose you win the jackpot (by getting sick) and you have a shopping list of nine possible health care expenditures, each priced at $1,500 (such as emergency department visit, first day in hospital, surgery, etc., on down to a few days of home health care). Table 5, below, shows how you might rank order the nine items by their value to you (what you would be willing to spend of your own money to obtain each). Now consider two different sets of rules governing winners of the game. If you receive the $13,500 in a lump sum cash distribution, you will buy all of the items on the list that are worth as much or more to you than the $1,500 asking price. You will buy up to the point where one more dollar of expenditure produces one more dollar of benefit (rehabilitative therapy in our Table 5 example). You will have climbed up on your output value curve to your "Point B." Once you have bought the five things on the list to get to this point, that will leave $6,000 that you will use to go to Hawaii. If, however, the rules of the game say that as soon as you make any $1,500 purchase (and only if you make it) you will be reimbursed up to a total of $13,500, you will go ahead and buy all nine things (because you can't touch any of the money not spent for these items). You are still happy, because you have the money you need for your health care and there is affirmative benefit from every item on the list. Your physician is happy because he or she got to practice "good medicine." The other nine people are not unhappy because, after all, they've had the peace of mind knowing that they were insured. Health insurance premiums might go up a little next year, but that is next year, and, besides, your employer pays the premium. Your employer is not too unhappy because the premium is deductible for tax purposes. So everybody wins. The only ones who lose are all of us, because resources were consumed for purposes of dubious value. If a patient is told he can stay an extra day in the hospital if he is willing to spend $400 of his own money, his decision will likely be different than if he knows his insurance pays for it.

Indeed, there is empirical evidence that patient choices change, depending on source of funding. The RAND Corporation conducted an 8-

Table 5. HEALTH CARE SHOPPING LIST

Service	Cost	Benefit
ER Visit and Diagnostics	1500	4300
Initial Hospitalization	1500	3450
Surgery	1500	2700
Hospital Days 2 - 3	1500	2050
Rehabilitative Therapy	1500	1500
Hospital Day 4 - 5	1500	1050
One Week of SNF and/or Home Health Care	1500	700
Hospital Days 6 - 8	1500	450
Hospital Days 9 -12	1500	300
	13500	16500

Section II.   The Content of Management

year study of patient sensitivity to price.[31] The study involved over 4,000 people who were placed into 13 groups that differed according to health insurance mechanism but were matched with respect to demographic characteristics (age, income, etc.). Twelve of the 13 groups got a maximum out-of-pocket exposure of $1,000 per family per year, with difficult deductible or copayment arrangements. One group, for instance, had a 25 percent copayment, and another had a 95 percent copayment (meaning they got 75 cents and 5 cents reimbursement for the first $4,000 and $1,053 dollars they spent, respectively). The thirteenth group had free care.

The results showed that the demand for health services is indeed price elastic (sensitive to price levels). For example, for every $2 of medical services (measured at billed charges) that the 95 percent copayment group bought, the 25 percent copayment group bought $3. They spent 50 percent more.[31]

The RAND study results suggest that people look at their own budgets and decide to forgo medical services they deem unnecessary so as not to incur large copayments and deductibles. But this might be penny-wise and pound-foolish, because they may have underlying illnesses that are not detected as early as they might have been, resulting in much larger expenses later on.

To address this concern, the RAND study continued to follow people for several years to see if they did, in fact, require larger quantities of medical care subsequently. No measurable effects were found among the payment groups. There were no statistically significant differences between or among any of the 12 partial-pay groups with respect to mortality, morbidity, or expenditures. When these 12 groups were compared with the one group that paid nothing, income distinctions became evident. For higher income families, there were again no differences between the payment and the free-care groups. For families that were at or below the poverty level, however, the poor in the free care group fared better than the poor in the other 12 groups. For example, those who were poor and needed glasses nearly always got them in the free care group; poor individuals who had to pay for them often did not. And, if an individual was poor and hypertensive and in the free care group, he was diagnosed and medicated much more frequently than an individual who was poor, hypertensive, and had to pay for care. There was even a slight increase in the actuarial life expectancy for the poor in the free care group.[32]

In addition to the RAND study, Medicare statistics on hospital utilization also suggest that (1) we have been operating closer to Point A than to Point B and (2) moving back toward Point B not only saves resources but can be accomplished without adversely affecting medical outcome. Subsequent to the initiation of the prospective pricing system in October 1983, there has been a 20-30 percent decline in the average length of stay of Medicare beneficiaries, with no attendant significant change in outcomes.[33]

The Medicare savings of the cost of an extra three or four days in the hospital is not a pure gain, of course. There is obviously a substitution of resources to provide alternative care outside of the hospital. That includes the opportunity cost to family members of having to provide some level of care or explicit out-of-pocket costs for providing home care services. While not saving 100 percent of the resources by shortening hospital stay, there is a significant saving nevertheless, and there has not been a significant change in morbidity or mortality statistics as a result of this dramatic reduction in hospital usage.[33]

Removing insurance's first-dollar-coverage insulation between the cost of resources consumed and the beneficiary of that resource use clearly works as a strategy for moving back from Point A toward Point B on Figure 5. The federal government's attempts to apply this lesson to the Medicare program have been largely frustrated by the political clout of the American Association of Retired Persons. Private-sector business, however, has been much more successful. Between 1981 and 1985, the average deductible and copayment for U.S. employees quadrupled as employers successfully bargained with unions, offering benefit reductions in lieu of layoffs in a weak economy.[34]

The second major way to use economic incentives to shift health care resources from Point A toward Point B is to focus on the provider. Deductibles and copayments place on the patient the cost of resources initially consumed. An alternative involves making the provider bear the cost of all resources consumed by and for the patient without benefit of cost pass-through to the individual patient. Both prepaid care mechanisms and rate regulation (e.g., Medicare's prospective pricing system) are examples of this approach. They place the provider at risk economically for actual resource consumption beyond average levels contemplated (or "budgeted") and incorporated in fixed rates set in advance for "packages" of care with are many individual "line items" of care.

The generic problems with these approaches are that they tend to maintain the cost/benefit insulation at the level of the patient. They therefore create the potential for patient/provider conflicts of interest, and/or they cause "cost-shifting," "unbundling," and a variety of other provider system-gaming.

Health Sector Trends

HMOs

Prepaid plans have about one-eighth of the national population enrolled and capture nearly six percent of national health expenditures. Enrollment growth since 1970 has been in excess of 14 percent per year

Section II.   The Content of Management

compounded; indeed growth exceeded a 20 percent annual compound rate for the 1984 to mid-1987 period. But nearly half of the 650+ plans are losing money in the late 1980s, bankruptcies are occurring, and growth has dramatically slowed from more than 25 percent per year to around 10 percent per year.[35,36] Minneapolis-St. Paul, the HMO showplace of the 1970s and early 1980s, actually showed a decline in the percentage of population enrolled from 43 percent to 42 percent during 1987.[37]

The potential for HMO/enrollee conflict of economic interest described in the previous section interacts with a number of other phenomena that may explain the slowing of the prepaid sector's growth. Increasingly, people prefer to choose not only a primary care physician, but also specialty providers episode by episode. Employers are claiming that they are not realizing significant cost savings from prepayment compared to managed care techniques applied to traditional payment mechanisms. The media have raised a variety of concerns about quality of care in prepaid settings and are also giving significant attention to HMO bankruptcies. Thus, HMOs of all types face significant challenges to their long-term viability in the years ahead.

Hospitals

Beyond HMO uncertainties, other broad trends are evident in the health care sector. The share of GNP that hospitals command has dropped from 42 percent to 39 percent over the past five years. Had hospitals not diversified away from pure acute care as a primary activity, hospital share would now be below one-third. With prospective pricing and HMOs giving hospitals economic incentives to reduce length of stay, with all payers having incentives to keep patients out of the hospital, and with concomitant advances in medical knowledge and technology, an increasing emphasis on outpatient treatment has emerged. Increasing numbers of minor surgeries are now being done without hospitalization. For instance, in the early 1980s, the average length of stay for an intraocular lens implant was 3 or 4 days. Today the hospital stay is zero days as the procedure is fully outpatient. As both economics and technology keep more people out of the hospital, those left in the hospital are, of course, sicker. Treatment costs more, but there are fewer cases.

The national average acute care utilization is just under 1,000 bed days per thousand population per year.[38] But this average also has a very high standard deviation. Medicare recipients use about 4,000 bed days per thousand per year; 5 to 14-year-olds use fewer than 150 days.[39] In New Orleans, the population uses 1,350 bed days per thousand per year. The Minneapolis-St. Paul area, which has approximately 70 percent more population than New Orleans, uses 650 bed days for 1,000 people, only half as many. Minneapolis-St. Paul's and New Orleans' different rates of acute care usage result from demographic, epidemiol-

New Leadership in Health Care Management

ogic, and economic reasons. Demographically, the population in New Orleans is older, blacker, poorer. Epidemiologically, while both are on the same river, something seems to happen as the Mississippi flows south. The highest rate of male bladder cancer in the U.S., for instance, is in South Louisiana, with the number of cases increasing as the river is followed from North to South. But, the biggest single explanatory factor is economic. In New Orleans, less than 5 percent of the population is enrolled in prepaid plans, while the Minneapolis-St. Paul figure is ten times larger. Enrollees in Twin Cities' prepaid plan spend fewer than 300 days per thousand in the hospital annually, some 70% fewer than the national average. Medicare enrollees in HMOs in the Twin City area use about 2,000 patient days per thousand per year, about half the national average for Medicare.[37] One hypothetical scenario for the year 2000 is as follows: The census bureau estimates the year 2000 population in the U.S. will be 268 million. If the entire country has achieved by then what Minneapolis-St. Paul has already achieved, 650 days per thousand per year (remembering, of course, that HMOs in those cities currently use less than 300 bed days per thousand per year), we will need 174.2 million bed days. That comes to an average daily census of about 477,260. Of course, more beds than that will be required, since there cannot be 100 percent occupancy (traditionally, 85 percent was considered "full"). Although average hospital occupancy has been in the 50-60 percent range recently, those percentages reflect licensed rather than staffed beds. It is likely that a 75 percent occupancy level is required for economic viability over a full asset life cycle. A 75 percent occupancy means that only 636,400 beds would be required nationally in the year 2000.

There are currently over 1,000,000 nonfederal, short-stay (acute) hospital beds, meaning we need to get rid of 37 percent of the hospital beds to meet our projected need in this scenario. This does not mean that 37 percent of the hospitals are going to close. It does mean that 37 percent of the beds currently licensed as medical/surgical are not going to continue to be acute care beds.

Physicians

With perfect geographical distribution by specialty, it would require only about 70,000 "active" admitters averaging one admission per day with a seven-day average length of stay to support a national average daily hospital census of 477,260 in the year 2000. In the extreme, that means only one of every 10 physicians would have admission privileges at a hospital.

In 1930 we had 141 physicians per 100,000 population, and by the late 1980s, 240-245 are expected.[40] By the year 2000 there will be approximately 260 physicians per 100,000 population. This includes the various supply sources (medical schools, foreign medical graduates) and accounts for expected retirements and deaths.[41]

Section II. The Content of Management

Two studies have addressed the issues of physician supply (both in aggregate and by specialty) and "need" for physician services in the United States. The Graduate Medical Education National Advisory Committee (GMENAC) issued a comprehensive report in 1980, based on 1974 data, which projected physician supply and "need" through 1990. In March 1986 the Public Health Service (PHS) issued "The Fifth Report to the President and Congress on the Status of Health Personnel in the U.S.," which revises the GMENAC projections and extends them to the year 2000, based on 1981 data.

A comparison of physician supply projections and a representative selection of specialties are shown in table 6, below, and table 7, next page. Internal medicine ranks first in popularity in the complete list of specialties, both now and in the future. General/family practice ranks second, general surgery third, and pediatrics fourth, with general surgery and pediatrics reversing order to fourth and third, respectively, by the year 2000.

In addition to variation in supply between specialties, there is wide variation in the geographic distribution within certain specialties. For example, at present there are, on average, 24 family practice physicians per 100,000 population nationally, but that average reflects a range from a low of 12 in Massachusetts to a high of 53 in North Dakota.[42]

Total growth of physician supply is anticipated to be outpaced slightly by the growth in primary care specialties, and considerably by that in other medical specialties such as dermatology, gastroenterology, and pulmonary diseases. Rates of growth in surgical specialties, in contrast, will not keep pace with the growth in total supply.[43]

The supply of female physicians is also projected to undergo substantial changes in the years ahead. In 1981 there were 55,800 female physicians, according to the PHS report. This number is expected to increase to 100,000 in 1990 and to 143,500 by the year 2000 to become 20.6 percent of all physicians. As recently as 1955, only 5 percent of all domestic medical school graduates were women; beginning in 1988, more than one-third are female.[44]

Estimates of total "excess" supply over requirements are made in both the GMENAC and the PHS reports (table 8, next page). The two models

Table 6. PROJECTED TOTAL PHYSICIAN SUPPLY

	GMENAC (1980)	PHS (1986)	
	1990	1990	2000
TOTAL	594,000	587,680	696,550
MDs	564,200	559,500	656,110
DOs	29,800	28,180	40,440
# PER 100,000 POPULATION	231.3	235.4	259.9

New Leadership in Health Care Management

Table 7. PROJECTED PHYSICIAN SUPPLY BY SPECIALTY (PHS)

	1981	1990	2000	% GROWTH 1981-2000
Internal Medicine	82,020	107,960	130,140	58.7
General/Family Practice	65,600	77,680	89,130	35.9
Cardiology	10,730	14,460	17,930	67.1
Pediatrics	32,590	45,020	56,750	74.1
General Surgery	37,990	41,930	44,140	16.2
Gastroenterology	4,600	7,170	9,850	114.2
OB/GYN	29,180	37,220	44,510	52.5
Ophthalmology	13,680	16,520	19,060	39.3
Othopedic Surgery	15,200	18,950	21,950	44.4
Plastic Surgery	3,370	4,740	5,940	76.2
Psychiatry	30,250	34,680	38,000	25.6
Public Health	2,250	1,900	1,270	-49.6
Diagnostic Radiology	8,820	13,570	18,110	105.4
Occupational Medicine	2,500	2,260	2,010	-19.4

Table 8. PROJECTED "EXCESS" SUPPLY (TOTAL)

	PHS (1981 Baseline)	GMENAC (1984 Revision)
1990	46,600	63,000
2000	77,800	137,000
% Increase	70%	117%

differ in their estimates of physician productivity to arrive at projections of "excess" supply. Although absolute numbers differ, both reports project an increase in the "excess" supply. Notable exceptions to this trend are psychiatry and preventive medicine, both of which are projected to experience a supply shortage by the year 2000.

What is worrisome about both the GMENAC and PHS models is their failure to include the possibility that physician life-styles may change toward more nonpractice time, a prospect made somewhat more likely by the increasing proportion of females among physicians; the compartmentalization of physician services; and the rapid expansion of physician substitutes, as well as their (or any model's) inability to forecast at least some significant events and trends.

Since GMENAC, AIDS has arrived; coronary bypass surgery has begun to be replaced by less invasive therapies; the rate of cesarean sections has escalated unabated, as has the use of test-tube fertilization; and organ replacement success and frequency have exploded.

Prepaid health plans (HMOs and CMPs) are another important factor, even though their growth has slowed. This is because prepayment is not going to go away and because the practice patterns of HMO physi-

Section II.   The Content of Management

cians differ dramatically from those observed among fee-for-service practitioners. A 1986 study of three HMOs using 1980-81 data found that HMO requirements for primary care physicians were significantly lower than that reported in the GMENAC study, with resultant 1990 estimated requirements being only 78 percent of the GMENAC projection for pediatrics and only 50 percent for adult health care.[45]

These substantially lower projections are not based on corresponding increases in physician productivity, however. On the contrary, in two of the three HMOs studied, the number of patient visits per physician was actually lower than in the GMENAC study. One explanation is that expanded use of physician substitutes, such as nurse practitioners and physician's assistants, enables the HMOs to provide services using fewer physicians. Another is that a kind of "productivity" factor is at work, such as physicians substituting telephone communication for face-to-face visits.[45]

In any event, HMOs are creating a "third compartment" of physicians (fee-for-service and public sector physicians comprising the other two), which employs a relatively fixed number of physicians, increasing the number only as patient enrollment grows. The need for outside fee-for-service physicians by members enrolled in the plan is minimal, for nearly all specialty services are included within the HMO.

Based on the PHS projected total physician supply of 696,550 by the year 2000, table 9, below, shows the differences possible between the "third compartment" and the rest of medical practice. In the year 2000, the nonfederal and federal sectors will have one physician per 339 patients while the prepaid group practice (HMO) sector will have one physician for 833 patients.[46]

The rapid expansion of physician substitutes will also alter the accuracy of the GMENAC and PHS models. The GMENAC study projected that eventually 12 percent of adult health care and 15 percent of child health care will be provided by nonphysicians. While physician substitutes

Table 9. U.S. POPULATION AND PHYSICIAN SUPPLY 1987 ACTUAL AND 2000 PROJECTED*

	1978	2000
Population (millions)		
Nonfederal and federal sectors	212	54
Prepaid group practices	7	214
Total	219	268
Physicians/100,000 population		
Nonfederal and federal sectors	173	295
Prepaid group practices	114	120
Average	171	260

*2000 based on 25% of the population enrolled in prepaid care and being served by 120 physicians/100,000 enrollees.

New Leadership in Health Care Management

have indeed been growing in number, Steinwachs believes these estimates are too large, in which case there will be a greater demand for
physician services and, in turn, a smaller excess of physicians.[45] By
contrast, the continued expansion in chiropractors, optometrists, podiatrists, and psychologists; the trend toward pharmacists being allowed to prescribe[47]; the proliferation of over-the-counter laboratory
tests; the ongoing emergence of nurses as independent practitioners;
and self-care sufficiency growing apace with the spread of general
medical knowledge through the population,[48] all tend to support the
GMENAC and PHS models' concepts of reduced need creating "excess"
supply.

But in mitigation are declining medical school enrollments (4 percent
fewer graduates in 1988 than in 1987[49]), physicians' personal desires for
more leisure time (requiring increased collegial "coverage" of patients),
expansion of the female physician cohort with its shorter expected
practice life (reflecting childbearing and child-rearing activity as nonpractice), the absorption of more physicians (particularly FMGs) in
currently underserved geographic areas domestically, the potential for
the export of physicians to an increasingly global economy, the emergence of AIDS and other as-yet-unidentified complex and intensely
resource-absorbing disease processes, the expansion of what is medically and surgically possible through new knowledge and technology,
and the expansion of the physician's domain to managerial and other
medically related roles. Indeed, a recent study has suggested that we
may be training too few of a variety of subspecialists.[41,50]

References

1. Wilensky, G. "Making Decisions on Rationing." *Business and Health*
3(1):36, Nov. 1985.

2. Pine, A. "Fixed Assets, or Why a Loan in Yap is Hard to Roll Over." *Wall
Street Journal*, Mar. 29, 1984, 1,24.

3. U.S. Department of Commerce, Bureau of Economic Analysis. *Survey of
Current Business*, July 1987.

4. *Economic Report of the President*, February 1988, Table B-43, p. 296.

5. Rettig, R. "The Politics of Health Cost Containment: End-Stage Renal
Disease." *Bulletin of the New York Academy of Medicine* 56(1):115-38, Jan.-
Feb. 1980.

6. Department of Labor, Bureau of Labor Statistics, *Work Life Estimate Effects
of Race and Education*, Bulletin 2254, Feb. 1986.

7. Evans, R., and others. "The Quality of Life of Patients with End-Stage Renal
Disease." *New England Journal of Medicine* 312(9):553-9, Feb. 28, 1985.

8. Abram, H., and others. "Suicidal Behavior in Chronic Dialysis Patients." *American Journal of Psychiatry* 127:1199-1204, Mar. 1971.

9. McKegney, F., and Lange, P. "The Decision to No Longer Live on Chronic Hemodialysis." *American Journal of Psychiatry* 128:267-74, Sept. 1971.

10. Schwartz, W., and Aaron, H. "Rationing Hospital Care–Lessons from Britain." *New England Journal of Medicine* 310(1):52-6, Jan. 5, 1984.

11. Lister, J. "The Politics of Medicine in Britain and the United States." *New England Journal of Medicine* 315(3):168-74, July 17, 1986.

12. Division of National Cost Estimates, Office of the Actuary, Health Care Financing Administration. "National Health Expenditures 1986-2000." *Health Care Financing Review*, Summer 1987, 1-36.

13. Greene, R. "What Price Is Life?" *Forbes* 140(5):42-5, Sept. 7, 1987.

14. Calculations by the author based on data from *World Development Report 1987*, p. 203.

15. Lubitz, J., and Prihoda, R. "The Use and Cost of Medicare Service in the Last Two Years of Life." *Health Care Financing*, Spring 1984, p.11-31.

16. *Source Book of Health Insurance Data–1986 Update*. Health Insurance Association of America, Table 3.2, 1986.

17. Calculated by the author from data provided by the Department of Commerce, Bureau of Economic Analysis, on GNP, and the Department of Health and Human Services, Health Care Financing Administration, on national health expenditures.

18. Calculated by the author from data provided by the Department of Labor, Bureau of Labor Statistics, on consumer price indexes, and the Department of Health and Human Services, Health Care Financing Administration, on national health expenditures.

19. Title 26, U.S. Code, Section 106, 1954.

20. Starr, P. *The Social Transformation of American Medicine*. New York: Basic Books, Inc., 1982, pp. 312-3.

21. *Source Book of Health Insurance Data–1986 Update*. Health Insurance Association of America, Tables 1.1 and 3.2, 1986.

22. Employee Benefit Research Institute's simulation of private health insurance coverage with full taxation of employer contributions to health insurance, 1979.

23. U.S. Congress, House Committee on Ways and Means. *Background Material and Data on Program within the Jurisdiction of the Committee on Ways and Means*. Committee print, 100th Congress, Second Session, March 24, 1988. Washington, D.C.: U.S. Government Printing Office, 1988, pp. 114, 810.

24. Household Economic Studies: Disability Functional Limitation and Health Insurance Coverage, 1984-85." *Current Population Report*. Bureau of the Census, Series P-70, No. 8, Dec. 1986.

25. U.S. Department of Labor, Bureau of Labor Statistics. "Current Labor Statistics." *Monthly Labor Review* 111(4):88(Table 15), April 1988, adjusted by author to include average cost of fringe benefits.

26. "Minimum Health Benefits for All Employees." *Congressional Record*, 100th Congress, 2nd Session, No. S1265, 1988.

27. Malloy, M. "Health, Canadian Style." *Wall Street Journal*, April 22, 1988, p. 21.

28. Iglehart, J. "Canada's Health Care System." *New England Journal of Medicine* 315(12):778-84, Sept. 18, 1986.

29. Iglehart, J. "Canada's Health Care System." *New England Journal of Medicine* 315(25):1623-8, Dec. 18, 1986.

30. Davis, J. "Defensive Medicine and Medical Malpractice." US Senate Hearing 98-1039, *Committee on Labor and Human Resources*, July 10, 1984.

31. Newhouse, J., and others. *Some Interim Results from a Controlled trial of Loss-Sharing in Health Insurance*. Santa Monica, Calif.: RAND Corp., Jan 1982.

32. Brook, R., and others. "Does Free Care Improve Adults' Health?: Results from a Randomized Controlled Trial." *New England Journal of Medicine* 309(23):1426-34, Dec. 8, 1983.

33. Tolchin, M. "22% Drop Is Found in Length of Stay in Hospitals in U.S." *New York Times*, May 25, 1988, p. 1,13.

34. Pear, R. "Companies Tackle Health Costs." *New York Times* , Mar. 3, 1985, p. F-11.

35. Southwick,. K. "Half of All HMOs Are Losing Money." *HealthWeek* 1(4):1,13, Sept. 28, 1987.

36. Freudenheim, M. "Prepaid Programs for Health Care Encounter Snags." *New York Times*, Jan. 31, 1988, pp. 1,17

37. Calculated by the author from data provided by InterStudy and the Metropolitan Council of the Twin Cities Area.

38. Calculated by the author from data provided by the U.S. Department of Commerce, Bureau of the Census, and *Hospital Statistics*, Chicago, Ill.: American Hospital Association, 1985-1987 editions.

39. Calculated by the author from data provided by the U.S. Department of Commerce, Bureau of the Census, and the Department of Health and Human Services, Health Care Financing Administration.

40. Starr, P. *The Social Transformation of American Medicine*. New York:

Section II.   The Content of Management

Basic Books, Inc., 1982, pp. 126, 422.

41. Iglehart, J. "The Future Supply of Physicians." *New England Journal of Medicine* 314(13):860-4, Mar. 27, 1986.

42. Data supplied by the American Academy of Family Physicians.

43. U.S. Department of Health and Human Services, Public Health Service, Bureau of Health Professions. *Fifth Report to the President and Congress on the Status of Health Personnel in the United States*, Table 3-46, March 1986.

44. U.S. Department of Health and Human Services, Public Health Service, Bureau of Health Professions. *Fifth Report to the President and Congress on the Status of Health Personnel in the United States*, March 1986.

45. Steinwachs, D., and others. "A Comparison of the Requirements for Primary Care Physicians in HMOs with Projections Made by the GMENAC." *New England Journal of Medicine* 314(4):217-22, Jan. 23, 1986.

46. Calculated by the author following the model advanced by Alvin R. Tarlov in "The Increasing Supply of Physicians, the Changing Structure of the Health Services System, and the Future Practice of Medicine," *New England Journal of Medicine* 308(20):1235-44, May 19, 1983.

47. Brannigan, M. "Pharmacists Will Soon Prescribe Drugs in Florida, to the Chagrin of Physicians ." *Wall Street Journal*, April 3, 1986, p. 29.

48. McGrath, A. "Just a Minute Doc." *Forbes* 136(5):132, Aug. 26, 1985.

49. Calculated by the author from 1987 and 1988 data provided by the National Resident Matching Program.

50. Schwartz, W., and others. "Are We Training Too Many Medical Subspecialists?" *JAMA* 259(2):233, Jan. 8, 1988.

Hugh W. Long, PhD, is Associate Professor of Health Care Management, A.B. Freeman School of Business, Tulane University, New Orleans, La.

CHAPTER 12

Cost/Quality Relationships:
A Generic Model for Health Care

by Robert B. Klint, MD, MHA, and Hugh W. Long, PhD

———

T he U.S. health care system is undergoing an unprecedented period of change precipitated by the interaction of major economic, social, and technological forces. The medical and managerial challenges wrought by these forces arrive, change, and disappear at a rapid pace. The health care sector, an incredibly complex aggregation of activities that has only recently begun to view itself as an industry, is often left in further confusion and inconsistency.

The introduction of prospective payment systems, establishment of captitated rates, increased monopsony power of some health care purchasers, ongoing efforts to reduce federal spending, and the growth of managed health care all tend to reduce the industry's inflow of dollars. Rising public and professional expectations for realizing the benefits of expanding medical technology, increasing provider operating expenses, rising capital needs, and unfulfilled health care expectations in some population segments all increase demand for services and their attendant funding.

As these social and economic forces vie for dominance, they do so in an environment characterized by an increasingly knowledgeable and assertive public, ever-increasing competition, growing provider networks and systems, the "corporatization" of health care, and an alleged oversupply of physicians. Questions of health care policy and social values are being asked. There is broadening public discussion of health care access, of divergent patterns of care and resource use, of the appropriateness of care for the terminally ill, and of the ethical and societal values at stake in all of these areas. There is increasing concern that "quality" will be compromised, even as that concept itself is altered and expanded beyond traditional boundaries. A new glossary is being developed; it includes "disquality," "undercare," and "cost-quality tradeoffs."

The fundamental characteristics of our future health care system depend in large measure on decisions being made now by leaders in

Section II. The Content of Management

health care, government, labor, and industry. The resource allocation and program decisions being made today by individual institutions, purchasers of health care, and designers of social and health care policy can be better formulated, implemented, and evaluated if we can develop a common framework and a common language that transcend the interests and viewpoints of particular constituencies.

This chapter presents a conceptual model for use by decision makers. The model is intended as a framework for discussing cost and quality, for allocating resources, for communicating between the many involved publics, and for clarifying some aspects of policy setting both at the institutional and at the system levels. The chapter explores the nature of the cost/quality relationship and offers a model for describing and explaining the major external constraints within which resource allocation decisions are made.

Quality

Some have proposed that the health care industry has used "quality" as its "miracle weapon" in defending its march toward a greater share of the gross national product. Justifications for the rising costs of care have been cloaked in a mysterious shroud understood only by medical professionals and health care managers.[1] Others have suggested that quality cannot even be defined; it is clearly recognizable only in its absence. "Disquality" was added to the glossary in 1986.[2]

Still others have assumed that major components of quality can indeed be identified if not fully quantified. Brook and Williams found that quality is directly influenced by synergism between the technology of care and the art of care, as modified by genetics, patient behavior, public health, and error.[3] Donabedian suggests that we judge quality by the degree to which the care given is capable, on the average, of producing the greatest improvement in health care that science can achieve.[4] The definition adopted by the American Medical Association additionally incorporates the patient's emotional status, effective use of resources, the medical record, health promotion, and promptness.[5] Affordability and accessibility are elements[6]; so are availability and client satisfaction.[1,7] Risk should be minimized[8]; harm should be avoided.[9] Evaluating both the process for delivering care and the structure that facilitates that process are additional ways of dissolving the shroud.

Medical measures of outcome such as mortality and morbidity may be less relevant as indicators of quality when the disease process itself and/ or other variables preclude a desired outcome. Similarly, a patient's satisfaction with a provider reflects both outcome and process (e.g., interaction with the provider) viewed relative to the patient's expectations. Thus, a patient's view of quality may also be an illusive marker if unrealistic expectations exist.

Garvin has suggested five approaches to defining product quality. These approaches were described in the context of manufacturing, yet may have direct application to the health care industry.[10] The transcendent approach views quality as some indefinable and innate excellence; the product approach identifies a measurable and specific ingredient or attribute possessed by the product; the user-based approach incorporates the notion of client satisfaction; manufacturing-based definitions are concerned with process, conformity with standards, and control measures; and value-based approaches define quality in terms of costs, worth, and "affordable excellence."[10]

Garvin's categorization of multiple quality definitions can be applied to health care and appears to be useful in bringing some order to the diverse and conflicting definitions frequently encountered. Outcome measures such as Donabedian's "greatest improvement in health" are currently viewed as central to defining quality and seem analogous to the product-based approach suggested by Garvin. Presumably no amount of courtesy, convenience, or availability can compensate for the avoidably poor outcome.

Refinements of quality definitions become increasingly important when outcomes in different provider settings are medically comparable. Such refinements may not assess outcome directly. They may be more indirect and more subjective, yet remain relevant ingredients in the evaluation process. These proxies for outcome include the processes by which care is delivered (a manufacturing set of definitions), the organizational structures and systems that support the process (also a manufacturing approach), and the patient's or purchaser's perception of the interaction (the user-based definitions).

Just as defining the quality of manufactured goods requires several approaches, so too does defining the quality of health care. Describing, defining, and measuring health care quality requires recognition of its multifaceted nature. Because no single approach is sufficient, both the definition and the systems used to monitor quality must encompass those major elements that individually represent input, process, and outcome. A quality assessment vector of eight major elements in that definition is described in the table on the next page.

Establishment of standards of care has been a major goal of the Joint Commission on Acreditation of Healthcare Organizations (JCAHO) and other accreditors, licensing bodies, peer review organizations, and professional associations. The prioritization and quantification of the component elements within the definitional matrix of the table on the next page have been elusive. Rank ordering of clients' perceptions of quality by Ware and Snyder suggests that there is a considerable overlap in the importance of physicians' "curing" and "caring" characteristics and that a relatively high importance is placed on availability, continuity, and access.[11] Categories of desirable attributes of medical clinics

Section II.   The Content of Management

Major Elements of a Health Care Quality Matrix

- Physician–Technical (input)

  Capabilities and characteristics of physicians as reflected by training, board certification, continuing education, liability history, medical records, and level of activity (numbers of procedures performed/diagnoses made)

- Hospital–Technical (input)

  Licenses, accreditation, and other official evaluations of institutional competence, such as JCAHO findings, university affiliation, currency of technology, nurse staffing ratios, level of activity (numbers of procedures performed), and liability history

- Physician–Art (process)

  "Art of care" characteristics of physicians as reflected by peer review findings, rapport with patients, availability, and listening and instructing capacities

- Hospital–Subjective (process)

  Hospital characteristics, including staff attitudes, service orientation, appearance, ambience, guest amenities, reputation, and empathy

- Continuity of Care (process)

  The degree to which a comprehensive spectrum of health care services exists, including services such as education, preadmission planning, discharge planning, and follow-up care, as appropriate

- Mortality (outcome)

  Patient outcomes resulting in death

- Morbidity (outcome)

  Occurrence of complications or other outcomes that are less than ideal, including hospital-acquired infections, returns to operating rooms within 24 hours, repeated procedures, lengths of stay of more than 2 standard deviations above the mean, or, if discharged, delayed returns to work or readmissions for the same diagnosis

- Customer Satisfaction (outcome)

  Evaluations (both subjective and objective) of patients' care from the perspective of lay parties such as patients and families and employers and other purchasers.

New Leadership in Health Care Management

have been ranked by administrators[11]; categories of physician actions by internists[12]; and characteristics of "good" hospitals by patients, medical staffs, and administrators.[7] A synthesis of physician characteristics revealed a high level of correlation between public and professional ranking of desirable and undesirable characteristics.[8]

Clearly, no universal or generally accepted ranking of the quality elements in the table, previous page, exists. However, we believe most clienteles or constituencies--patients, purchasers, physicians, nurses, administrators--would agree on a list of attributes such as these characterizing "good" quality care. We also believe that these same clienteles might well differ as to the rank ordering or relative importance of the elements in table at left. Further, we aver that different providers demonstrate varying amounts of the listed characteristics, as well as varying degrees of achievement relative to each element, and that, ultimately, such provider achievements are measurable.

It is also important to realize that the notion of "quality" can be observed and perhaps measured from a variety of foci. For the purposes of this chapter, we identify three such foci:

- Individual--What is the quality of care received by a particular patient (either generally or in a specific episode of care)?

- Micro-Aggregate--What is the quality of care received by all patients of Doctor X? What is the quality of care received by all DRG 127 patients at Hospital Y?

- Macro-Aggregate--What is the quality of care for newborns nationally?

Cost

Associated with any output, (good or service) of whatever quality are two types of costs. The first of these is the out-of-pocket quantity of cash required or credit incurred to command, directly or indirectly, the resources used to produce the output. The second type of costs comprises foregone opportunities, if any, to create additional wealth (cash flow), opportunities lost because of the very nature of the resources and process employed to generate the output.

Out-of-pocket costs, while apparently a straightforward concept, are often difficult to identify in practice. For example, producers of output have a complex task of determining the relevant cost where (1) significant fixed or capacity costs are spread over large quantities of output over varying lengths of time, (2) it is very expensive to measure accurately the actual incremental or variable costs associated with each output among many, and (3) use of resources is shared among many activities (e.g., overheads). Allocation among those activities is necessarily subjective. Similarly, purchasers of output for others (e.g., employers' payments for health services for employees) may have a difficult time identifying their costs relative to an employee's illness when a fixed number of dollars not tied to current output has been paid into a risk pool, especially when future payments (premiums) are influenced by current resource consumption. It should also be noted that out-of-pocket costs necessarily include indirect costs such as salaries of staff in the Health Care Financing Administration (HCFA) for the Medicare program, liability (malpractice) insurance premiums paid by health care providers, and the local HMO's advertising expenditures to gain market share. These are all real costs, even if distant from hands-on patient care.

Opportunity costs are no less complex, ranging from alternative uses of direct resources themselves to the lost interest on prepaid premiums, to productivity foregone because of illness and absenteeism, to attendant tax revenues lost, and to marginally lower living standards reflecting excess mortality and morbidity.

Relationship of Quality to Cost*

Cost/Quality Viewpoint

The precise elements of a definition of quality as well as the rank order of importance of those elements may vary by clientele. It is equally true that costs differ by party. The opportunity cost to a physician of expending additional time with a patient or members of the patient's family is quite different from the direct cost to a hospital of the resources consumed in the carrying out of the doctor's orders occasioned by that extra time spent understanding the patient's needs. The cost to the hospital for those resources is quite different from what the hospital may receive from an external payor: billed charges, discounted charges, cost plus or minus, or a regulated rate such as a Medicare prospective payment using the DRG system, none of which is likely to match the actual premium plus deductibles and copayments paid by that patient or that patient's employer currently or in the past.

Thus it is necessary to specify not only a quality focus (individual, micro-aggregate, macro-aggregate) but also a cost/quality viewpoint that must identify the clientele whose perspective is to be examined. The potential viewpoints include many divergent possibilities such as patient, taxpayer, employer, Office of Management and Budget, HCFA, shareholder, nonprofit hospital administrator, attending physician, patient's family, PRO, malpractice insurer, and more.

*The elements of this model are based on a presentation by Professor Long to the faculty and students of the Hospital Administration Program in the School of Public Health at the University of Michigan in 1973. Since 1975, Professor Long has used this model as part of his presentation in the "Physician in Management" seminars sponsored by the American Academy of Medical Directors and originally funded by a grant from the Robert Wood Johnson Foundation.

Cost/Quality Interactions

A number of generalizations that transcend both viewpoint and focus can be made with respect to cost/quality relationships. For example, the maximalist school would suggest that additional quality will always result from additional resources dedicated to health care. Traditionally, many physicians have behaved in ways consistent with this view. The hypothetical relationship is illustrated by Curve A in figure 1, below. At polar extreme would be the minimalist school, represented by some religious sects that believe no intervention is best and that any use of resources reduces quality of life and spirit. Curve B in figure 1 would represent such a position.

The optimalist school states that quality increases only to a finite maximum as more and more resources are applied, and declines thereafter (Curve C in figure 1, below). The extra laboratory test, the sixth stool guaiac, and the additional respiratory therapy treatment increase costs but may add little to the certainty of the diagnosis or to the likelihood of recovery. Their elimination may have no signifcant adverse effect on morbidity or mortality,[13,14] and their inclusion provides no salutary

Figure 1. FAMILY OF COST/QUALITY RELATIONSHIPS

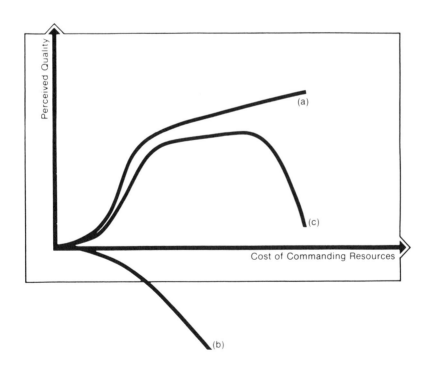

Section II. The Content of Management

results. Indeed, quality ultimately declines because of iatrogenic outcomes, nosocomial events, or physical discomfort. Perceptions of quality may decrease because of psychological reactions to cost or to the environment in which diagnosis or treatment is administered. The family of cost/quality relationships must also embrace the spectrum of unnecessary surgery, improper prescriptions, and incorrect treatment where the patient is compromised or harmed even as costs increase. It is in this broader context that we offer Curve C in the figure.

This curve conceptually incorporates elements of all of the relationships decribed above. We suggest that such a curve must ultimately describe all cost/quality relationships, regardless of viewpoint or focus, particularly as public awareness of cost/quality relationships and provider competition increase.

For any cost/quality viewpoint, resource allocation decisions are made that result in cost/quality combinations within the area under Curve C. These decisions are subject to two major constraints. The first constraint relates to quality and establishes a lower limit below which activity simply cannot consistently occur over the longer term without system failure (Line A in figure 2, below). Depending on viewpoint, this absolute floor is largely set by such activities, entities, or conditions as licensure, accreditation standards, the legal (tort) system, public accountability, reputation, professional review organizations, union contracts and competitive labor markets, medical standards, the referral

Figure 2. CONSTRAINTS TO COST/QUALITY COMBINATIONS

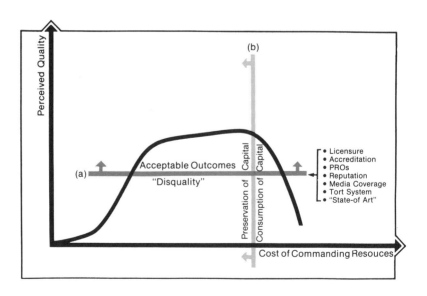

marketplace, morbidity and mortality outcomes, and ethics. It represents the product-based notion of acceptable outcomes. The position of the quality floor may be moved higher on the quality axis upon the initiative and at the discretion of decision-makers having a particular viewpoint (e.g., physicians, managers, Congress, JCAHO).

The second major constraint is financial. From the economist's point of view, this constraint represents the point between the preservation and the consumption of capital. In a more immediate sense, it represents the crossover between solvency and insolvency (Line B in figure 2). Whatever the source of funds (fees, revenue, appropriations, gifts, grants, etc.) for a particular viewpoint, there is some level of cost so large that there is no possibility of its being covered by incoming funds. To incur costs beyond what can be so covered is again to ensure system collapse within its respective funding cycle and asset life.

Government rate regulation of some or all of the marketplace (e.g., Medicare's prospective pricing system or New Jersey's all-payer mechanism), of course, defines the position of the solvency constraint along the cost axis. It is immediately apparent, of course, that centrally planned manipulation of this constraint in the name of "cost control" may simultaneously affect "quality control" by denying the market at least some higher levels of quality.

The area under that portion of the cost/quality curve above and to the left of the acceptable quality and solvency constraints represents all apparently feasible cost/quality combinations, which are redepicted in figure 3, next page. The cost/quality curve itself is the upper boundary of the area and corresponds to Garvin's notion of affordable excellence. It describes the maximum quality that can be achieved for a given expenditure of resources and the minimum cost at which a given level of quality can be realized. The curve further represents the maximum achievable cost/quality efficiency within each focus, and as such can be viewed as a process or technology constraint. As knowledge and technology expand, of course, we would naturally expect this boundary of "the possible" to shift upward and to the left, presenting an ever-moving cost/quality efficiency target. Any point within the area bounded by these three contraints (acceptable quality, solvency, and technology) represents less efficiency and less than achievable quality for the resources expended.

Cost/Quality Efficiency and Cost-Effectiveness

Regardless of viewpoint, a major goal for all decision-makers is to make cost-effective choices. If each of the points labeled "A" through "H" in figure 3, represents a cost/quality combination within the feasible area XYZ, certain obvious guides for decision-makers emerge. Primary among these is the "northwest quadrant rule." Any cost/quality combination to the left of or above a given combination (i.e., to the "north-

Section II.   The Content of Management

Figure 3. FEASIBLE COST/QUALITY COMBINATIONS AND THE NORTHWEST QUADRANT RULE

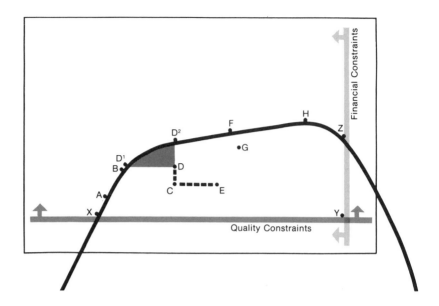

west") is said to dominate the given combination. A combination due "west" of the given combination offers "identical" amounts of quality for less cost and is, therefore, obviously preferred; one due "north" of the given combination offers higher quality for identical cost and likewise dominates any choice between the two. Any combination both "north" and "west" of the given combination offers both higher quality and lower cost and hence dominates any comparison with the given combination. Thus in figure 3, G is dominated by F; E by B, C, and D; C by B and D; and Z by F and H. D is inferior to any combination in the shaded area of figure 3 and is ultimately dominated by the D' to D" portion of the cost/quality curve that bounds the shaded area. Hence, only X, A, B, D', D", F, and H are undominated.

It is in this context that we can appreciate the statements of some[15,16] that "quality costs no more" or that "quality is cheaper--doing it right the first time costs less." These are certainly true statements if the starting point is one of cost/quality inefficiency. They do *not* lead to the conclusion, however, that there is no relationship bewteen cost and quality.

Indeed, the set of efficient cost/quality combinations that constitute the cost/quality curve is that relationship. The characteristic shared by combinations X, A, B, D', D", F, H, and all other points on the cost/quality curve to the left of H (representing maximum attainable quality)

New Leadership in Health Care Management

is that no point on that boundary is dominated by any other. Each is "economically efficient" in cost/quality terms, and collectively they represent the efficient cost/quality frontier running from X through H.

Doubilet et al. have cautioned against the misuse of the term "cost-effective," suggesting that its use be restricted to those instances where obtaining the additional health care benefit is worth the additional cost.[17] We cannot concur. In the context of our model, a cost-effective decision is any decision that moves the provider toward greater cost/quality efficiency, i.e., any northwest-moving choice. Once the technological boundary is reached and cost/quality efficiency is attained, the term "cost-effective" is no longer meaningful. Cost cannot be reduced without also reducing quality, and quality cannot be enhanced without incurring additional cost. There cannot be a meaningful cost/quality tradeoff unless cost/quality efficiency has already been achieved (through a series of cost-effective decisions); once true tradeoffs are required, cost-effectiveness as a criterion must be supplemented by the judgments of the various clienteles who bear the resulting costs and enjoy the resulting benefits.[18]

As suggested above, increased public awareness of cost and quality considerations, combined with increased competition for market share within the health care sector, should ultimately force the system from the interior of the feasible region to the efficient frontier, as decision-makers follow the dictates of the northwest quadrant rule.

Cost/Quality Tradeoffs

What are ultimately more interesting, of course, are decisions that involve moves to the northeast (Should additional cost be borne to increase quality?) or to the southwest (Should quality be lowered to reduce costs?) when cost/quality efficiency has been achieved.

Indeed, the entire concept of an efficient frontier having more than a single cost/quality combination gives lie to the mythology of "a single class of care." Market segmentation can easily be defined as targeting distinct cost/quality combinations, and the choice of *where* in a particular focus one wants to be along the cost/quality frontier is a question of great economic and political significance.

Thurow[19] raised this question, suggesting a multitiered system reflecting the notion that, systemwide, patients will receive the quality they are capable of bargaining or paying for. An expansion of this notion is shown in figure 4, next page. Note that this depiction is from the viewpoint of an economist looking at quality and cost with a macro-aggregate focus and should *not* be interpreted to suggest that any *individual* provider entity would apply differential resources to patients based on expected payment from or on behalf of the patient.

Section II.   The Content of Management

Figure 4. POTENTIAL MULTI-TIERED SYSTEM BASED ON PURCHASING POWER

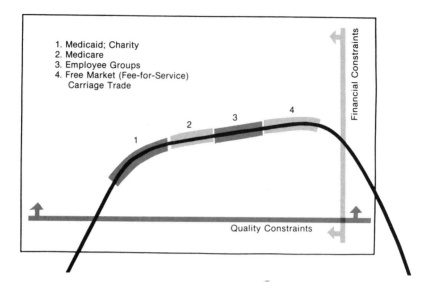

1. Medicaid; Charity
2. Medicare
3. Employee Groups
4. Free Market (Fee-for-Service)
   Carriage Trade

Financial Constraints

Quality Constraints

Figure 5. SATISFACTION INDIFFERENCE CURVES FOR TWO DIFFERENT MARKET SEGMENTS

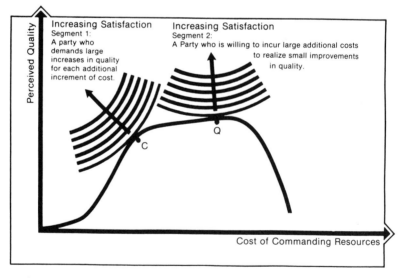

Perceived Quality

Increasing Satisfaction
Segment 1:
A party who demands large increases in quality for each additional increment of cost.

Increasing Satisfaction
Segment 2:
A Party who is willing to incur large additional costs to realize small improvements in quality.

C

Q

Cost of Commanding Resources

Rather, individual providers may well be advised to choose a market niche that targets one of these market segments and to abandon the strategy of attempting to be all things to all patients. Economic reality suggests that it is only reasonable to concentrate on that portion of a market that will be satisfied on a reasonably consistent basis with a particular range of efficient cost/quality combinations.

Figure 5, previous page, depicts satisfaction indifference curves for two very different market segments. Segment 1 may represent the payment mechanisms society puts in place for the medically indigent. This societal perspective tends to be highly cost-adverse, constraining covered services, and is most "satisfied" at point C on the cost/quality curve. Providers choosing to serve this market must tailor their activities to the social, economic, and medical characteristics of this segment.

By contrast, Segment 2 might reflect the "carriage trade," quality-seekers who are willing to pay for the search and who achieve maximum satisfaction at cost/quality combination Q. Some providers will undoubtedly choose to function in this market to the exclusion of others, reflecting the market's prestige as well as its economic attributes.

Conclusion

Many cost containment efforts in health care have been based on utilization review. The use of preadmission certification, second surgical opinions, and length-of-stay reviews largely applies the northwest quadrant rule, relying on an assumption that excessive resources are being consumed for a given quality level. The attention thus paid to cost may have been somewhat successful in controlling the rate of increase in health care costs, but questions about the resulting quality effects are being raised.[1,20-23] Quality of care is the single most important factor in deciding where to go for health care,[24] yet there is clear evidence that the health care system already has multiple tiers, which are distinguished by the relative importance different quality care elements are given and/or external fiscal realities.[19]

Our conceptual model should serve as a useful tool in communicating these market realities to numerous publics. Figure 4 suggests that selected marketplace segments may be arrayed in different positions along the cost/quality efficient frontier based on the cost/quality trade-offs that have been made, either explicitly or implicitly. Policy-makers at both institutional and national levels should be aware that all parties to the decision-making process may be forced to choose from among those segments as resources become more constrained.

For example, taken in isolation, the Medicaid reality may well be as shown in figure 6, next page, where welfare or "social safety net" policy depresses the quality constraint and/or state-level constitutional requirements for balanced budgets shift the fiscal constraint to the left. This would contrast with figure 7, next page, depicting Medicare reality. The American Association of Retired Persons (AARP) is possibly the most powerful political lobby in Washington. Its influence with both the Congress and the Executive Branch probably elevates the quality constraint by, for example, insisting that Medicare extend the range of covered services to include organ replacement. Simultaneously, the AARP pushes against the fiscal constraint by opposing draconian reduc-

Section II.   The Content of Management

Figure 6. INFLUENCES ON QUALITY CONSTRAINTS: STATE GOVERNMENT POINT OF VIEW

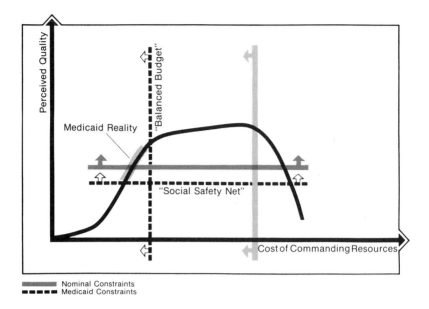

Nominal Constraints
Medicaid Constraints

Figure 7. INFLUENCES ON QUALITY CONSTRAINT: CONGRESSIONAL POINT OF VIEW

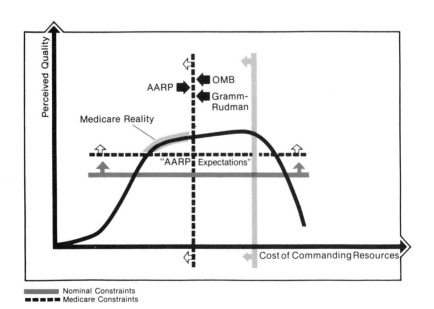

Nominal Constraints
Medicare Constraints

tions in payments to providers. This is mitigated by a Gramm-Rudman philosophy or a Reagan OMB fiscal policy in which deficit reduction objectives override health policy and attempt to move the fiscal constraint to the left.

Limitations and Directions for Further Research

By observing the effects of adding or withdrawing resources, one can estimate where a provider has been positioned along the cost/quality efficient frontier or within the feasible region at a previous point in time. Objective determination of current cost/quality position is more difficult than ex post analysis unless there is a known historical "track." Even if absolute positions can reasonably be estimated, however, ascertaining position relative to the technological boundary (cost/quality efficient frontier) may be problematical. Not only is the shape and position of the entire boundary hard to estimate for a given provider, but, at best, the points on that boundary in our figures represent only central tendencies of distributions. These distributions often exhibit significant dispersion in both the cost and the quality dimensions, reflecting the natural range of disease processes, and human response to them as well as to their treatment.

Nonetheless, applying this model at the micro-economic level, where expectations and values can be better assessed, can provide important input for provider positioning in the marketplace. While application at the macro-economic level suffers from the weaknesses of all generalizations, it should serve as a means of communicating with the numerous publics affected by public policy decisions.

Additional research into the quantification and measurement of quality is needed. Finding agreement on the elements of quality and their relative importance will be important, at least within each clientele's viewpoint and at each level of focus. If quality is the manageable aspect of health care suggested by Ellwood[20] and if quality continues to appear as a major variable in employer health service purchasing, in provider marketing, and in public policy discussions, then agreement on its component parts and on their relationships to cost will be critical to achieving cost/quality efficient health care within our society.

References

1. Reinhardt, U. "Quality of Care in Competitive Markets." *Business and Health* 3(8):7-9, July-Aug. 1986.

2. *Illinois PRO Objective Summary.* Peoria, Ill.: Mid-State Foundation for Medical Care, Inc., 1986.

3. Brook, R., and Williams, K. "Quality of Health Care for the Disadvantaged." *Journal of Community Health* 1(2):132-56, Winter 1975.

Section II.   The Content of Management

4. Donabedian, A. "What is Quality?" Lecture, Center for Health Services and Policy Research, Northwestern University, Evanston, Ill., Oct. 6-7, 1986.

5. Billmeyer, D., and others. "Quality Care." *JAMA* 256(8):1032-4, Aug. 22-29, 1986.

6. Rose, J. "Americans Call for Affordable, Accessible, Quality Health Care." *American Family Physician* 33(4):97, April 1986.

7. Elbeik, M. "Perceptions of Hospital Care." *Health Management Forum* 7(1):70-8, Spring 1986.

8. Donabedian, A. *The Definition of Quality and Approaches to Its Assessment.* Ann Arbor, Mich.: Health Administration Press, 1980, pp. 8-64.

9. *The Genuine Work of Hippocrates*; translated from the Greek by Francis Adams. Baltimore, Md.: Williams and Wilkins, 1939.

10. Garvin, D. "What Does Product Quality Really Mean?" *Sloan Management Review* 26(1):25-43, Fall 1984.

11. Ware, J., and Synder, M. "Dimensions of Patient Attitudes Regarding Doctors and Medical Services." *Medical Care* 13(8):669- 82, Aug. 1975.

12. Sanazaro, P., and Williamson, J. "A Classification of Physician Performance in Internal Medicine." *Journal of Medical Education* 43(3):389-97, Mar. 1968.

13. Neuhauser, D., and Lewicki, A. "What Do We Gain from the Sixth Stool Guaiac?" *New England Journal of Medicine* 293(5):226-8, July 31, 1975.

14. Zibrak, J., and others. "Effect of Reductions in Respiratory Therapy on Patient Outcome." *New England Journal of Medicine* 315(5):292-5, July 31, 1986.

15. Winchell, J. "Reduced Costs Can Improve Care." *Health Care* 27(7):15-20, Oct. 1985

16. McClure, W. "Buying Right: How to Do It." *Business and Health* 2(10):41-44, Oct. 1985.

17. Doubilet, P., and others. "Use and Misuse of the Term 'Cost-Effective' in Medicine." *New England Journal of Medicine* 314(4):253- 56, Jan. 23, 1986.

18. Russell, L. "Balancing Cost and Quality: Methods of Evaluation." *Bulletin of the New York Academy of Medicine* 62(1):55-60, Jan.-Feb. 1986.

19. Thurow, L. "Medicine Versus Economics." *New England Journal of Medicine* 313(10):611-14, Sept. 5, 1985.

20. Ellwood, P., and Paul, B. "Commentary: But What about Quality?" *Health Affairs* 5(1):135-40, Spring 1986.

21. Rettig, P. "Value, Not Just Costs, Need to Be Considered for Quality Managed Care." *Business and Health* 4(6):64, April 1987.

22. Jensen, J. "More Consumers Are Willing to Pay Higher Price for Quality Healthcare." *Modern Healthcare* 16(17):48-9, Aug. 15, 1986.

23. "Medicine: A Special Report: Declining Quality of Care for the Elderly Is Hinted in New Studies, Which Blame Cuts in Medicre for the Situation." *Wall Street Journal* 210(37):1, Aug. 20, 1987.

24. "HMQ Survey: A Mandate of High-Quality Health Care." *Health Management Quarterly*, pages 3-6, Fourth Quarter 1986.

Robert B. Klint, MD, MHA, is Executive Vice President of SwedishAmerican Hospital, Rockford, Ill. Hugh W. Long, PhD, is Associate Professor of Health Care Management, A.B. Freeman School of Business, Tulane University, New Orleans, La.

Section II.   The Content of Management

Marketing As a Necessary Function In Health Care Management: A Philosophical Approach

by Eric N. Berkowitz, PhD

T he changing competitive climate of health care during the past decade has led to a greater sophistication in the management of medicine. One business function that has received greater attention in health care has been marketing, a traditional management tool.

The Evolution of Marketing

Common to many hospitals today is a director of marketing position. Yet as late as 1976, fewer than 10 hospitals in the United States had marketing directors. While marketing is now more common, the marketing philosophy is not as well appreciated. Hospital and medical philosophy can be viewed as evolving to a marketing orientation over three phases.[1]

Phase 1--The Production Orientation. Through the 1970s and for many hospitals today, the hospital has been a production-oriented institution. It might best be characterized by a mission statement such as: "We are a hospital providing high-quality medicine to the community. We must have physicians and nurses to provide it, just as we need administrators to keep the books."

The focus of a hospital at this stage of its philosophical evolution is on the provision of "high quality." Providing high-quality services is the key force dominating all other hospital planning and strategy considerations.

Phase 2--The Sales Era. Of late, far more hospitals have moved to a second stage of philosophical evolution, sales. Hospitals have grown to recognize that there is competition for patients. Other hospitals, medical groups, and prepaid plans are but some of the providers striving to satisfy the medical needs of the community. At this point of organizational consciousness, the philosophical mission of the hospital could be paraphrased as: "We are a hospital providing a number of medical services to the market. We must have a first-rate public relations effort to encourage physicians in the community and patients to utilize our services to their fullest capacity."

At this stage of evolution, the issue is one of capacity utilization. The goal is to fill beds. It is not marketing that is occurring at this point, it is sales. The hospital develops an effective public relations effort to the community and provides staff breakfasts or orientations for the medical staff. All efforts are to stimulate demand to fill beds.

Phase 3--The Era of Marketing. While many hospitals have marketing directors, there are in fact few hospitals at this stage of philosophical evolution. It might best be described as: "We will assess the health care needs of the market and meet them."

The focus of the organization is not on capacity to fill by attracting referrals. It is on attracting referrals through the provision of a needed service. In the third phase, the philosophical focus of the organization has shifted subtly, but importantly. Recall that in the first phase (production), the organization's purpose was to provide medical care. In the second stage (sales), the organization develops strategies to fill its beds. In the last phase of philosophical development (marketing), the organization exists to meet the health needs of the market. It is not the beds that are sold to the community. The health needs of the market determine the configuration of beds.

The Planning Process

To best understand the impact of a marketing philosophy on a hospital, it is important to consider the planning process undertaken by most health care groups. The typical hospital or group practice follows the nonmarketing planning approach described below.[2]

Nonmarketing Plan. Regardless of the industry, most organizations follow a similar planning sequence. Just a few words are usually dissimilar, which tends to make it appear that planning in one industry might be truly different from another. Consider the long-range planning process of a hospital. Figure 1, at right, portrays the typical sequence in a nonmarketing planning approach. The first step is designating the mission. In most hospitals, the mission is global, such as, "provide high-quality medicine to the community regardless of race, creed, religion, or ability to pay." The nonmarketing planning process really begins at the second step--specifying the strategy. Before discussing this stage, we will digress to consider the composition of those who define the hospital's strategy.

> **Figure 1.**
> **NONMARKETING PLANNING SEQUENCE**
>
> Mission/Goals
> ↓
> Strategy
> ↓
> Tactics
> ↓
> Implementation

Section II.   The Content of Management

Most hospitals have a long-range planning committee. Typically these committees are composed of a few members of the hospital board, the senior hospital administrator, and a department head or two. A few people are often more influential than others. These individuals might be termed the "hallway politicians." They are very effective at going door-to-door within the hospital, lining up votes for their programs or ideas.

The hallway politicians begin to exert their influence at the strategy stage. Strategy meetings are the crucial point at which the hospital must decide which two or three programs or areas will receive the attention and focus of management and, often, financial resources for the next few years. Several ideas are discussed at these sessions--starting a preferred provider organization (PPO), increasing the capacity of the laboratory to become one of regional stature, or building new facilities.

Within this scenario, a physician rises and proclaims his long-standing loyalty to the hospital. He notes that he has never admitted a patient to another facility. He may even cite his growing national stature as a futurist in the field of medicine. To him, the strategy for the future is clear, it is sports medicine (although any program can be substituted). It also happens that this physician is an orthopedic surgeon.

Not everyone in the room may be as clear on this path for the future. Yet this physician had lined up his votes beforehand. The vote is 7 to 5 in favor of sports medicine. The hospital will commit its physical, financial, and personnel resources to establishing a sports medicine program in the ambulatory care wing of the hospital.

Tactics are the next stage of the planning process. This is when the hospital realizes there is no one in-house with expertise in sports medicine. A search firm is hired to scour the country for a director of sports medicine. A director is hired and conflict occurs. Any hospital has finite resources. New programs demand start-up dollars, and other departments find that their budget increase requests are put on hold. In many facilities there is a space shortage. The appearance of a new program means that another department's space is reduced. Space and budget are two key sources of conflict in any hospital.

The fourth stage of the nonmarketing planning model is implementation. Before implementation occurs, however, an unsettling question suddenly arises in the administrative suite of most hospitals. "Where are the patients going to come from?" The hospital's public relations department is reminded that sports medicine is opening in 30 days, and a community open house is needed. The public relations director prints invitations and places an advertisement in the local newspaper announcing an open house for the new sports medicine program. The open house is held on a Sunday. Three people show up.

New Leadership in Health Care Management

Four months later the hospital finance committee meets to review the utilization of sports medicine relative to projections. It is discovered that sports medicine is not meeting expectations. Two explanations quickly surface. The first reason proposed for failure is simple. Public relations did a poor job, and there was not enough advertising. Occasionally, depending on the amount of capital invested and the size of the budget deficit, a second explanation is given. The director who was hired to run the program is not generating enough referrals. The question before the group is how to get rid of the director.

Both of these explanations are possible, but a third, competing explanation rarely is voiced. There is no need in the community for a sports medicine program. People who suffer sports-related injuries are satisfied with the treatment provided by their primary care physicians and by referrals to physical therapists. Physicians who treat sports-related injuries see no advantages in referrals to a program beyond what they are presently using. Alternatively, two or three sports medicine programs already exist in the area. The hospital's program is in no way different from (or better than) existing providers. The program will not make it.

Marketing-Based Planning. The alternative approach is one in which the impact of marketing can be seen. The two approaches are similar in many respects (Figure 2, below). The first step is the same. Every organization, whether it is a hospital, a free-standing laboratory, or an automobile manufacturer, determines its own mission.

The influence of marketing is felt in the second step. In the previous model, a group within the hospital determined the strategies. In a market-based approach, the next step is to assess the needs of the market. This market could consist of physicians, patients, third-party payers, or corporations. Rather than to decide on an *a priori* basis to enter sports medicine, the purpose is to identify areas of need and to generate a significant competitive advantage over other providers.

For example, in many areas several endocrinology services are available for physician use. As the director looks for new opportunities, the

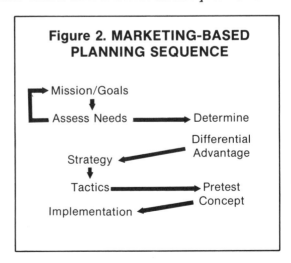

Figure 2. MARKETING-BASED PLANNING SEQUENCE

Mission/Goals → Assess Needs → Determine Differential Advantage → Strategy → Tactics → Pretest Concept → Implementation

Section II.   The Content of Management

question to pose to prospective referring physicians is "What don't you like about the endocrinology group you now use?"

In a nonmarket-based planning model, the chief of endocrinology may act in the same way as the hallway politician described in the previous example. The chief may assume that he or she knows what the market needs or how it might want a service delivered. In a market-based approach, the users and buyers of the service provide the direction. For example, for sports medicine, a market-based approach might find that existing satisfaction with the providers or alternatives for sports-related injuries is high. Sports medicine then might be an area with little opportunity for establishing a differential advantage. The hospital might still decide for other reasons, such as maintaining the loyalty of the orthopedic surgeons, to enter sports medicine, but the expectations for the services must be reduced. In this case, the marketing-based planning model might uncover little opportunity for sports medicine but a significant interest in the corporate community for an industrial medicine component with a strong toxicology program.

The third step in the market-based model is tactics. The assessment step would have defined the tactic, if the identified need (industrial medicine) matches the mission of the organization--high-quality medicine. In this case, an industrial medicine program would be consistent. Now the tactic is an internal challenge. Can the hospital put together an industrial medicine program that meets the market's expectations?

Figure 2 illustrates a second difference in the marketing model after the tactics stage. Before the hospital gets to full-scale implementation, the service must be pretested. Pretesting a service is more difficult than pretesting a product, where a company can make a prototype to test consumer reaction. Pretesting in a service industry entails pretesting the concept.

The provider meets with a group similar to the potential purchaser of the final service and in great detail describes how the service will be delivered, its price, and how the service can be accessed. The question to be proved with potential users is whether the described service is what they meant when they talked about laboratory outreach or industrial medicine and if they will buy it.

The foundation of this marketing-based planning approach is that the market, not the individuals internal to the organization, dictates the direction in which the organization will go.

The marketing-based approach establishes the price of the service. In the "assessment of needs" and pretesting stages, the market must be measured in terms of how the market wants the service delivered. What location or hours are convenient for buyers?

The last stage of the marketing-based model is similar to the previous approach--implementation. Unlike the nonmarketing planning approach, there is less need for an open house to find the patients who might use the service. It is known at the implementation stage that the service is needed and that it has been configured the way the market wants in terms of delivery and price. The key remaining challenge is to inform the market that the service is available--to promote the service to the market.

In this conceptualization of the marketing-based planning approach, the definition of marketing becomes clearer: "Marketing is the process of identifying the market's need, of planning and developing a service to meet those needs, and of determining the best way to price, promote, and deliver the service."

This definition contains the four components of marketing that are common to all organizations whether they are for-profit or not-for-profit--product (service), price, promotion, and distribution. These four components, the basis for the tactics in any marketing plan, are referred to as the marketing mix and are described in greater detail at the end of this chapter.

Why Marketing Now?

Why is marketing an important issue among health care providers? Fifteen or 20 years ago, there was no need for a marketing orientation in a hospital or medical group. Until recently in many communities, when a hospital service was offered, there was a need. In the past few years, however, more competitors have appeared in the marketplace. They have come from proprietary organizations, free-standing independents, and doctors' offices. Moreover, offering a new service can represent a significant investment in terms of expensive technology. Fifteen or 20 years ago, when a hospital or clinic offered a service that was not successful, the director or long-range planning committee summed up the failure as a "good learning experience." Fewer and fewer organizations can afford too many such learning experiences with today's financial and competitive realities.

Marketing-based planning does not guarantee success. Surveys can be reliable; pretesting can be conducted. Yet in the time intervening from conceptualization to final offering, conditions can change. Marketing cannot guarantee success, but it can reduce the probability of failure. The nonmarketing planning model places tremendous pressure on the director of the clinical laboratory to be an extremely accurate forecaster of market needs. Although many successes have undoubtedly been built on just this type of forecasting, most would agree that the probabilities of success are probably higher for creating a service that someone wants by first asking them what they prefer.

Section II.   The Content of Management

Risks of Marketing

The delineation of these two approaches to planning should reveal the potential advantages of a marketing approach. Fully understanding the differences between these two philosophies also reveals why marketing has been defined as advertising. Marketing is dangerous. Many professionals feel that, because they are professionals, they know what is best for the market. With a marketing-based approach, the professional does not want to hear the answer regarding the desired service or the way in which a service should be configured, if this market preference goes against his or her view. It is safer to translate marketing as advertising. "Marketing" then becomes promoting the service the provider wants to offer. If the service fails to generate demand, marketing is at fault. The possibility that the service did not meet the market's preferences is not raised.

The difference between these two approaches to planning, coupled with the definition of marketing, should lead to an understanding of the differences between marketing and advertising. Marketing is not advertising, but advertising is one element of the marketing mix.

In health care, there is always an easy challenge to marketing. The needs assessment is done, and there is a clear understanding of how the market wants the service delivered, but the market's preference is counter to the professional's preference. The professional can always cite quality as the reason a service cannot be offered according to the market's preferences. Offering a service according to market preference would destroy the quality of care.

Consider this scenario. Twenty years ago, if a woman asked her obstetrician whether her spouse could be in the delivery room, the almost universal response was "no." Few lay people would argue with the reason given: it would destroy the quality of care. Over time, women would not accept this argument in the case of a routine delivery. Furthermore, enough women desired this arrangement so that eventually some obstetricians met the need. Today if you visited a delivery room, the spouse and possibly siblings would be present. Grandparents are occasionally allowed in, along with someone to run the video camera. In many communities, the only person missing is the obstetrician, who has been replaced by a nurse midwife. The lesson is clear. No organization has to bend to market demand provided that no competitor rises up to meet the need. In many hospitals today, volume has dropped dramatically as more services can be provided in physicians' offices without the accompanying overhead charges. The risks for marketing are clear, but the costs of ignoring the market in today's competitive environment may be greater than most health care organizations can afford.

The Consumer Perspective

Inherent in the marketing-based planning process is the need for the organization to go outside to assess needs in the marketplace. Central to effective marketing is defining the product or service not from the provider's perspective but from the market's view. To more clearly address this issue, consider the decision on hospital selection.

When a patient is faced with hospitalization, the physician plays a major role in selecting the facility. The attending physician may have privileges at two or even three facilities where the technical capabilities are such that the procedure could be performed. The physician will indicate at which hospitals he or she has admitting privileges and then ask the consumer if there is a preference. In this case, the consumer is making a purchasing decision.[3] Figure 3, below, depicts the hospital selection decision from the consumer's perspective.

The diagram has two components. One is labeled the primary product. The primary product is the technology within the hospital and the medical expertise of the staff. The primary product is the portion of the service that must exist for the organization to even be considered a reasonable alternative. For example, if a hospital does not have the technology or staff to do liver transplantation, it lacks the primary product and would not be considered as a competitor.

The second component of Figure 3 is labeled the offered dimension. This dimension represents the attributes that the consumer uses to judge the hospital in terms of service quality--attitude of the nursing staff, patient procedures, admitting process, and layout of the facility.

This aspect of marketing often troubles the health care professional. The previous explanation indicates that the primary product, the di-

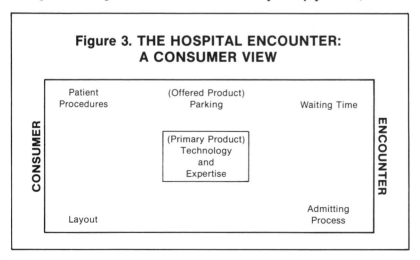

Figure 3. THE HOSPITAL ENCOUNTER: A CONSUMER VIEW

Section II.   The Content of Management

mension most professionals view as the real "quality" aspect of the service, is taken for granted. Furthermore, the consumer is not judging on quality but instead on soft dimensions such as attitude, friendliness of staff, or waiting time in the emergency department. This perspective does not undermine the importance of quality. Rather, quality is not a source of a differential advantage but instead is the cost of entry for being a competitor.

In fact, the primary product component is important to the consumer in selecting between providers when the technical or expertise dimension can be observed or documented. The difficulty in health care is the specialty and even subspecialty nature of knowledge in areas such as internal medicine, endocrinology, nephrology and clinical laboratory medicine. In most cases only an internist can truly judge whether another internist is proficient in terms of primary product knowledge. The only individual capable of judging whether a clinical laboratory is truly high in terms of its primary product quality (its technology and staff expertise) may be the director of another clinical laboratory.

Figure 4, below, shows this same perspective in the selection of a clinical laboratory by a physician. As with consumer's selection of hospitals, many physicians can choose among several clinical laboratories. When physicians select one laboratory over another, they have purchased a product. This product has two dimensions: a primary and an offered component. Again, the primary product is technology and expertise. Yet the typical physician cannot differentiate among laboratories on this critical component. How do they differentiate among laboratories in deciding that one is better than another? The offered components of speed, cost, detail of report, reliability of pick-up, and drop-off service play the key roles. These dimensions can be observed and judged by the physician.

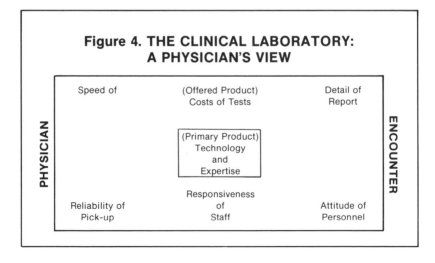

Figure 4. THE CLINICAL LABORATORY:
A PHYSICIAN'S VIEW

New Leadership in Health Care Management

This discussion may lead one to question the importance of the primary product, medical expertise and technology, in health care marketing. Judgment of services on the offered product components does not mean that the expertise of the physicians is unimportant, but rather that most services exist within a reasonable range of primary product quality. In fact, one might describe the quality of medical care as a bell-shaped curve with the tail ends of the curve representing truly exceptional quality--either good or poor. Few providers operate on either end. The ability to perceive *real* differences on primary product quality for services within the middle range is difficult for consumers and physicians.

If one assumes a bell-shaped curve of medical quality, quality is less a point of difference. Quality becomes a given, the initial cost of entry to compete in the marketplace. In order to make the primary product a point of difference, the buyer must notice a difference. Because the challenge is difficult in health care, services are judged on the offered product components.

Components of Marketing Strategy

In discussing the sequence of a marketing planning approach, the four components of strategy were identified as the service (product), the price, the location (place), and the promotion. These elements have been referred to as the four Ps of marketing. While space constraints do not allow significant discussion of any one element, the remainder of this chapter will highlight each "P."

The Product

The essential element of any marketing program is a service that is desired by the market *and* configured in the manner that the market wants. The early testing stage for a service is critical, in that promoting a service not designed to market specifications may be a fast way to kill its demand. It is very difficult to restore a base of referrals if early physician experience with a service is negative.

In developing the marketing effort for any medical service, the concept of the product life cycle is useful. All services may be viewed as existing in one of four stages, depicted in Figure 5, next page. This graph shows a generalized life cycle. Time is represented on the x-axis and revenue or patient volume on the y-axis. Marketing objectives vary over the course of these stages.

In the first stage (introduction), a new service, such as an arthritis program, is introduced. The major marketing objective is to generate awareness. At this stage, promotion, particularly in the form of mass advertising, is important. Product quality is important in order that first-time referrers have a positive experience. In early stages of a service's

Section II.   The Content of Management

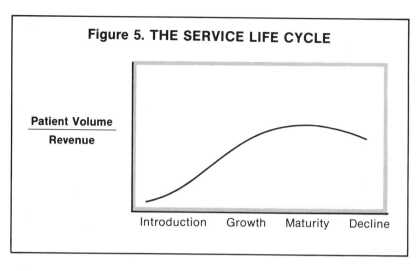

Figure 5. THE SERVICE LIFE CYCLE

Patient Volume
Revenue

Introduction   Growth   Maturity   Decline

offering, it is also helpful to keep the number of alternatives within the program limited in order to help maintain product quality.

The second stage of the life cycle is growth. It is at this point that competitors enter the market. The key objective at this stage is to lock up the flow of referrals. For example, the arthritis program may sign capitation contracts with HMOs to be the treatment source for arthritis. Also, at this stage it is beneficial to offer additional varieties of the program to expand the market. For example, a specialized arthritis program for children might be considered as a way to expand market presence.

The third stage of the life cycle is maturity. As the curve indicates, demand is leveling off. The marketing objective at this point is maintenance. Any referrals lost at this stage cannot be replaced with new referrals. It is at this point that commitment must be made to develop new services to get back to the early stages of a life cycle.

Decline is the last stage of the life cycle. A service often declines for reasons beyond the control of the provider. Demographic changes have led to the decline of many hospitals' pediatric units. Technology has virtually eliminated polio wards. This stage is often the most difficult for an institution to address. It can be emotional. Often it is hard to shut down a service on which a clinic built its early reputation. Services in the decline stage, however, tend to consume a disproportionate share of management time or financial resources. In medicine, declining services often cannot be closed down because of their link to the offering of other more profitable offerings. Yet the fiscal and personnel support of these declining services must be closely maintained.

Place

The place component of marketing is the distribution element. This comprises offered components such as location and hours the service is offered. Location is often an important issue for specialty services that are offered in university settings or other large tertiary facilities. In this instance, access may be particularly difficult for the patient. The distribution strategy may entail having on-campus overnight accommodations, an out-of-town visitors' office, or, if possible, satellite offices.

For referral physicians, distribution is often defined as scheduling access. The primary product quality can be high, but the physician must be able to get a patient in to be seen. In an interesting distribution strategy, the Mayo Clinic is setting up a telecommunications satellite link with its three facilities. Physicians at locations distant from Rochester can talk to and see specialists at the main facility. This strategy is a great advantage in terms of access.

Price

The price component for medical services for many years was of little importance, because insurance coverage made it a non-issue. The appearance of large-scale contractual buyers, such as HMOs, however, has increased price consciousness. From a marketing perspective, there are two components to price. One component is the floor. This represents the internal cost of delivering the service and is determined through basic cost accounting. Marketing strategy, however, is concerned with the ceiling or the price the market is willing to pay. If the floor is higher than the ceiling, no amount of promotion can make the service acceptable to the market. It is the difference between the ceiling and the floor that represents the margin to the institution. An important aspect for early stage market research is determination of the ceiling price among insurers, HMOs, and consumers for a proposed service offering.

Promotion

While marketing is not sales, sales is a part of marketing. Promoting a service can be done through personal selling, advertising, and publicity.

Historically, medical services have relied on publicity to get information on their services to the public. Publicity consists of news stories on television and in the print media. This component is valuable for its appearance of credibility and because there is no direct cost for the time or space. The disadvantage of this method is the lack of control. Mass advertising overcomes this disadvantage, although there is a sizable direct cost involved. Figure 6, next page, shows the selection trade-offs for the various promotional media.

Section II.   The Content of Management

Figure 6. SELECTION TRADEOFFS WITH ALTERNATIVE MEDIA

	Cost of Placement	Selectivity	Message Quality	Lead Time
Newspapers	Relatively expensive.	Little selectivity except in major metro areas. By zip code or region.	Poor photo reproduction. Person can spend time with message.	Easy to obtain space with short notice.
Magazines	Relatively expensive	Great selectivity by lifestyle, interest. Reasonably good selectivity by area (particularly metro).	Excellent photo reproduction. Person can spend time with message.	Often requires contracting for space for a month or more prior notice.
Direct mail	Relatively inexpensive	Excellent selectivity on criteria required by organization.	Excellent as function of dollars spent in printing.	Little required except to produce mail piece.
Radio	Inexpensive	Reasonable selectivity.	Must be short, simple. Difficult to hold attention.	Little advance notice required to run a commercial.
Television	Expensive.	Reasonable - a function of time of day and show selected	Excellent for sight and sound. Relatively short messages required. Hard to hold attention.	Often requires substantial lead time with station for time.
Outdoor	Relatively inexpensive.	Little selectivity except by location of billboard.	Requires short, simple message.	Space availability often requires long lead time.

Reprinted from: Steven G. Hillestad and Eric N. Berkowitz.
Health Care Marketing Plans: From Stategy to Action, Dow Jones-Irwin, Homewood, Illinois, 1984, p.118.

Prerequisites for Effective Marketing

Understandably, the transition to becoming a marketing-oriented organization has been difficult for many hospitals and medical groups.[4] Some get bogged down because they either do not understand--or have not yet met--four prerequisites for becoming marketing-oriented. These four prerequisites are illustrated in Figure 7, below.

■ *Pressure to be marketing-oriented.* This first condition refers to a view that must be shared and accepted throughout the organization

Figure 7. PREREQUISITES FOR EFFECTIVE MARKETING

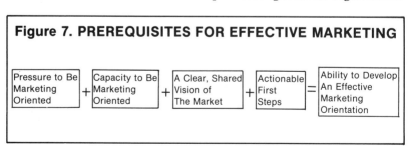

| Pressure to Be Marketing Oriented | + | Capacity to Be Marketing Oriented | + | A Clear, Shared Vision of The Market | + | Actionable First Steps | = | Ability to Develop An Effective Marketing Orientation |

New Leadership in Health Care Management

concerning the need for an improved marketing orientation. Not only must senior management feel pressure and want to become more marketing-oriented, but peer pressure must be strong throughout the organization to understand and respond to customer needs. In addition, information and reward systems must recognize the value of a customer orientation, and department or program marketing objectives and measurement systems must be tied to progress on this front.

- *Capacity to be marketing-oriented.* This second component refers to the capabilities and depth of hospital management staff. The hospital must have enough staff members who are not only experienced and adequately trained, but also devoted to improving the hospital's marketing effort. To begin with, management and staff must be receptive to ideas on how to become more marketing-oriented. In addition to having appropriate people and management depth, and recognizing that significant time must be devoted to improving marketing efforts, an understanding must be developed as to how these efforts fit with other hospital priorities.

- *A clear, shared vision of the market.* Many questions must be answered to develop an awareness and understanding of the marketplace. Who are the key customers and stakeholders? What are their needs? What changes must the hospital make to become marketing-oriented and meet the needs of these core constituencies? How is this organization going to differentiate and distinguish itself from others?

- *Actionable first steps.* Once the first three components are in place, the organization must develop an understanding of how daily marketing decisions and tasks must change. This effort requires a clear and complete set of written action plans and implementation programs. It also demands well-defined mechanisms to track progress and address minor difficulties in implementation before they become major ones.

Summary

Marketing has been presented not only as a functional dimension of management, but also as a philosophy to guide strategic planning. Advertising, in spite of common misperceptions, is only one dimension of a marketing strategy that begins with a needs assessment. The historical approach to developing health care services has been an inward process that results in looking for demand. In today's increasingly competitive marketplace, the goal is to identify a differential advantage for a service needed by a defined target group. The challenge for the health care organization is to use the marketing mix to meet the need.

References

1. Berkowitz, E. "Marketing: Its Meaning and Application in Rehabilitation Medicine" in *A Primer on Management for Rehabilitation Medicine*. Philadelphia: Hanley Belfus, Inc., 1987), pp. 247-256.

2. Berkowitz, E. "Marketing the Clinical Laboratory: An External Perspective." *Clinical Laboratory Management Review* 1(3):133-45, May/June 1987.

3. Berkowitz, E., and Flexner, W. "The Market for Health Services: Is There a Non-Traditional Consumer?" *Journal of Health Care Marketing* 1(1):25-34, Winter 1980-81, and Berkowitz, E. "Marketing the Hospital of the Future." *Proceedings*, 1981 Executive Symposium, University of Iowa, pp. 17-33.

4. Diamond, S., and Berkowitz, E. "Building a Marketing Orientation for Hospitals." Presentation at Academy for Health Care Marketing, American Marketing Association, March 1987.

Suggested Readings

Berkowitz, E., Kern, R., and Rudelius, W. *Marketing*. St. Louis, Mo.: Times-Mirror Mosby, 1986

Flexner, W., Berkowitz, E., and Brown, M. (Eds.). *Strategic Planning in Health Care Management*. Rockville, Md.: Aspen Systems, 1981

George, W., and Compton, F. "How to Initiate a Marketing Perspective in a Health Services Organization." *Journal of Health Care Marketing*. 5(1):29-37, Winter 1985.

Hillestad, S., and Berkowitz, E. *Health Care Marketing Plans from Strategy to Action*. Homewood, Ill.: Dow Jones -Irwin, 1984

Rathmell, J. *Marketing in the Service Sector*. Cambridge, Mass.: Winthrop Publishers, 1974.

Zallocco, R., Joseph, W., and Doremus, H. "Strategic Market Planning for Hospitals." *Journal of Health Care Marketing*. 4(2):19-28, Spring 1984.

Eric N. Berkowitz, PhD, is Chairman and Professor, School of Management, University of Massachusetts, Amherst.

CHAPTER 14

Maintaining Quality
in a Cost-Conscious Environment

by Alex R. Rodriguez, MD

"...I will prescribe regimen for the good of my patients according to my ability and my judgment and never do harm to anyone. To please no one will I prescribe a deadly drug, nor give advice which may cause his death...I will not cut to stone, even in a patient in whom the disease is manifest; I will leave this operation to be performed by practitioners in this art...."--Hippocratic Oath (5th Century B.C.)

At the very foundation of the principles and practice of medicine lies a professional commitment to quality. In becoming a physician, the emerging practitioner assumes a personal responsibility to abide with the ethical charge to heal whenever possible but never to do harm. Thus, the most basic component of the historical health care covenant between the physician and the patient has been based on a personal and professional contract, which in turn has been based on the abiding social, legal, and scientific parameters of the time and place. Physicians have been either supported or limited in their capacities to provide effective health services within these prevailing parameters, as much as the patient's physical, emotional, and intellectual status provide a conditional influence on quality.

Evolutions in modern Western medicine have altered these boundaries dramatically. More recent developments in technology, specialization, and financing of health services have further changed a once-dyadic interaction into one involving many parties having a stake in the health contract.

Out of this modern version of the primordial soup has emerged the physician executive, representing a unique evolutionary fusion in health care roles. This evolution has been neither random nor routine. It represents a natural balance in the emerging influence of nonprofessional factors upon the traditional autonomy of the physician-patient contract. The physician executive thus represents an evolutionary mechanism for professional control over quality, and continuation of a basic value foundation in medicine. In the present and future, health

Section II.   The Content of Management

care quality control will further emerge as the major focus and distinctive charge of the physician executive. This chapter will focus on quality control as an essential historical phenomenon that will influence the continuity of medicine as a profession and of improved public health.

Modern Medicine and the Quest for Quality Control

Despite a number of technical advances in Western medicine during the latter part of the nineteenth century and the relative excellence of care in a few urban settings, U.S. health care in the early twentieth century was largely a combination of folk remedies, quackstery, and the poor efforts of physicians limited in training and resources. The American Medical Association's Council on Education, concerned about the uneven quality of training in U.S. medical schools, spurred the Carnegie Foundation to conduct a study and make recommendations for improvements. The ensuing effort was summarized in the historical Flexner Report,[1] which served as a springboard for significant national changes in medical curricula and credentials. Subsequent efforts by Wetherill,[2] Codman,[3] and Bowman[4] led to development of hospital and surgical standards. These reflected serious efforts by the medical profession to assume professional responsibility for improving quality-effectiveness of health services through professional standards and monitoring activities.

Over time, quality impositions on health services have come from many specific initiatives and through many imperatives, including the following:

- The establishment of the Joint Commission on Accreditation of Hospitals (JCAH) in 1951 by the American Hospital Association, American College of Surgeons, and American College of Physicians.

- Promulgation of the Medicare and Medicaid programs in 1965 by the federal government, which required facilities seeking reimbursement under those programs to conduct various quality assurance activities, such as restrospective utilization and quality reviews.

- Subsequent establishment in 1972 of Professional Standards Review Organizations by the federal government to monitor hospital and physician services under Medicare and Medicaid, according to predetermined quality and utilization guidelines.

- Federal funding of hospital development through the Hill-Burton Act and of medical education through grant programs.

- Federal stimulation of biomedical research through intramural (e.g. National Institutes of Health) and extramural research.

- More stringent individual and cooperative state roles in medical licensing and monitoring.

- Medical-legal sanctions and legislative requirements establishing legal parameters for quality in health services.

- Growth in health benefits and insurance, which has stimulated the availability of increasingly more technically sophisticated, more comprehensive, and more resource-intensive health services.

- Growth of the consumer movement, which has spurred the accepted roles of patients in becoming better informed about, and involved in, clinical decisions.

These developments have resulted in both positive and problematic consequences related to quality control by the physician. Most prominently, there now is an unprecendented "greed for life and health"[5] by Americans, which reflects a profound demand-side sense of entitlement to ideal quality outcome. This has been fueled by the success of the health care system in achieving historic gains over disease and illness and in making services accessible and affordable, as well as by sociological phenomena that are associated with the assumption of "rights" in free societies. That physicians and hospitals fall short of these increasing expectations is the grist for unprecedented lawsuits, soap operas, and serious professional inquiry.[6-8] Compounding the difficulties that drive physicians to work within the externally imposed demand for optimal outcome ("quality") services are the combined internal demands of professional ethical dictates and a reinforcing economic dialectic stirred up by reimbursement systems. All of these make it very difficult for a physician to say "no" to a patient[9] or to adequately manage quality in an autonomous, controlled fashion. These accumulated initiatives and imperatives have also massed together to contribute to the upward spiraling of health costs, for which there is an established national consensus that a crisis of some proportion exists. It is this economic-financing crisis that frames the environment of contemporary quality management.

Paying For Quality

The financing of equitable and adequate quality health services looms as an ultimate challenge of the next 20 years for U.S. society and the medical profession. How this will be accomplished in an environment in which cost containment now predominates health benefit and services policy is not clear. However, it should be clear that physician practitioners and managers will need to be as critically and collaboratively involved in decisions about cost restraint as any party involved in the socioeconomic agenda-setting.

The driving forces in setting the quality of care agenda are global and national economic trends and priorities, the health care provider acting

Section II.   The Content of Management

as a professional and economic unit, the consumer of health services, and the payer.[10] Certainly, the emerging range and depth of roles of payers in dictating conditions for reimbursement have had a profound impact upon the practice and management of health care services.[11-14] They have also spurred other developments:

- A change in the basic concept of quality in health services from one of a pure quest for excellence in the structure, process, and outcome of care to that now represented in the Accreditation Manual for Hospitals--"the greatest achievable health benefit, with minimal unnecessary risk and use of resources, and in a manner satisfactory to the patient."[15]

- A highly evolved scientific literature on quality, utilization, and risk management, based in the health services research and clinical realms.[16-21]

- The need for clinical specialists, dually and expertly trained in both established medical specialties and in quality-utilization-risk management, to conduct clinical case management functions in clinical settings.[22]

Physician Management of Quality

Specific roles for physicians involved in quality, utilization, and risk management activities are now being elaborated in contemporary clinical services provided under the scrunity of complex cost-driven structures.[23]

- *Advocate:* pleading the cause for the patient or other complainant.

- *Technical specialist:* using special knowledge of the subject or business of the organization.

- *Trainer-educator:* teaching and instructing.

- *Collaborator in problem solving:* working jointly with others to find solutions.

- *Alternative identifiers:* finding, creating, or stating choices.

- *Fact finder:* searcning for and discovering the bits of information that establish the real events of the case.

- *Process specialist:* creating and supporting a series of actions leading to problem resolution.

- *Reflector:* giving back stated options and alternatives for continued consideration.

In addition to these clinical case management roles, quality management requires the support and direction of physician executives involved in administrative direction of clinical programs.

While the "eight basic role tasks" of the physician executive identified by the American Academy of Medical Directors in 1980 explicitly included "improving the quality of patient care," each of the other roles can also be viewed as clinical quality management[24]:

- Determining and improving medical practices used in patient care.

- Dealing with problems or differences between physicians.

- Evaluating physician care provided in the organization.

- Advising, counseling, and/or otherwise motivating physicians.

- Recruiting physicians to the organization.

- Dealing with outside medical organizations and societies.

- Improving own professional knowledge and skills.

The physician executive, as a quality manager, should be seen as a major factor in paying for quality. Moreover, the physician executive will require increasingly more technical and administrative knowledge-skills in order to adequately manage the "essential elements of quality,"[25] which is care that:

- Produces optimal improvement in the patient's physiologic status, physical function, and emotional and intellectual performance, consistent with the best interests of the patient.

- Emphasizes the promotion of health, the prevention of disease or disability, and the early detection and treatment of such conditions.

- Seeks to achieve the informed cooperation and participation of the patient in the care process and in decisions concerning that process.

- Is based on accepted principles of medical science and the proficient use of appropriate technological and professional resources.

- Is provided with sensitivity to the stress and anxiety that illness can generate and with concern for the patient's overall welfare.

- Makes efficient use of the available technology and other health system resources needed to achieve the desired treatment goal.

- Is sufficiently documented in the patient's medical record, to enable

Section II.   The Content of Management

continuity of care and peer evaluation.

The physician executive will need to be familiar with the complex of theories and techniques that will allow effective strategic planning and operational effectiveness in the "shifting paradigm" that characterizes the current market environment of health care and that poses a challenge to quality management.[26] To do so, the physician executive must be clinically competent and have more in-depth familiarity with such technical areas as:

- Health care systems and institutions.

- Performance review methods and systems.

- Information systems.

- Organizational theory: systems, management, change.

- Health economics.

- Health law.

- Institutional environmental health and safety.

- Learning systems and instructional methods.

A number of course and degree offerings in these subject areas are being developed by such professional organizations as the American Academy of Medical Directors and the American College of Utilization Review Physicians. The market demand for physicians to assume clinical case and systems management roles can only increase as the demand by payers to restrain costs and maintain quality continues. This demand will pose challenges for individual physicians and professional organizations to respond by becoming actively involved now in developing management skills in the many physicians who will be required to define and manage cost-effective care. It should be obvious that anything less than a current and highly proactive level of training of physician executives will result in further incursions by nonmedical personnel into the management of both physicians and of quality of care decisions.

Technical, Professional Issues in Quality Management

Quality management is rapidly becoming highly technical. Standards and criteria are being evolved daily through both professional consensus development and data analysis.[27,28] Structured technology and therapeutic assessment activities are directed by third-party payers (e.g., Health Care Financing Administration, Blue Cross and Blue Shield plans), professional associations (e.g., American Medical Association, American College of Physicians), foundations, government entities (e.g.,

Office of Technology Assessment), and other organizations (e.g., private corporations, trade associations), utilizing various expert in-house and contracted resources. Such activities have an already significant effect upon costs and quality of health care[29,30] and clearly will assume an even greater role in the future. The emergence of clinical decision analysis as a basic clinical skill will also follow the increasing need of health systems managers to turn to physician executives for direction on more scientifically derived medical necessity determinations.[31,32] The future efficiency and effectiveness of these clinical technical developments is already being shown to be critically dependent upon the sophisticated data systems being established at every level of the modern health care system. These systems will continue to provide one of the major vehicles for monitoring, reshaping, and reimbursing physicians' clinical decisions.[33]

Professional issues abound for physician practitioners and managers in the current and future era of cost restraint. Physician executives must often wear the dual cloaks of allowance and restraint in managing resources related to quality structure, process, and outcome. Committing resources for professional education and monitoring is often a difficult responsibilty when peers view such activities as unnecessary or unwarranted intrusions into their autonomy and when financial managers see such activities as marginally justified or too expensive to support in a competitive market. Such physician executives must deal with their own ambivalences about being the organization's "hired gun" and seemingly abrogating professional charges to be primarily a "patient advocate."[34,45] Ethical issues also arise with the specter of rationing and gatekeeping functions, especially when financial and entrepreneurial incentives charge the quality and utilization decision made by the practitioner and physician executive.[36,37] The American Medical Association has attempted to establish professional standards in regard to quality and professional compensation through its *Current Opinions of the Council on Ethical and Judicial Affairs*[38]:

Costs

While physicians should be conscious of costs and not provide or prescribe unnecessary services or ancillary facilities, social policy expects that concern for the care the patient receives will be the physician's first consideration. This does not preclude the physician, individually or through medical organizations, from participating in policy-making with respect to social issues affecting health care. (Section 2.09)

Unnecessary Services

Physicians should not provide, prescribe, or seek compensation for services that are known to be unnecessary or worthless. (Section 2.17)

Economic Incentives and Levels of Care

Section II. The Content of Management

The primary obligation of the hospital medical staff is to safeguard the quality of care provided within the institution. The medical staff has the responsibility to perform essential functions on behalf of the hospital in accordance with licensing laws and accreditation requirements. Treatment or hospitalization that is willfully excessive or inadequate constitutes unethical practice. The organized medical staff has an obligation to avoid wasteful practices and unnecessary treatment that may cause the hospital needless expense. In a situation where the economic interests of the hospital are in conflict with patient welfare, patient welfare takes priority. (Section 4.04)

The American Medical Association has also established guidelines for quality assurance activities that should serve as professional markers for physicians involved in quality, risk, and utilization management activities[39]:

1. *The general policies and processes to be utilized in any quality assurance system should be developed and concurred with by the professionals whose performance will be scrutinized, and should be objectively and impartially administered. Such initial involvement and commitment with ongoing objectivity is critical to assuring continued participation and cooperation with the system.*

2. *Any remedial quality assurance activity related to an individual practitioner should be triggered by concern for that individual's overall practice patterns, rather than by deviation from specified criteria in single cases. Because of the inherent variability of patients and biological systems, judgment as to the competence of specific practitioners should be based on an assessment of their performance with a number of patients and not on the examination of single, isolated cases, except in extraordinary circumstances.*

3. *The institution of any remedial activity should be preceded by discussion with the practitioner involved. There should be ample opportunity for the practitioner to explain observed deviations from accepted practice patterns to professional peers, before any remedial or corrective action is decided upon.*

4. *Emphasis should be placed on education and modification of unacceptable practice patterns rather than on sanctions. The initial thrust of any quality assurance activity should be toward helping the practitioner to correct deficiencies in knowledge, skills, or technique, with practice restrictions or disciplinary action considered only for those not responsive to remedial activities.*

5. *The quality assurance system should make available the appropriate educational resources needed to effect desired prac-*

New Leadership in Health Care Management

tice modifications. Consistent with the emphasis on assistance rather than punitive activity, any quality assurance program should have the capability of offering or directing the practitioner to the educational activities needed to correct any deficiencies, whether they be peer consultation, continuing education, or self-learning and self-assessment programs.

6. **Feedback mechanisms should be established to monitor and document needed changes in practice patterns.** Whether conducted under the same auspices or separately, linkages between quality assurance activity and a quality assessment system should allow assessment of the effectiveness of any remedial activities instituted by or for a practitioner.

7. **Restrictions or disciplinary actions should be imposed on those practitioners not responsive to remedial actitivies, whenever the appropriate professional peers deem such action necessary to protect the public.** Depending on the severity of the deficiency, such restrictions may include loss of medical and medical specialty society membership, loss or revocation of specialty board certification, restriction or rescission of hospital staff privileges, third-party payment denials, or suspension or revocaton of licensure.

8. **The imposition of restrictions or discipline should be timely, consistent with due process.** Before a restriction or disciplinary action is imposed, the practitioner affected should have full understanding of the basis for the action, ample opportunity to request reconsideration and to submit any documentation relevant to that request, and the right to meet with those considering its imposition. However, in cases where those considering the imposition deem the practitioner to pose an imminent hazard to the health of patients, such restrictions or disciplinary actions may be imposed immediately. In such instances, the due process rights noted above should be provided on an expedited basis.

9. **Quality assurance systems should be structured and operated so as to assure immunity for practitioners conducting or applying such systems who are acting in good faith.**

10. **To the degree possible, quality assurance systems should be structured to recognize care of high quality as well as to correct instances of deficient practice.** The vast majority of practicing physicians provide care of high quality. Quality assurance systems should explore methods to identify and recognize those treatment methodologies or protocols that consistently contribute to improved patient outcomes. Information on such results should be communicated to the professional community.

Section II.   The Content of Management

The urgency of payers' demands for changes in the costs and related structures of health care systems is placing tremendous pressure on organized medicine to respond to physicians' needs for support and direction in both absorbing externally imposed changes and providing proactive input into alterations and continuity in health care services. Professional association will increasingly broaden their scope of activities to include more data collection and analysis, standards-criteria development, and basic research and technology assessment on the efficacy of medical evaluations-treatments, as well as traditional educational, public education, and lobbying activities. Moreover, the heightening scrutiny of medicine[40] could either lead such associations into defined union activities or will likely cause physicians to form unions. This could create much more tension in the physician-patient relationship, as it already has between physicians and payers and hospitals.[41] The sum of these tensions will become one of the major potential burdens or avenues of contribution involving physician executives.

The Future of Quality

There have been few surprises during the 1980s in developments related to financing, organization, and management of health services[42] and their import for the future. The consequences of "glut,"[43] oversupply of physicians,[44] and high costs of medical education[45] against a backdrop of an epochal economic roller coaster since 1973 have profound implications for future medical practice and the health status of the nation. Future medical practice will follow current trends[46,47] and alternative future scenarios related to world and national geographical and socioeconomic events.[48] At the heart of all of these changes will reverberate the quest for quality. In a democratic system, public interest will express itself in legal and legislative ways as necessary public policy regarding the right to, and affordability of, high-quality health services. In a recent commentary on the immediate future,[49] Otis Bowen, MD, Secretary of Health and Human Services, has affirmed the following points:

- "The physician's healing touch must be tempered by the limits of society's resources."

- Rising health care costs are a primary priority of public policy.

- Health is fundamental to the pursuit of happiness and basic to the strength and vitality of a nation.

Dr. Bowen underscores that the nation's "supreme challenge" is to contain costs without limiting equitable access to high-quality care. To achieve this end, greater emphasis must be placed on developing better quality assessment and management tools, legal protections, professional incentives for quality outcome "productivity," and broader, more effective preventive efforts. Research commitments must be maintained to ensure greater efficacy and cost-effectiveness in health services. Information systems must be developed that will provide meaningful data for practitioners to make effective treatment decisions and for cost management decisions to be made. To accomplish these ends, the health professions should assist public and private payers and consumers of care in developing consensus and systems for cost-effective, quality care. Dr. Bowen believes this can be accomplished to effect a balanced system that is rendered "competitive" through improved public information, yet accommodating to "personal preferences" of patients. This is an inspiring "challenge and opportunity" that will surely require a continuing, if not substantially increased, federal effort, more than some politicians have been committed to in recent years. Unfortunately, the politician's perceptions of "willingness of the taxpayer to be taxed" will continue to weigh heavily in budget allocations that too often fail to assure quality for an unacceptably large number of Americans. The future of quality in health services will, then, hinge largely upon the public's continued demand for high-quality care, its willingness to assert that demand through public policy and payments commensurate with other publicly and privately financed priorities (e.g., transportation, luxury items, national defense).

Several contemporary writers have voiced opinions about how quality could be provided practically in an era of cost restraint and how it must be preserved as a matter of national health and social policy. Albert N. May, MD, proposes five criteria that can be used to build a consensus for defining, delivering, documenting, and promoting quality in a competitive marketplace[50]:

- *Availability:* full range of integrated health services, including preventive, tertiary, and long-term.

- *Accessibility:* immediacy and proximity of services.

- *Affability:* compassionate, service-oriented attitude and capability.

- *Affordability:* for patients and third-party payer.

- *Accountability:* effectiveness of quality and utilization management.

Paul M. Elwood, Jr., MD, a leading architect of alternative delivery systems and competitive health strategies in the United States, has noted "several disquieting signs" emerging from the rapid development of large vertically and horizontally integrated health systems[51]:

- Difficulty in getting the concept of managed care to certain communities because of lack of product differentiation, consumer distrust, and consumer willingness to bear higher out-of-pocket costs to maintain freedom of choice.

Section II. The Content of Management

- Difficulty in setting up managed care operations in certain areas because of lack of physician support, in turn tied to their disquietude over administrative burdens, diminished revenues, loss of autonomy, and ethical conflicts.

- Belief by some health plans and third-party administrators that cost controls and quality assurance can be effectively provided through utilization review, not requiring the actual structure of managed care.

- Lack of emphasis on quality control (structures, delivery, assessment, documentation, reimbursement) and marketing in managed care systems.

Dr. Ellwood believes the "third generation" of managed care programs will be successful if they can address the following problem areas:

- Manage and market quality.
- Cope with the physician revolt.
- Differentiate services.
- Influence physician and hospital selection.
- Cover the uninsured.

A major obstacle to the quest for quality is that so much of health care occurs in the tertiary sector. Too much suffering is unnecessary[52] and requires complex, intensive services at the points of more highly evolved pathological states. Clearly, too much of human disease and illness is related to life-style and other preventable circumstances.[53] Future quality and cost management will require more emphasis on health promotion and disease prevention efforts[54] such as:

- Economic incentives and disincentives that steer health plan beneficiaries toward healthier behaviors.

- Health education and other health promotion (e.g., risk assessment, early detection, behavior interventions, and illness monitoring) programs--worksite, schools, media, etc.

- Increased provider skills and interventions, coupled with allowable reimbursements, for disease prevention and health promotion efforts.

If anything might be both right and wise in health care at the present time, a major national push toward preventive programs in the future would certainly seem indicated, based on the substantial experience to date of preventive efforts.[12-14,52,53] An intelligent approach that addresses psychological and stress-related variables in both actual illness and misdirected health services utilization could significantly reduce (as much as 50 percent) the costs attributed to physical disease and illness.[52,55] Any view of quality in health care services must thus consider the unnecessary losses in health status and productivity that could be

New Leadership in Health Care Management

prevented. This will become one of the major areas of opportunity and activity for physician executives involved in quality management in the future.

A Footnote on Quality

Quality is at once a subjective and objective state. It is a major component in demand-side and supply-side health economics and in health delivery systems. As quality structure, process, and outcome measurements are achieved, so they soon also elude even the skilled physician practitioner and physician executive. They are both real (measurable, controllable) and apparitional in any given patient or patient population, due to the limitations in the control anyone really ever has over disease and health. Nevertheless, quality is the major policy issue facing consumers, payers, providers, and regulators of health care in the future. Its provision will serve as a measure of American economic and management prowess, as well as an index of social priority. In the ongoing assessment of policy commitments to quality in health care, we may discover the ultimate bottom line. And in the ongoing responsibility to manage quality, the physician executive will daily face the ultimate professional challenge.

References

1.   Flexner, A. *Medical Education in the United States and Canada: A Report to the CarnegieFoundation for the Advancement of Teaching*. New York: Arno Press, 1972.

2.   Wetherill, H. "A Plea for Higher Hospital Efficiency and Standardization." *Surgery, Gynecology, Obstetrics* 20(6):705-707, June 1915.

3.   Codman, E. *A Study in Hospital Efficiency as Demonstrated by the Case Report of the First Five Years of a Private Hospital*. Boston: Thomas Todd Publishers, 1916.

4.   Bowman, J. "Hospital Standardization Series--General Hospitals of 100 or More Beds: Report of 1919." *Bulletin of the American College of Surgeons* 4(1):3-26, January 1920.

5.   Abram, M. Address to Blue Cross and Blue Shield Association--Medical Director's Conference, Chicago, Sept. 6, 1984.

6.   Mechanic, D. "Public Perceptions of Medicine." *New England Journal of Medicine* 312(3):181-183, Jan. 17, 1985.

7.   Cousins, N. "How Patients Appraise Physicians." *New England Journal of Medicine* 313(22):1422-1424, Nov. 28, 1985.

8.   Brody, D. "The Patient's Role in Clinical Decision-Making." *Annals of Internal Medicine* 93(5):718-722, Nov. 1980.

Section II.   The Content of Management

9. Daniels, W. "Why Saying No To Patients In the United States Is So Hard: Cost Containment, Justice, and Provider Autonomy." *New England Journal of Medicine* 314(21):1380-1383, May 22, 1986.

10. Rodriguez, A. "Quality Assurance: An Introduction." *Handbook of Quality Assurance in Mental Health.* New York: Plenum Press, 1988.

11. Mechanic, D. "Cost Containment and the Quality of Medical Care: Rationing Strategies in an Era of Constrained Resources." *Milbank Memorial Fund Quarterly–Health and Society* 63(3):453-475, Summer 1985.

12. Fox, P. *Synthesis of Private Sector Health Care Initiatives.* Office of Assistant Secretary for Planning and Evaluation (U.S. Department of Health and Human Services); Washington, D.C., March 1984.

13. Fielding, J. *Corporate Health Management.* Menlo Park, Calif.:Addison-Wesley Publishing, 1984.

14. Fox, P., and others. *Health Care Cost Management.* Ann Arbor, Mich.: Health Administration Press, 1984.

15. *Accreditation Manual for Hospitals.* Chicago: Joint Commission on Accreditation of Hospitals, 1987

16. Donabedian, A. "An Introduction to Quality Assessment and Assurance," Course on Quality in Health Care, National Institute on Health Care Leadership and Management of the American Academy of Medical Directors, Tucson, Ariz.; Nov. 17, 1987.

17. Donabedian, A. "Twenty Years of Research on the Quality of Medical Care." *Evaluation and the Health Professions* 8(3):243-265, Sept. 1985.

18. Donabedian, A., and others. "Quality, Cost and Health: An Integrative Model." *Medical Care* 20(10):975-992, October 1982.

19. Donabedian, A. "The Epidemiology of Quality." *Inquiry* 22(3):282-292, Fall 1985.

20. Bausell, R. "Quality Assurance: An Overview." *Evaluation and the Health Professions* 6(2):139-41, June 1983.

21. Williamson, J., and others. *Principles of Quality Assurance and Cost Containment in Health Care: A Guide for Medical Students, Residents, and Other Health Professionals.* San Francisco: Jossey-Bass, 1982.

22. Rodriguez, A. "The Emerging Specialty of Clinical Outcome Management." *Quality Assurance and Utilization Review: Current Readings in Concept and Practice.* Sarasota, Fla.: American Board of Quality Assurance and Utilization Review Physicians, 1987.

23. Ziegenfuss, J. "Toward a Definition of Roles for Physicians in Quality Assurance." *Quality Assurance and Utilization Review* 2(2):36-41, May 1987.

24. Slater, C; "The Physician Manager's Role: Results of a Survey." *The*

Physician in Management. Tampa, Fla.: American Academy of Medical Directors, 1982.

25. Burns, J. "The Quality of Medical Care: The Employer's Perspective." Course on Quality in Health Care, National Institute on Health Care Leadership and Management of the American Academy of Medical Directors, Tucson, Ariz. Nov. 18, 1987.

26. Kaufman, R. "Dealing with a Shifting Paradigm." *Physician Executive* 13(3):10-14, May-June 1987.

27. Donabedian, A. "Criteria and Standards for Quality Assessment and Monitoring." *QRB* 12(3):99-108, March 1986.

28. *Measuring Quality of Care: A Resource Guide.* Chicago: Department of Health Care Review, American Medical Association, Oct. 1987.

29. Shaffarzick, R. "Health Care Technology and Quality of Care." *Quality Assurance and Utilization Review* 2(3):84-89, Aug. 1987.

30. Steinberg, E. "Techniques for Influencing Clinical Decision-Making. Course on Quality in Health Care, National Institute on Health Care Leadership and Management of the American Acadmey of Medical Directors, Tucson, Ariz., Nov. 20, 1987.

31. Pauker, S., and Kassirer, J. "Decision Analysis" *New England Journal of Medicine* 316(5):250-258, January 29, 1987.

32. Sox, H. "Decision Analysis: A Basic Clinical Skill." *New England Journal of Medicine* 316(5):271-272, January 29, 1987.

33. Meyer, H. "Are You a Good Physician: New Data Systems Inspect M.D. Performance." *American Medical News* 30(23):1, 35-7, June 19, 1987.

34. Warshaw, L. "The Role of the Physician as the Patient's Advocate." *New York Business Group on Health Newletter* 7(5):1,8, May 1987.

35. May, W. "On Ethics and Advocacy." *JAMA* 256(13):1786-87, Oct. 3, 1986.

36. Relman, A. "Antitrust Law and the Physician Entrepreneur." *New England Journal of Medicine* 313(14):884-5, Oct. 3, 1985.

37. Relman, A. "Dealing with Conflicts of Interest." *New England Journal of Medicine* 313(12):749-51, Sept. 19, 1985.

38. *Current Opinions of the Council on Ethical and Judicial Affairs.* Chicago: American Medical Association, 1987.

39. *Guidelines for Quality Assurance.* Chicago: American Medical Association, 1987.

40. Scheier, R. "Can Medicine Bear the Scrutiny?" *American Medical News* 31(1):1,22, Jan. 1, 1988.

Section II.   The Content of Management

41. Burda, D. "Governing Board Creating Physician-Hospital Rift." *Modern Healthcare* 18(4):42, Jan. 22, 1988.

42. Kralewski, J. "The Physican Manager and the Evolving Health System." *The Physician in Management.* Tampa, Fla.: American Academy of Medical Directors, 1982.

43. McClure, W. "Buying Right: The Consequences of Glut." *Physician Executive* 13(5):7-10, Sept.-Oct. 1987.

44. Tarlov, A. "Shattuck Lecture–The Increasing Supply of Physicians, the Changing Structure of the Health Services System, and the Future Practice of Medicine." *New England Journal of Medicine* 308(20):1235-44, May 19, 1983.

45. Council on Long-Range Planning and Development. "Health Care in Transition: Consequences for Young Physicians." JAMA 256(24):3384-90, Dec. 26, 1986.

46. Relman, A. "The Changing Climate of Medical Practice." *New England Journal of Medicine* 316(6):333-34, Feb. 5, 1987.

47. Geyman, J. "Future Medical Practice in the United States: A Choice of Scenarios." *JAMA* 245(11):1140-43, March 20, 1981.

48. Goldschmidt, P. *Health 2000.* Baltimore, Md.: Policy Research Institute, 1982.

49. Bowen, O. "Shattuck Lecture–What Is Quality Care?" *New England Journal of Medicine* 316(25):1578-80, June 18, 1987.

50. May, A. "Cost Pressures Will Force Sharper Definitions of Quality." *Physician Executive* 12(5):6-8, Sept.-Oct. 1986.

51. Hinz, C. "New Forecast: Emphasis to Shift Back to Quality." *American Medical News* 30(6):3,48, Feb. 13, 1987.

52. *Closing the Gap: The Burden of Unnecessary Illness.* New York: Oxford University Press, 1987.

53. *Promoting Health/Preventing Disease: Objectives for the Nation.* Washington, D.C.: Public Health Service, U.S. Department of Health and Human Services, 1980.

54. Marcarelli, J. "The Foundation for Future Health Care." *Physician Executive* 13(3):19-20, May-June 1987.

55. Institute of Medicine-National Academy of Sciences. *Behavior, Health Risks, and Social Disadvantage.* Washington, D.C.: National Academy Press, 1982.

Alex R. Rodriguez, MD, is Senior Vice President, Professional Affairs, Preferred Health Care, Ltd., Wilton, Connecticut.

CHAPTER 15

Commitment and Discipline

by Sandra L. Gill, Eric W. Springer, Esq., and Andre L. Delbecq, DBA

I t is becoming clear that health care managers are at risk for all professional activity that takes place under their jurisdiction. The disruptive professional or egregious coalition creates obstacles and stress that few health care organizations can afford in this era of rapid change and competitive forces.[1] Health care leaders need to make timely decisions consistent with legal decisions and sound management principles[2] in their development of commitment and discipline. The focus of this article is on the process of organizational commitment to norms and the application of disciplinary policies and procedures, consistent with recent legal decisions and social psychological research.

Legal and Managerial Perspectives

Professional conduct is no longer considered apart from the impact of one's behavior on others. As Skillicorn has stated, "Behavioral incompetence can be as detrimental to patient care as professional incompetence."[3] Legal decisions have clearly established "that the hospital's legal responsibility for the quality of patient care embraces the quality of medical care as well, and that the hospital, therefore, has not only the right but the duty to establish and enforce standards of competence in physicians who practice in the hospital. The quality of care cannot be divorced and therefore the hospital must require that physicians, no less thn hospital employees and visitors, meet reasonable standards of personal behavior in the hospital."[4]

Managerial and social psychological studies have also established the link between individual behavior and organizational circumstances and events.[5] Organizations are known to be powerful influences upon the behavior of new members,[6,7] just as individual behavior of one member may affect others in the same setting.[8] There are managerial interventions, however, that could, if used wisely, preclude the necessity of formal legal actions regarding the behavioral competence of health care practitioners. Regardless, management should develop and review with legal counsel the organization's bylaws, policies, and procedures re-

Section II.   *The Content of Management*

garding the expected behavior of health care practitioners.

The Psychology of Rewards and Punishment

One of the consistent findings in social psychology over the past 20 years is that punishment is rarely effective in the long run.[9] Individuals who perceive their leaders to be rewarding and capable of recognizing constructive behavior and commitment show a willingness to be influenced by the leader, express higher rates of attraction and commitment to the organization, engage in more self-motivated problem-solving and constructive behavior, become more self-disciplined, and have less need for formal control because informal norms maintain high performance.[10] At best, punishment tends to cause a temporary "lull" in the unacceptable behavior and may simply result in more covert acts, or in more egregious behavior that challenges the authority of the leader.

Managerial and social psychological research have long examined the process of organizational commitment. More recently, legal decisions have also addressed the issue of behavioral competence among health care practitioners. Most cases have dealt with the "disruptive" person, the individual whose behavior interferes with what may otherwise be acceptable--if not superior--clinical competence. Legal precedents support the managerial need for a clear code of professional conduct, e.g., by-laws that include the specification of consequences for noncompliant behavior.

Developing Commitment

The contemporary health care leader needs to establish and employ three key factors that build commitment to organizational goals and norms: volition, visibility, and irrevocability.[11]

First, once credentials and character have been determined to meet organizational standards, the professional must perceive a sense of free choice to join the organization and behave in a compatible way.[12,13]

Second, visible leadership and mentoring should provide ongoing reinforcement of constructive organizational behavior.[14,15] Symbolic rewarding of individuals who meet organizational standards of excellence is a visible and dynamic way to increase others' sense of commitment to the organization.[16]

A second leadership act to promote the development of "fit" between individual values and organizational philosophy is visible, symbolic communication.[9] As symbolic communicators, health care leaders need to continually provide articulation of the philosophy, vision, and long- and short-term goals of the organization. They also need to provide examples of desirable conduct and standards of excellence. Explicit statements and symbolic actions provide a benchmark for emerging leaders and other members to reinforce desired behavior patterns.

The leadership acts of engaging in problemsolving, establishing priorities, readjusting to new circumstances around key projects, and linking priorities to organizational goals and norms remain effective strategies for developing commitment to organizational philosophy, inasmuch as they are used for discussion and clarification.[17]

Third, a system of conformance must be established to provide restraint against disruptive, noncompliant acts. The irrevocable consequences of failing to observe the established behavioral norms should be delineated in a clear code of conduct.[10] A growing body of legal decisions support the view that a record of disruptive conduct is not different from a record of substandard clinical performance.[4] Health care organizations, especially the medical staff component, must become much more serious and consistent in the timely application of appropriate disciplinary sanctions to behaviorally disruptive professionals. Professionals who voluntarily choose to practice in health care organizations must be held to the same standards of professional conduct as those who are employed. They should be recognized and rewarded for their constructive competence as well.

Diagnostics for Disciplinary Interventions

What can health care leaders do if faced with instances of noncompliant behavior, evidencing lack of commitment to the organization's protocols and practices? Even the leader who rewards constructive performance will need to diagnose an appropriate response to undesirable behavior. In the workplace, individual behavior is a function of perceived role(s) and individual style or preference (figure 1, below). Managerial intervention must consider not only the behavior but the rights of the individual who may exhibit stylistic or idiosyncratic behav-

Figure 1. DISCIPLINE CATEGORIES

Task Outcomes

		Instrumental	Stylistic
O b s e r v a b i l i t y	Public	1 Sanction Discipline Steps	2 Give Information
	Private	3 Cite Norms Obtain Data	4 Avoid

Section II.   The Content of Management

iors that do not affect professional competence.[18]

Two questions may be used to help select an appropriate leadership intervention in the face of apparently disruptive behavior:

- Is the behavior role-related, or is it a matter of personal style that does not detract from the individual's professional competence?

- Is the behavior observable, i.e., can it be corroborated?

In the following section, four specific protocols for intervening in hypothetical, conceptually distinct, behavioral events are provided. These guidelines are consistent with both social psychology and legal findings.

Case #1: "Public" Role-Related Behavioral Infractions

When infractions of clearly role-related expectations are corroborated, the imposition of negative sanctions is a managerial imperative. Social psychological studies have demonstrated that a "laissez-faire" style of leadership, in which normative and overt deviance is tolerated, contributes to an unproductive, neurotic organizational climate.[19] When there is clear evidence that misconduct has occurred, sanctions should be imposed as soon as possible after the event to optimize the corrective impact. Such interventions should be decisive, specific, and clear in terms of both consequences for the present misconduct and future consequences for any additional misconduct (figure 2, below).

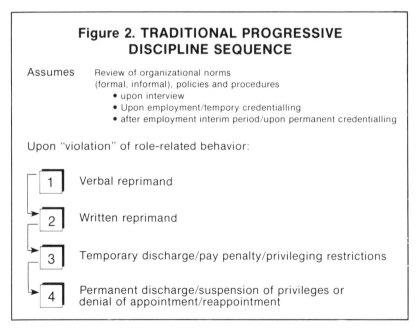

Figure 2. TRADITIONAL PROGRESSIVE DISCIPLINE SEQUENCE

Assumes   Review of organizational norms
(formal, informal), policies and procedures
- upon interview
- Upon employment/tempory credentialling
- after employment interim period/upon permanent credentialling

Upon "violation" of role-related behavior:

1   Verbal reprimand

2   Written reprimand

3   Temporary discharge/pay penalty/privileging restrictions

4   Permanent discharge/suspension of privileges or denial of appointment/reappointment

This is not an easy decision to make, because the hospital is at risk whatever action it takes.[2] If it does nothing in the face of disruptive behavior, it contributes to a "laissez faire" atmosphere. On the other hand, if managerial action is taken, legal counteraction may be threatened or pursued. However, the courts have dealt with and upheld intervention regarding a variety of disruptive behaviors in hospitals that most likely would apply in any health care setting. Among the specific behaviors covered in legal cases are impertinent and inappropriate comments written (or "cute" illustrations drawn) in patient medical records or other official documents; impugning the quality of care in the hospital or attacking particular practitioners, nurses, or policies[20]; sexual harassment of nurses, other hospital employees, or patients[21]; refusal to accept medical staff assignments or to participate in committee or departmental affairs on anything but one's own terms, or to do so in a disruptive manner[22]; rude or abusive conduct to nurses or other hospital employees[23]; and threats and/or physical assaults on physicians, employees, or others on hospital property.[24]

The courts have upheld hospital decisions to act in cases of disruptive practitioners. A series of cases has established the right of the hospital to deny initial appointment to the medical staff on evidence of or reasonable doubts about an applicant's prior conduct.[25] However, bylaws language should be clear on the issue of behavioral competence to defend against the inevitable suits that will emerge from denied applicants.

Courts also have upheld denial of reappointment of disruptive health care practitioners: "Every court which has reviewed a hospital's denial of reappointment due to the physician's disruptive behavior has found such misconduct to be a sufficient basis for the decision not to reappoint."[2]

When disruptive behavior occurs during the term of appointment, both wisdom and decisive action are required. A single episode of disruptive behavior, which might not appear to warrant revocation of privileges, may actually be one in a series of episodes that render the practitioner's continued presence in the hospital intolerable. In fact, practitioners may well claim that the absence of previous intervention precludes consideration of their history in current decisions. However, "no court has yet held that, by failing to take action at some particular point in a continuing course of disruptive conduct, the hospital has, in effect, waived earlier incidents and is therefore foreclosed from considering them in revoking an appointment."[26]

What about the single episode of disruptive behavior? Can summary suspension be invoked? The courts have supported suspension in single episodes of clinical misbehavior, but decisions are split regarding disruptive behavior. Presumably, the imposition of summary suspension would have to show that the practitioner's continued presence

Section II.   The Content of Management

imposed a severe threat to patient safety or directly impaired the orderly operation and management of the organization.[27]

In summary, individual disruptive behavior that impairs the competence of the health care practitioner, or that burdens the effectiveness of others, requires decisive disciplinary intervention. The protocols for handling these situations should be clearly stated by the organization in all appropriate documents. While policy publication and decisive action may not, by themselves, curb the disruptive behavior of the individual, they do protect the hospital and serve to reinforce its obligation to provide high-quality medical care free from either clinical or behavioral incompetence.

Case #2: "Private" Role-Related Behavioral Infractions

A hospital is at risk for all professional activity that takes place under its jurisdiction. While this risk may support hospital management's efforts to rid itself of disruptive practitioners, the nature of legal proceedings requires a full, often tedious and redundant, development of evidence to support an allegation of disruptiveness. Thus, the managerial imperative to intervene may be outweighed by the potential of a court battle for injunctive relief and money damages for wrongful charges. One result is a kind of institutional paralysis in all but the most obvious cases. Maintaining fundamental due process and a full and fair opportunity for allegedly disruptive practitioners to avoid onerous discrimination is as important in the management of discipline and sanctions as the appropriate imposition of disciplinary action.[2]

Perhaps nowhere does the dilemma become as challenging as in the situation in which a role-related allegation of misconduct is made but is not immediately corroborated. The leader is advised to restate institutional bylaws, policies, etc. that have allegedly been violated, along with the penalties for such behavior. In this fashion, information is dispersed and the opportunity for volitional self-correction is provided. Of equal importance, such immediate action reinforces the grounds for the work group to intervene with corrective action, in the event such an infraction is inadvertent.[28]

If the severity of the allegation is great, e.g., a threat to patient safety or to other hospital practitioners and employees, an immediate investigation may be appropriate. If a reasonable doubt exists regarding an individual's competence, further actions may be taken, e.g., suspension. It is particularly important that no individual be subjected to unreasonable treatment or castigations, lest it create a "witch-hunt" atmosphere and consequent threat of wrongful charge litigation.

Case #3: Individual Style vs. Conformance: Respecting Rights

Respecting the practitioner's due process rights is perhaps most clearly illustrated in cases where the behavior at question is a matter of individual style that does not interfere with clinical or behavioral competence. Management must respect the rights of practitioners who are "different" to the same extent that they invoke action in the case of disruptive individuals. Expressing unorthodox opinions, displaying unusual tastes, or manifesting alternative life-styles are often a seductive arena of inappropriate--and risky--management intervention. While the formal leadership of the organization may represent a majority whose preferences run counter to those of the offending individual, the organization has a positive obligation to treat such practitioners with the same degree of tolerance and acceptance it affords the "regulars." As long as personal idiosyncrasies do not affect the ability of others to do their jobs or do not impinge on others' rights to complete their business free of burdensome harassment, and the practitioner continues to perform well professionally, negative sanctions should not be involved.[2]

What course of action is appropriate? Such a circumstance requires a combination of mentoring and constructive feedback to solicit the voluntary cooperation of the individual.[29] First, in meeting with an individual whose preferences are "different," a clear statement of the issue is required. This includes what is not at issue, i.e., the individual's clinical or professional competence. In fact, a statement of his value to the organization is recommended to provide a testament to the true context of the meeting.

Second, a specific behavioral description of the event should be given, e.g., seemingly impatient or curt telephone manner, a pattern of interrupting co-workers or subordinates in meetings, or a manner of making comments that seems cynical or particularly harsh. Along with this specific description of behaviors should follow a description of the impact of such conduct, e.g., apparent anger, embarrassment, hurt, etc. on the immediate and indirect participants in the situation. The unintended consequences of the conduct should be discussed, e.g., alienation of and lack of cooperation from others in the organization.

Finally, an opportunity for problem-solving and follow-up support or coaching should be offered.

The purpose of feedback is not to change behavior through coercive action. Rather, it is to provide accurate, unambiguous information about the consequences such behavior has on the organization and an opportunity for the individual to engage in more compatible behaviors. Of utmost importance is the element of volition in this event, because the individual may decide that the price of conformity is too great.

Case #4 "Private" Behaviors: Avoid Interventions

Organizational leaders may well be tempted to intervene when co-workers and subordinates appear to be experiencing personal prob-

Section II.   The Content of Management

lems or when rumors imply that "someone ought to be concerned." Common examples include marital difficulties, family distress, and age-related life transitions. At the risk of seeming less than nurturant, it is our advice that organizational leaders can ill afford the role confusion or ambiguity[30] that may accompany such noble concerns. As leadership interventions, such acts often contribute to the recipient's confusion about the intent, credibility, or capacity to provide appropriate help. Further, it may confuse the role relationship should subsequent events require disciplinary action. While one's intent may be to be helpful and friendly, the cost to subsequent credibility and capacity to maintain appropriate role authority is often quite high.[10] Professional staff, special programs, and counseling services may be more appropriate and usually are better equipped to manage such potentially complex situations.

Summary

Court decisions have established that hospitals, and presumably other health care organizations, are at risk for all professional acts, whether clinical or behavioral, that occur within their jurisdiction. Inappropriate action and failure to take appropriate action are both part of the complex context of risk affecting contemporary hospitals and medical centers.

In this chapter, we have provided a brief review of social psychological research and legal precedents for an integrated managerial strategy that enhances organizational commitment and maintains appropriate standards for behavioral competence. Commitment derives from free choice and volition, visible examples of constructive role-related behaviors, and irrevocability, i.e., a compliance system of bylaws, policies, and procedures for the maintenance of high-quality care and an orderly institutional environment.

Four circumstances for managerial interventions have been described, along with protocols for leadership actions that are consistent with recent court decisions. Beyond these guidelines, the development and review of corporate bylaws with adequate legal counsel was advocated to provide a bulwark against legal entanglements.

Finally, it should be noted that a variety of leadership development strategies have already been established to augment our recommendations. Training in role clarification and negotiation[31]; appraisal interviews[32]; feedback and effective communications[33]; and problem-solving techniques[34] are already available for leaders. These guidelines should be supplemented with annual leadership development programs, which include a review of current and emerging legal and disciplinary issues affecting health care organizations.

References

1. Whetton, D. "Understanding and Preventing the Innovation Retarding Effects of Organizational Decline." Paper presented at the Academy of Management Annual Meeting, August 1980, Detroit, Mich.

2. Springer, E., and Casale, H. "Hospitals and the Disruptive Health Care Practitioner--Is Inability to Work With Others Enough to Warrant Exclusion?" *Duquesne Law Review* 24(2):377-423, Spring 1985.

3. Skillicorn, S. "Peer Group Committee Tackles Physician Behavior Problems." *The Hospital Medical Staff* 10(7):2-6, July 1981.

4. Horty, J. "The Disruptive Physician." *Hospital Law* 2(12):1, Dec. 1984.

5. See Reis, M., "Surprise and Sense Making: What Newcomers Experience in Entering Unfamiliar Organizational Settings," *Administrative Science Quarterly,* 25(2):226-51, June 1980; Van Maanen, J., and Schein, E., "Toward a Theory of Organizational Socialization," in *Research in Organizational Behavior,* Vol. 1, 1976, pp, 209-264; Van Maanen, J., "Breaking In: Socialization to Work," in *Handbook of Work, Organization and Society,* Chicago: Rand McNally, 1976, pp. 67-130; and Brim, O. Jr., "Socialization Through the Life Cycle," *Socialization After Childhood: Two Essays,* New York: J. Wiley, 1966, pp. 1-49.

6. Milgram, S. "Behavioral Study of Obedience," in *Psychological Foundations of Organizational Behavior,* Santa Monica, Calif.: Goodyear, 1977, pp. 246- 257.

7. See Collins, B., and Raven, B. "Group Structure: Attraction, Coalitions, Communications and Power" in *The Handbook of Social Psychology,* Reading, Mass.: Addison-Wesley, 1968, Vol. 4, pp. 102-105; Pitts, J., "Social Control: The Concept," in *International Encyclopedia of the Social Sciences,* New York: MacMillan and Co. and The Free Press, 1968, Vol.16, pp. 381-396.

8. See Kerr, S., and Slocum, J. "Controlling the Performance of People in Organizations" in *Handbook of Organizational Design,* New York: Oxford Press, 1981, pp. 115-134; O'Reilly, C., and Weitz, B., "Managing Marginal Employees: The Use of Warnings and Dismissals," *Administrative Science Quarterly,* 25(3):467-84, November 1980; Chopra, K., and others, "The Effect of Constructive Confrontation on the Rehabilitative Process," *Journal of Occupational Medicine,* 21:749-52, 1979; Huberman, J., "Discipline Without Punishment Lives," *Harvard Business Review,* 53:6-8, 1975; Huberman, J., "Discipline Without Punishment," *Harvard Business Review,* 42:62-8, 1964.

9. See Delbecq, A., ibid, p. 189; Luthans, P., and Kreitner, R., *Organizational Behavior Modification,* Glenview, Ill.: Scott Foresman, 1975. For an opposite view see O'Reilly and Weitz, ibid., pp. 479-80.

10. Delbecq, A. "Influence of Professional Behavior: The Management of Norms and Behavior" in *The Physician in Management,* Tampa, FL; American Academy of Medical Directors, 1980, pp. 179-92.

Section II.   The Content of Management

11. See Angle, J., and Perry, J. "An Empirical Assessment of Organizational Commitment and Organizational Effectiveness," *Administrative Science Quarterly,* 26(1):1-14, March 1981; Salancik, G., "Commitment and the Control of Organizational Behavior" in *New Directions in Organizational Behavior*, Chicago: St. Clair Press, 1977, pp. 1-54; Kiesler, C., *The Psychology of Commitment; Experiments Linking Behavior to Belief,* New York: Academic Press, 1971.

12. See Calder, B., and Staw, B., "The Self-Perception of Intrinsic and Extrinsic Motivation," *Journal of Personality and Social Psychology,* 31:71-80, 1975; Ross, M., "Salience of Reward and Intrinsic Motivation," *Journal of Personality and Social Psychology,* 32:245-54, 1975.

13. O'Reilly, C., and Caldwell, D. "The Commitment and Job Tenure of New Employees: Some Evidence of Postdecisional Justification." *Administrative Science Quarterly,* 26(4):597-616, Dec. 1981.

14. See Van Maanen, J., op. cit.; Glaser, B., and Strauss, A., Status Passage, Chicago: Aldine Press, 1971; Berlew, D., and Hall, D., "The Socialization of Managers: Effects of Expectations of Performance," *Administrative Science Quarterly,* 11(11): 2-7,223, September 1966.

15. O'Reilly, C. "The Creation of Corporate Culture: Lessons from Cults and High Technology Firms." Presentation at Santa Clara University Executive Seminar in Corporate Excellence, February 1985.

16. See Brozovich, J., and Shortell, S., "How to Create More Humane and Productive Health Care Environments," *Health Care Management Review,* 9(4):43-4, Fall 1984; Timmel, N., and Brozovich, J., "Managing Through Values," *Hospital Forum,* 24:31-9, May-June 1984; Deforest, C., and others, "Enhancing the Spirit of a Hospital Through Focus on Organizational Values," presentation at "Managing Change in Health Care: Strategies for an Age of Limits," Monterey, CA, 1982.

17. French, J., and Raven, B. "The Bases of Social Power" in *Group Dynamics.* Evanston, Ill.: Row Peterson, 1960, pp. 607-23.

18. Springer and Casale, ibid; see also *Rosner v. Eden Township Memorial District,* 58 Cal. 2d 592, 375 p. 2d 431 (1962) and *Leonard v. Board of Directors, Prowers County Hospital Dist.,* 673 P 2d 1019, (Colo. 1983).

19. *Ladenheim v. Union County Hospital,* 76 Ill. App. 3d 90, 394 N.A. 2d 770 (1979).

20. *Leonard v. Board of Directors, Prowers County Hospital Dist.;* supra note 33; supra note 34.

21. See *Belanoff v. Grayson* 98 A.D. 2d 353, 471 N.Y. Supp. 2d 91 (1984); Bolling v. Baker, 671 S.W. 2d 559 (Tex. App. 1984).

22. *Laje v. R.E. Thompson General Hospital,* 564 F. 2d 1159 (5th Cir. 1979); *Meredith v. Allen County War Memorial Hospital Commission,* 397 F 2d 33 (6th Cir. 1968); *Robbins v. Ong* 452 F. Supp. 110 (S.D. Ga. 1978); *Glass v. Doctors Hospital,* 213 Md. 44, 131 A. 2d 254 (1957); *Clair v. Centre Community*

Hospital –Pa. Super– 463 A. 2d 1065 (1983); *Grodjesk v. Jersey Medical Center,* 135 N.J. Super. 393, 343 A. 2d 489 (1975).

23. *Robbins v. Ong, supra note 39; McMillan v. Anchorage Community Hospital*–Alaska–646 P. 2d 857 (1982); *Eidelson v. Archer*–Alaska– 645 P. 2d 171 (1982); *Even v. Longmont United Hospital Association,* 629 P. 20 1100 (Colo Ct. App. 1981) (1982); *Ladenheim v. Union County Hospital, supra* note 34; *Spencer v. Children's Hospital*–La. App.–419 So. 2d 1307 (1982), rev'd on other grounds–La.–432 S. 2d 823 (1983); *Akopiantz v. Board of County Commissioners of Otero County,* 65 N.M. 125, 333 P. 2d 611 (1959); *Ponca City Hospital v. Murphree*–Okl.–545 P. 2d 738 (1976); *Ritter v. the Board of Commissioners of Adams County Public Hospital District No. 1,* 96 Wash. 2d 503, 637 P. 2d 940 (1981) *enbanc.*

24. *Robbins v. Ong, supra* note 39. For a discussion of cases involving disruptive physicians, see Horty, J., "The Disruptive Physician", *Hospital Law,* 2:1, Dec. 1984.

25. For cases in which courts have upheld a hospital's denial of initial appointment because of disruptive behavior of the applicant, see *Sosa v. Board of Managers of the Val Verde Memorial Hospital,* 437 F. 2d 173 (5th Cir. 1971); *Silver v. Queen's Hospital,* 63 Hawaii 430, 629 P. 2d 1116 (1981); *Ladenheim v. Union County Hospital District, supra* note 34; *Hagen v. Osteopathic General Hospital of Rhode Island,* 102 R.I. 717, 232 A. 2d 596 (1967); *Sussman v. Overlook Hospital Association,* 95 N.J. Super. 418, 231 A. 2d 389 (1967); *Huffaker v. Bailey,* 273 Or. 273, 540 p. 2d 1398 (1975); *Rao v. Auburn General Hospital,* 19 Wash. App. 124, 573e P. 2d 834 (1974).

26. *Supra* note 32; 277 Pa. Super. 363, 419 A. 2d 1191 (1980).

27. *McMillan v. Anchorage Community Hospital; supra note 36; see also Ritter v. Board of Commissioners of Adams County Hospital District No. 1, supra note 42.*

28. O'Reilly and Weitz, *ibid.*

29. Delbecq, A., and Ladbrooke, D. "Administrative Feedback on Behavior of Subordinates." *Administration in Social Work* 3(2):153-66, Summer 1979.

30. Katz, D., and Kahn, R. *The Social Psychology of Organizations,* 2nd Edition. New York: J. Wiley, 1966, pp. 204-8.

31. Harrison, R. "Role Negotiation: A Tough-Minded Approach to Team Development" in *The Social Technology of Organization Development.* La Jolla, Calif.: University Associates, 1972, pp. 84-96.

32. See Levinson, H., "Appraisal for What Performance?" *Harvard Business Review,* 54(4):30, July-August, 1976; Koontz, H., "Making Managerial Appraisal Effective," *California Management Review,* 15(2):46-55, Winter, 1972.

33. Delbecq and Ladbrooke, ibid; Gordon, T. *Leader Effectiveness Training,* New York: Wyden Books, 1980.

34. See Ulschak, F., and others, *Small Group Problem Solving,* Reading, Mass.:

Section II.   The Content of Management

Addison-Wesley, 1981; Delbecq, A., and others, *Group Techniques for Program Planning: A Guide to Nominal Group and Delphi Processes,* New York: Scott Foresman, 1975.

Sandra L. Gill is President, Performance Management Resources, Inc. a health care leadership development firm. Eric W. Springer, Esq. is Principal in Horty, Springer, and Mattern, P.C., a Pittsburgh law firm in hospital and health care law. Andre L. Delbecq, DBA., is Dean, Leavey School of Business and Administration, Santa Clara University.

CHAPTER 16

Groups and Decision-Making:
Getting the Most Out of Meetings

by Sandra L. Gill

G roups are distinguished by six characteristics, most notably described by Knowles.[1]

- A group requires a *"definable membership,"* i.e., members must know who belongs and who does not.

- A group has a *"consciousness"* of itself as a single entity. Members of the group have a sense of identification with one another.

- A group has a sense of *shared* purpose, goals, or ideals.

- There must be *interdependence* among the group members. They must need one another to satisfy the group's goals.

- A group is distinguished by the *interaction* of its members, by the way they communicate, influence, and interact with one another.

- A group acts as a *single entity* rather than as a collection of individual actors.

Especially under conditions of conflict, many physicians withdraw from collective activity and act independently of their colleagues[2]. They have been described as "tough battlers," who single-mindedly pursue an individual goal. In the face of conflict, physicians often fight more aggressively or abandon public efforts to exert person-to-person influence. Thus, the physician executive is faced with individuals who only occasionally behave interdependently.

Types of Groups

Knowing the varieties of groups is helpful in understanding a difficult situation as well as in knowing how to direct an effort that requires collective action.

Section II. The Content of Management

Work Groups

The most obvious type of professional group is the work group. Work groups have been distinguished from other types of groups by their commitment to a primary task. Often, work groups are inhibited from task completion by unconscious, collusive behaviors, commonly referred to as "basic assumptions."[3] Because of basic assumptions, a group acts as if it had a purpose other than accomplishing its primary task. For example, a group may act as if it is dependent on someone inside the group (the leader, perhaps) or outside the group (the chief of staff, hospital CEO or board, or society) to complete its work. The group then engages in procrastination, scapegoating, and helplessness, acting as if it needs some additional power or force to achieve its goals.

A second type of basic assumption is "fight-flight." In this case, a group fails to accomplish its task because its members are preoccupied with fighting or avoiding some imagined force. For example, a group may create a scapegoat and spend the meeting time castigating the imagined scapegoat rather than designing effective strategies to achieve its goals.

A third kind of basic assumption is "pairing." In this case, two of the group members pair to create a sense of hopefulness among the other group members that someone will absolve the group of its task.

Basic assumptions continually distract leaders from the primary task. They occur because group members prefer to create fantasies rather than face the often difficult realities of getting a job done. Fundamentally, basic assumptions serve to preserve the status quo. Specialists in basic assumption groups point out that all group leaders are susceptible to such tendencies and that recognizing one's own tendencies regarding basic assumptions can be helpful in preventing them from diverting attention from primary goals and tasks.[4] As Rioch states "...in the mature work group, which is making a sophisticated use of the appropriate basic assumptions, the leader of the dependency group is dependable; the leader of the fight-flight group is courageous, and the leader of the pairing group is creative."[5] Thus, an awareness of basic assumptions in groups can enhance group productivity.

Reference Groups

Reference groups may be the result of formal or subjective decisions.[6] For example, the physician who is elected to the hospital governing board may perceive his or her role as representing the medical staff on the board rather than identifying with the governing board. The physician board member subjectively acts under the influence of the Medical Staff. In many cases, reference group membership does conflict with the goals of the actual group, and role clarification will be required.

Abstracted Groups

Abstracted group membership is important because it tends to establish expectations and behaviors for future group function. A group member may use a previous group experience as his or her role model for the current actual group. For example, an aggressive, combative role model from a previous hospital medical staff may be abstracted to the current medical staff, where conflict is normally smoothed over or avoided. The abstracted group model would violate current medical staff norms (expectations), and the group member would likely be perceived as a difficult colleague. The deviations from the current group's model of behavior may create discomfort or conflict within the current group.

Hangover Groups

The term "hangover group" is used by Napier and Gershenfeld[6] to refer to the impact of unresolved conflicts and anxieties in previous groups on current groups. For example, growing up as the youngest child may have been a "sink or swim" situation in a large family, with combative, aggressive, and stubborn fighting to get "one's own." If this perception carries over into groups in adult life, usually at an unconscious level, the individual acts as if he or she is in the same situation. The difficulty with this, of course, is that group members then make decisions on the basis of historical events and perceptions rather than current realities. Leaders are particularly inhibited in such situations, because members are not relating to current events that may be controlled.

Groups may be categorized in as many different ways as they have purposes. Groups are influenced heavily by members' past experience, and effective group leaders must be sensitive to the unconscious efforts among group members to act out previous experiences and assumptions. Leaders have a unique responsibility to provide clarification of the group purpose while at the same time not succumbing to group tendencies to become dependent on the leader for achievement of the group task.

Leadership for Group Development

There are numerous models of group development; indeed, different kinds of groups develop at different rates. Tuckman[7] provides a memorable conceptual model of group development derived from a variety of small group studies.

The first stage of Tuckman's model is called "forming." During this stage, the primary leadership task is to clarify purpose and task for the group. Leaders can expect to be challenged and tested during this stage, as group members attempt to discover and react to the task and to the ambiguity of achieving a goal effectively. Group members expect guidance and support from the leader in structuring this new situation

Section II.   The Content of Management

and in achieving this first task of group development. Leaders can assist the group by providing a well-planned agenda, which includes attention to group discussion, brain--torming, and techniques for making decisions.

It is usually very helpful to start the first meeting with a brief overview of the purpose, time frame, available resources, constraints, and strategy for developing a working plan. Certainly, the leader should attend to careful introductions of each of the group members, including the reason they were selected or appointed to the work group. The leader should also clarify his/her role and solicit reactions from the group regarding the leadership tasks needed to achieve the task. In the absence of such discussion, many erroneous assumptions are likely to be made and the possibility for group dependency on the leader is created. Group leaders need to be very clear about their own limits early in the development of groups. Most groups assume their leaders have much more time, energy, and resources than they actually do, and so come to be dependent on the leader.

It is especially important at this stage that the leader clarify shared values and interests to create an opportunity for group cohesion. In the absence of overtly discussed common values, small groups have a tendency to split into smaller cliques rather then function as a single entity. The group leader has to pay particular attention to this tendency and should reiterate at frequent intervals why it is important for the group to function as a single unit, preferably motivated by a common interest. In the absence of a common vision, a group can be expected to fragment and engage in conflicts.

Soon after the group's formation, the second stage of its development begins, which Tuckman calls "storming." The novelty of the new group wears off, and the reality of the task begins to create tensions. Often, the formal group leader is challenged in an overt or covert fashion. Members may disagree over how their work is to be done, and over who should do what.

At this point the leader's role shifts to that of a statesperson who facilitates problem-solving. The leader should acknowledge the conflicts and provide suggestions for a means to resolve the differences. Often, "active listening" is sufficient to displace the tension and redirect the group to productive discussions. However, the leader may also need to exert formal authority and make strong recommendations. General guidelines for this stage include the leader's attention to the following: clarification and description of specifics, rather than making general judgments; a focus on changeable, do-able ideas rather than fixed limitations and complaints about them; and a concern with the present situation and potential solutions rather than historical, unchangeable circumstances.

It is at the second stage that many groups succumb to basic assumptions and attempt to move away from the group goal into more entertaining distractions (e.g., depending on the leader to make all decisions, solve all problems, etc.).

If the second stage is successfully developed, most groups move into establishing rules and protocols for getting their work done. This third stage is called "norming." Norms are expectations, most often unstated, that group members have of one another. Frequently the norms of the group and its members are in conflict. Thus, clarifications of basic working procedures is a crucial task in group development.

Usually, groups determine quite readily what resources are needed, and how to access them. In essence, the group must decide how to decide. However, this may not be so. Until a group determines its procedures for solving problems, a great potential for unnecessary conflict is ignored. Leaders who address these developmental issues early on will benefit from more functional behavior in later stages.

Tuckman then describes groups as moving into a more mature stage, i.e., "performing." Coordination of delegated assignments, frequent briefings and information exchanges, and achieving closure on intermediate issues are of paramount concern here. Effective leaders attempt to anticipate group concerns by raising issues before they become a crisis; developing problem-solving methods; and providing group members recognition and support for jobs well done.

Group leadership is much more than task analysis, intuition, or social grace. A group leader must be sensitive to the needs of group members as individuals and as organizational representatives. Clarification of the group purpose, of individual roles within the group, and of decision-making alternatives, and provision of recognition and professional support are ongoing tasks for group effectiveness. Leaders often draw upon various group members to provide appropriate contributions in each of these areas. It becomes the group's task to manage itself, where the leader facilitates and enhances the development of the group.

Decision-Making Guidelines for Group Leaders

Two of the most critical elements for effective group functioning are the leader's attention to agenda development and rehearsal in a variety of decision-making techniques.[8] Agenda planning and development can preclude numerous group dysfunctions. Armed with a variety of decision-making methods, group leaders can obtain decisions even when time and circumstance are less than optimal (figure 1, next page).

Purpose/Outcome

Leaders have their greatest impact when they clarify the purpose and ex-

Section II. The Content of Management

Figure 1. MEETING PLANNING GUIDE

Purpose/Outcome: (write down major result in verb-noun phrase) _____

Date/Time/Place: _____ # Participants: _____

Seating Arrangements: (alter seating to achieve key objectives)

Special Issues/Constraints: _____

Orientation to Participants: _____

_____

_____

....

Routine Information Items: Est. time   Leader   Topic

    Seating:

    A-V needs:

Action Items: Est. time   Leader   Topic   1st, 2nd Decision Mtd.

    Problem Solving:

    Negotiation:

Outcomes/Results:

Summary:

Next Action Steps:

Reminders:

Evaluation of Meeting:

    Results:

    Process:

pected outcomes of meeting in the first two minutes (when the quorum is present). The specific task of the group should be stated in terms of outcomes rather than beginning steps so that a shared vision and mind-set for the group is formed. There are often many ways to achieve a task;

the leader should focus more on results than on the methods for achieving them.

Date/Time/Place

While date, time, and place are often known, reiteration rarely hurts.

Number of Participants

The size of the group has a dramatic impact on group functioning.[9] Essentially, any group larger than a dozen participants will require careful, assertive leadership to prevent dysfunctional cliques from forming and, potentially, subverting the group goal.

Seating Arrangements

Effective group leaders know that the stage is a crucial prop in the conduct of effective meetings and pay careful attention to seating arrangements. Most leaders intuitively know that round and rectangular tables facilitate group discussion. Theater seating enhances didactic presentations where group attention is focused toward the front. For many meetings, leaders may wish to start out with theater seating for briefings, announcements, short presentations, etc. Then, after a break, they may direct the group to rearrange tables and chairs for small group discussion, brainstorming, etc.

Orientation to Participants

Group leaders should tell members how they can be helpful. For example, if the leader wants to present a series of quick announcements and doesn't want to be interrupted, members can be asked to withhold their questions until the end of the announcements. Asking members for helpful behavior provides a clear orientation and creates a constructive group norm.

Agenda Planning

For each item on a topical agenda, the speaker/leader for each topic should be identified. It is a simple orientation to participants and listeners and helps cut down on potential disorganization. A time estimate for the topic discussion is a crucial addition. In the absence of time estimates, most speakers consume two to three times the amount of meeting time that they do if given a time increment. How the time estimate is established depends on the nature of the group. Informal time estimates from participants are usually adequate. The leader may need to reduce original estimates to keep within the stated time frame of the meeting. I typically prefer that the group reduce time estimates so that the leader is not placed in an adversarial role with the group. Regardless of how time estimates are obtained and developed, they are

Section II. The Content of Management

Figure 2. A QUICK SUMMARY ON DECISION MAKING METHODS

You have 3 basic choices:

	PUBLIC METHODS	PRIVATE METHODS

Concensus (All agree)	Voice vote
	Show of hands
	Other
	  "Vote with your
	  feet, knuckles
	  win," signed
	  memo or report
		Ballot card
		Closed Chamber
		  or panel

Majority rule	Voice vote count
	Count of hands
	  Thumbs up-down
	Other
	  item selection
	  or purchase, etc.
		Ballot card
		Forced choice
		Estimate submitted
		  in writing, then
		  tabulated

Minority rule	Charisma
	"Marshall Law"
	Benevolent dictatorship
	  or abdication of leaders
	Fiat/divide and rule
	Mob action
		Covert divide and rule
		Character assassination
		  and backbiting
		Coups and creating chaos

Recommendations:

Use concensus to make, affirm simple decisions - makes people feel good to occasionally "all agree"

Use majority rule to negotiate issues between factions, with "due process" structure; use estimates for aggregating judgements.

Use minority rule, i.e. exercise authority, in crisis situations and inform people of your decisions with requests for their cooperation due to the crisis.

---

critical to the timely completion of most meetings.

It is also extremely helpful to have a timekeeper in each meeting. Leaders are often engaged in the substance of discussion, and the presence of a collegial timekeeper makes a substantial contribution to the management of the meeting. A group member may volunteer to give each speaker several minutes' "warning" before time expires and to call time when it has expired. While this may sound strict or harsh, most groups quickly adopt this technique as a very effective mechanism for meeting management.

The agenda will identify both routine items and action items. Routine items would include brief announcements, noncontroversial reminders, etc., that require no group action beyond simple clarification. Action items require some kind of group decision-making and need more strategic planning. Action items need to be prepared with a primary and a backup decision-making method so that if time expires

New Leadership in Health Care Management

and the group fails to make a decision with its preferred method, a backup decision-making technique has been identified to move the group through the roadblock.

Some action items will require creativity and brainstorming. Others will require more forceful negotiation and tradeoffs (figure 2, previous page). Effective group leaders must be clear about the kind of decision needed because these are two very different procedures.[10,11]

A third item is for the recording of meeting outcomes and results. This section provides an ongoing record of progress for the participants, especially if recorded during the course of the meeting on a flip chart or overhead transparency. Provided as a visual aid, it keeps group members focused on the topic; it also enables latecomers to enter discussions without referring to all previous discussions. Probably the most helpful aspect is that it can provide a quick summary for meeting minute preparations. Some Medical Staffs have formulated actual memoranda with similar headings preprinted for the completion of departmental meeting minutes as required by JCAH.

Evaluation of Meeting

Most group leaders do not evaluate their meetings. However, should you chose to do so, it is recommended that you distinguish meeting results from the process dynamics of the session. Aggressive personalities, shy individuals, or people with high needs for control may artificially inflate or deflate evaluation results because they are dissatisfied with the process dynamics, even though they accept the results of a particular meeting (figure 3, next five pages). Interval scales, letter grades, or words may be used to elicit participant responses.

Summary

Decision-making is the essence of an effective group. The precursor to effective-decision making is agenda planning and strategy. Consideration of the meeting room; arrangement of table(s), chairs, supplies, and audiovisual aids; and participant orientation are important. Clarification of the purpose of the meeting and alternative strategies for making decisions are essential.

Developing responsible helpers, especially a timekeeper and a recorder/facilitator, from the decision-making group is important. Group leaders are then able to engage in substantive discussions without fear that the agenda will be abandoned.

The suggestions presented here have been summarized from a decade of experience with medical staffs and health care organizations. In the contemporary realm of health care leadership, management of groups and decisions is a basic survival skill. These basic guidelines are but a

Section II.   The Content of Management

starting point.

An exceptionally wide literature is available to group leaders. The dynamics of small groups, meeting management, and decision-making protocols are widely published; videotapes, 35-mm films, and books-on-tape are also abundantly available for further skill development.

Figure 3. SELECTED TROUBLE-SHOOTING GUIDE TO MEETING DYNAMICS

Participant Problems	Possible Causes	Prevention	Action Rx
Angry Outbursts	Person needs group or place to express deep feelings, concerns. Person may need security or control over outcomes; becomes provoked when meeting creates ambiguity.	Talk before meeting to solicit concerns and ventilate feelings, and reach agreement on behavior in meeting.	Use breaks, caucuses, or established guidelines for time and behavior management. Review Coping with Difficult People (Bramson) for additional steps.
People talking at same time or past each other.	Lack of listening skills, knowledge of meeting process or competing issues.	Develope and review discussion protocols with group; use round-robin speaking or writing to get all ideas out; assign person to help paraphrase or moderate discussion.	Invoke agreed upon rules for discussion. Ask moderator or recorder to restate previous issues. Cite sequence of speakers, and provide re-statement of their concerns. Cite time limits for representative of key positions to make summary statements.

Participant Problems	Possible Causes	Prevention	Action Rx
Person says or implies ideas are hopeless and dampens morale or enthusiasm.	Person may be "negative" or "complainer" with need to resist corrective actions or desire to block new approaches.	Meet with person ahead of time to review his/her needs and views. Identify impact of negative behavior and ask for contributions. Be prepared to excuse person from meeting or otherwise control judgemental comments.	Set ground rules for separating creativity from evaluation comments; use silent writing to solicit evaluations. Ask people to identify "strength and modification to improve" vs. "weakness". Avoid commiseration or apology.
Many people talking about different issues at same time.	Lack of common agreement on decisionmaking and discussion protocols; conflict of ideas or leadership or meeting. Unclear outcome or goal to discussion.	Set up step-by-step design for meeting process; review agenda and meeting process with facilitator to assist with managing agenda process, if you are content specialist.	State all agenda items in verb-noun outcome terms. Clarify each person's role in meeting before start. Clarify protocols for discussion. If seems necessary, break up larger issue into subcomponents and focus on each part in some agreed upon order. Consider assigned task forces for simultaneous discussions and subsequent reports back to group as whole, for voting or action planning.

Section II.   *The Content of Management*

Participant Problems	Possible Causes	Prevention	Action Rx
Dispute over major values, e.g., what's right, wrong.	Value conflict; need to be right; fear of unknown or lack of accurate information.	Identify some common values everyone holds, then work back to lower-level agreements or options. Use "shuttle diplomacy" to create common ground in more protected format than large or public meeting.	Appeal to common vision or common enemy to motivate sense of shared concerns. Agree to disagree and try to move on, with concerns appropriately noted. Use caucus or break to meet with principals or key representatives. Restate person's value to group to encourage search for solution. Consider use of outside facilitator or provide new insight.
"Broken record" repetitive discussion or adversarial positions.	People stuck on position vs. interests. Lack of perceived options. Emotional tie which is stronger than influence of new or different information.	Identification of interests, vs. positions through brainstorming, scenario writing, personal discussions with friendly group.	Use Negtiation Model. Use brainstorming for set period of time, during which no evaluation is allowed. List options and use 3 X 5 cards for individuals to assign priorities or number values to their personal choices in nonthreatening way.

Participant Problems	Possible Causes	Prevention	Action Rx
Conversation dominator	Feels he has more or better information on issues; feels need to be heard or need to be right.	Set up agenda with time estimates and identification of who talks when at outset of meeting. Meet with person ahead of time to review your methods for conducting meeting and managing discussion.	If necessary, interrupt person, thanking him/her for comments and asking others for discussion; be prepared to accurately restate person's comments along with agenda structure and participation rules you have set with group. Be prepared to identify sequence of speakers you will allow to make comments to give all time to speak.
Person casts blame or incites other(s) in meeting.	Person wants to deny his/her responsibility or role, transfer blame or views onto others; may want to divide group against itself. Or, person may feel defensive and unfairly treated in meeting.	Meet with parties ahead of time to have them focus on behaviors instead of attribution of motives and blame. Establish rules for interrupting or restating issues if they become accusative vs. descriptive.	Review rules and intent to interrupt or restate if accusations occur. Establish rule for managing questions, rebuttals, e.g., each party has time limit to make statements without interruptions to present full, descriptive case. Be prepared to restate each party's interests and concerns rather than positions.

Section II.   The Content of Management

Participant Problems	Possible Causes	Prevention	Action Rx
Group not able to stay on time during the meeting.	Unclear assignment of available time and order of agenda; insufficient leadership authority or confusion over who's in charge; lack of clarity on what is action item and what is information only.	Assign time keeper and alert group to this ahead of meeting.	Review time estimates for each agenda item and role of time keeper. Ask group to determine priority among agenda items and decide what and how to attend to entire agenda.
Mountain-out-of-molehill sniping about minor point.	Commitment to personal needs beyond interest in group issues. Lack of experience in larger group.	Meet with person ahead of time to solicit views and ask for helpful meeting behavior.	Review protocol for productive meeting. Place issue in overall perspective. Ask to note and then set issue aside to achieve larger goals.
Lack of participation.	Anxiety; fear of being wrong or inappropriate. Lack of adequate information or experience; perceived status difference.	Brief members ahead of time; ask for specific input or help ahead of time. Review meeting format to reassure person.	Use round-robin recording or ballot cards to get input in systematic fashion. Break large group into 5-7 person groups, or into self-selected dyads for brief discussion periods. Ask for straw vote or show of hands on clearly stated options.

References

1. Knowles, M., and Knowles, H. *Introduction to Group Dynamics*. New York: Cambridge Books, 1959. Revised Edition. New York: Association Press, 1972.

2. Delbecq, A., and Gill, S. "Justice as a Prelude to Teamwork in Medical Centers." *Health Care Management Review* 10(1):45-51, Winter 1985.

3. Colman, A., and Bexton, W. (Editors). *Group Relations Reader*. Sausalito, Calif.: GMEX, 1975.

4. Gill, S. "Guidelines for the Management of Temporary Task Force Teams" in *Managing Human Services*. Davis, Calif.: International Dialogue Press, 1977.

5. Rioch, M. "Group Relations: Rationale and Technique." *International Journal of Group Psychotherapy* 20(3):340-355, July 1970.

6. Napier, R. *Groups, Theory, and Experience*, Second Edition. Boston: Houghton Mifflin Co., 1981, pp 47-92.

7. Tuckman, B. "Developmental Sequence in Small Groups." *Psychological Bulletin* 63(6):384-99, June 1965.

8. Thompson, J., and Tuden, A. "Strategies, Structures and Processes of Organizational Decision," *Comparative Studies in Administration*. Pittsburgh, Pa.: University of Pittsburgh Press, 1987, pp. 194-216.

9. Shull, F., and others. *Organizational Decision Making*. New York: McGraw-Hill Book Company, 1970, pp 127-168.

10. Zander, A. *The Purposes of Groups and Organizations*. San Francisco: Jossey-Bass Publications, Inc., 1985.

11. Fisher, R., and Ury, W. *Getting to Yes: Negotiating Agreement Without Giving In*. New York: Penguin Books, 1983.

Sandra L. Gill is President of Performance Management Resources, Inc., a health care leadership development firm.

CHAPTER 17

Communication As A Tool Of Influence

by Pat Heim, PhD

T he ability to influence others is at the core of being an effective executive. The vehicle of the influence process is communication. There are few things in our lives with which we have as much experience as communication. We start communicating the day we are born and do not stop until we die. At the same time, few things are as confusing to us as communicating effectively. In fact, most managers cite effective communication as their most significant problem. In this chapter we will address communication as a tool of influence:

- Communication and the leadership process.
- Common barriers in communication.
- What you say is what you get (the verbal message).
- What you see is what you get (the nonverbal message).
- Chip theory (building your influence base).

Recently, a well-known professor of management, Warren Bennis, published a book, Leaders, describing some of America's top leaders.[1] Specifically, Bennis was looking for the common thread among these individuals. He interviewed, and in some cases lived with, 90 leaders from both the public and the private sectors.

After concluding the interviews and before writing the book, Bennis found himself in a quandary. He expected certain commonalities--possibly dress-for-success attire, verbal agility or the like--but seemed to find none. In the end, the similarity Bennis found among the 90 was that all had visions of where they were going. They knew where they were going and what it would look like when they got there. Second, each of the leaders was able to communicate his or her vision to others. Bennis refers to this critical communication as the "management of meaning."

Recently, Steve Jobs, the cofounder of Apple Computer and founder of the new computer company Next, Inc., was interviewed on television. When asked if he is driven to succeed, there was a long thoughtful pause, "No...no, I'm not *driven*. My people and I are *pulled*...pulled as if by a magnet toward this exciting picture of the contribution we know we can make. We're almost running toward the picture." Jobs is a master of vision. He creates a reality that does not exist and then motivates his people by the excitement of that future.

The ability of executives to influence others and have others follow them lies in their capacity to communicate a picture of the future. And to communicate it in a way that causes others to want to join in achieving that goal. But what is actually involved in communicating vision? The two primary components are liturgy and redundancy. Liturgy is essentially a "stump speech." The same message is communicated repeatedly in a consistent fashion. Eventually, the message becomes more than an idea--it becomes the goal people are working toward.

It is a rare occasion when others quickly and accurately embrace our ideas. Some fear change, others are cynical, and still others just aren't listening. If you want the support of others, you must have a consistent liturgy about the future you want, and you must be redundant communicating it. You will think, "I've said this before a million times. Aren't they getting tired of it?" But it is the consistent repitition through different communication channels, rituals, and media that brings others to support the future you propose and allows them to see how they can contribute to making it become reality.

Barriers to Communication

A cardinal rule of communication is that you cannot *not communicate*. Even if you choose not to communicate about an issue, you are still sending a significant message. Others will read into your lack of response what they believe to be there. And the more influential your position, the more others will take notice and interpret your lack of communication. What's more important is that you are no longer in control of how the message will be understood. Recently a manager said to me, "I don't know what they are so upset about. I haven't even responded to the memo yet." What he didn't understand was that lack of response is a response. Choosing to take no action is a decision, a decision to which people will attribute meaning.

So it becomes crucial that you manage your communication so that the message that you want others to receive is in fact what they come to understand. If you don't take an active part in this management of meaning, others will assign meaning by default.

In the communication process there are some predictable distortions that will occur. We can be better communicators by proactively managing these potential distortions.

Section II. The Content of Management

We each have filters through which we see the world. These filters distort what we see and therefore what we believe is "reality." For instance, if you had been bitten by a large dog when you were a child, there is a good chance that today, as an adult, you would be frightened of large dogs. What other people see as a cuddly family member you see as a potentially harmful animal. Whether these memorable incidents have been positive or negative, they will shade what is seen.

Additionally, our personal demographics become filters. Which part of the country you grew up in, whether it was an urban or rural setting, the kind of school you attended, the size of your family, and your religious upbringing (or lack of) all become filters. We have no choice about seeing with our filters. A good manager will know his or her filters and how they may distort what he or she understands.

Health care practitioners develop their own filters. Physicians and administrators frequently have very different filters and therefore see the same situation very differently.[2]

Administrators:

- Are hired as general managers.

- Are multidisciplinary.

- Must control individuals.

- Must establish rules of conduct.

- Must serve many interests concurrently.

- Make decisions on the basis of policy (consensus).

- View hospital cost control as high priority.

- Are realists.

- Represent organizations.

Physicians:

- Are entreprenuerial capitalists.

- Are specialists.

- Resist being controlled.

- Resist rules.

- Are oriented to one group (patients).

- Must make their own decisions.

- View hospital cost control as restrictive.

- Are idealists.

- Represent themselves.

Is it any wonder that physicians and administrators have a tendency to see the other as wrong? The filters that they bring to the management arena are very different.

Effective communicators will focus on understanding their own filters and the filters of those whom they are attempting to influence. For example, the administrator may interpret your suggestions through a financial filter, the director of nursing may see them through a patient care filter and your colleagues may view them with their specialty filters, group practice filters, or the like. Your job is to address each of these views. It's a tall order, but ignoring the filters only magnifies problems and diminishes your effectiveness as a leader.

A second barrier to communication is our natural tendency to categorize. Every day we are faced with this big, booming, buzzing world. We must put some order to it, and the way we do that is by categorizing. Every time we encounter a new person, we immediately begin to categorize him or her--age, sex, height, weight, profession, position, power, effectiveness, and more. The process of categorizing another person takes less than four minutes and the result often remains static for years.[3]

We also categorize the behavior of others on the basis of our past experiences. For instance a high-level executive told me that when he was hired as a new graduate, he often found that the days available to him as vacation were inadequate. So when he needed an extra day off, he would call in sick. Today he is an executive in a large corporation, with responsibility for more than 500 employees. When one of them calls in sick, he believes the employee is just taking an extra day off. Like most of us, he explains actions in the present based on his personal past experiences. At the executive level this can lead to serious misunderstandings.

Because categorization is natural and normal, what we must do is override it. There may be times in dealing with an individual with a particular specialty, for example surgery, when you may incorrectly categorize the person or his or her actions. We have no choice about whether we do this. But we do have a choice about which categories we choose and about when and how often we revise how we see

Section II.   The Content of Management

someone. The key is being aware of this natural categorization process and managing it.

The third barrier to effective communication is our tendency to notice what's important to us. Think about the day you took possession of the car you now own. Let's say it's a blue Buick. Remember how many Buicks suddenly were on the road that day? And a disproportionate number of blue Buicks! That was because suddenly, on that day, blue Buicks became important to you.

A physician who works for a pharmaceutical company told me that she frequently finds herself "tuning out" at meetings. But at the mention of the word "clinical," she quickly focuses back on the discussion. Again, because clinical issues are of great concern to her. At meetings you chair or attend, you may notice various individuals tuning in or out at words such as "financial," "patient care," or "HCFA."

Our ability to manage others fairly and effectively can be hampered by our tendency to notice what is important to us. Some behaviors and characteristics we tend to especially notice, and others we miss altogether. For instance, if someone who works for you is from the same part of the country or was educated at the same institution as you, you will have a natural tendency to notice him or her more than other people. And if you like that person, you will often notice the good things he or she do disproportionately. On the other hand, you may not notice similar accomplishments of others. Conversely, if you have been having a problem with one individual, you will unconsciously be on the lookout for when he or she does "it" again. And you may not even notice the person's positive behavior or the problem behaviors of others whose behavior is not as significant to you.

If you find that some of these examples strike home, that's a good sign-- you are human. But to be an effective leader, you must manage each of these natural tendencies. They are some of the most common barriers in the communication process.

The Verbal Message

To this point we have been looking at some of the communication barriers that are a result of the perceptual process. Now we are going to focus on the verbal component of the message.

Often, it seems to us that we have been very clear, but those other people just didn't catch on. Below are some examples of message problems from actual medical records.[4]

"The patient has chest pains if she lies on her left side for over a year."

"On the second day the knee was better, and on the third day it had completely disappeared."

"By the time she was admitted to the hospital, her rapid heart had stopped, and she was feeling much better."

"If he squeezes the back of his neck for four or five years, it comes and goes."

"Discharge status: alive but without permission."

Luckily, most of our errors are not this extreme. But the words that you choose create the "reality" of your vision in the minds of others. Because you must be able to communicate your ideas to others if you want them to follow you, you need to be strategic with your message.

First, each message we send has three parts: what we intend, what we say, and what they hear.

What you intended: I'm concerned about our ability to financially support this new piece of equipment.

What you said: Have you verified the financials on that new equipment?

What was heard: He doesn't think I can handle financial decisions.

How do you deal with the three-part message? The key is Receiver-Oriented Communication. This means designing your message in such a way that the words you choose make sense to the receiver rather than are most meaningful and logical to you--words that will allow the receiver to paint the picutre in his or her head that you have in yours.

Often we focus on the accuracy of the message. This is far less important than the receiver-oriented focus. You have probably known a couple who have been married for decades. If he asks her to bring him the "thing-a-ma-gig" from the kitchen, she knows exactly what he wants. His communication has been effective. He got what he wanted. In fact, if he had used the precise culinary term, she may have been confused. On the other hand, if he communicates the same message to you or me, we will be totally lost. Meaning is not in words. Meaning is in people.

When we share a common language with others with whom we work, we often feel more a part of what they are doing. When we don't share the language, we don't feel part of the team. As a leader, you must note whom you have included on committees and other teams. Those from different disciplines, specialties, and departments, who "don't speak the language," may not participate as full members of the team.

Section II.   The Content of Management

The Knowledge/Communication Gap

Another frustration in communication arises from the Knowledge/ Communication Gap. The gap occurs when we are telling someone about something with which we are very familiar. The better we understand a topic, directions, or information of any kind, the poorer we are likely to be in explaining them to another.

When we are knowledgeable, we unconsciously presume a similar amount of base knowledge in the person with whom we are communicating. We leave gaps in the message that others will fill in, often inaccurately. This is not a problem when others share our background and knowledge, for example, someone in the same specialty, but that is rare. The gap becomes even more important when you begin to communicate conceptual ideas, such as your vision. A good rule of thumb is to over-communicate by explaining with more detail, examples, and analogies than seems necessary. This is why the redundancy in your communication is important to its success.

The Nonverbal Message

Whenever we communicate, there are always two layers to the messages we send: the verbal layer and the nonverbal layer. When we are concerned about others understanding us, we usually focus on the verbal component. We tend to be far more aware of the verbal message and assess it for accuracy, meaningfulness, and the like. But if the verbal and nonverbal messages differ in what they are comunicating, it is the nonverbal message that we will believe. At the same time, this nonverbal layer is almost invisible to us.

Some authors have indicated that there is a one-to-one meaning in the nonverbal cues we send. If my arms are crossed, it indicates that I don't like what you are saying. It may mean that, but it also may indicate that I'm cold or it may be the most comfortable way for me to sit at this moment. To accurately assess the meaning of a nonverbal cue, we must always look at the patterns that we see and the context within which the nonverbal cue is communicated. There is never a one-to-one meaning.

Nonverbal cues are not new to you. You have been sending them since you were born, and others have been unconsciously interpreting them. Additionally, you have been unconsciously interpreting the nonverbal cues of others.

What our body says. How we stand tells others a great deal about our comfort and confidence at a given time. When we feel powerful and sure of ourselves, we have a natural tendency to pull our body up and to spread our arms and legs out. Conversely, when we feel vulnerable, we will pull the body down and in.

Let's say that you are making an important presentation to a very powerful and influential group. One member of the group begins to vehemently attack your ideas. The natural inclination is to pull in and down, to back away from the attacker. The powerful approach is to do the opposite. Become more erect, open up and move toward the individual. This can be a very effective way of disarming without a confrontation.

In the process of leading and influencing others, we must look as if we are sure of what we are saying even when we are not. One way we cue others is whether our posture is open or closed.

Another way we unconsciously signal discomfort is with gestures known as adaptors. Adaptors are rubbing, patting, and scratching, which we use to make ourselves feel comfortable. You may be wondering if you have ever seen any of these adaptors before. Go to the nearest busy freeway or expressway during rush hour. You'll see plenty of adaptors--people running their hands through their hair or rubbing their necks, faces, ears, etc.

Recently I was asked to work with an executive who felt very uncomfortable doing performance appraisals. When I met him, I was surprised that he had this discomfort, because he held a very senior position and seemed to exude confidence and power. But as soon as we began the practice session, he rubbed the back of his left hand with his right thumb and didn't stop throughout the appraisal! Afterward I mentioned the adaptor. Although we had previously talked about this nonverbal cue, he was totally unaware of how he had communicated his discomfort.

Height also affects how we are seen by others. Research has found that, up to 6'8", a man is more likely to hold a higher position in an organization and make more money the taller he is. I'm not going to advocate putting lifts in your shoes, but one can manage the issue of height. When having an important meeting or discussion, notice if you must look up to the other individual. If so, you may want to invite the person to sit down to discuss the issue as a way of equalizing the power. On the flip side, others may find you very intimidating if they must look up to you when conversing.

If your goal is to be perceived as powerful and credible, stand when giving a presentation. If the goal is to make others feel comfortable, sit down and speak eye to eye. Be cautious of those who will manipulate the situation to diminish your feeling of power. I once met with a health care executive who had just been promoted to the executive suite. In fact, I was one of the first people to meet with him in his new executive office with its new executive furniture. I sat down in the chair he indicated, which was directly across the desk from him. After we were both seated he realized that I was looking down at him. He stood up,

Section II.   The Content of Management

turned over his chair, cranked it up, turned it back over, sat down, saw that he was now looking down at me and said, "Now let's talk."

Managing territory. I was once told that the definition of a hospital is "a set of independent kingdoms connected by a common heating system." Each department has its territory and often feels that the equipment, patients, or personnel within that department belong to it rather than to the hospital at large.

If you have a dog, you have seen territoriality in action. You can also do an experiment that will give you an idea of how territorial humans are. When you're having lunch with someone, imperceptibly push the salt shaker onto his or her half of the table. The person will most likely push it back. Move the shaker again, and they are likely to return it to your side. Try doing this as many times as you like. At the end of lunch, ask if your lunch companion noticed anything unusual. Typically, the person will not have noticed a thing. We are very territorial and yet unaware of how it affects us.

A supreme example of the management of territory was given by Jack Anderson, who once wrote of former Chief Justice Burger: "He has now annexed to his personal offices the court's conference room, the inner sanctum, where the justices meet to thrash out their decisions. He has even installed a desk so there can be no mistaking that the court convenes in Burger's lair."[5]

In arranging an important meeting with others, a strategic decision to make is, whose territory? If they meet on your territory, they will usually feel a bit uncomfortable and awkward, and the converse is true. You may want to choose a neutral territory so none of you feels disadvantaged.

Where one sits at meetings may also influence the outcome. We tend to give power, and often leadership, to the person who sits at the end of a rectangular table. So you may want to get to meetings early and sit at the end of the table when you would like to have more influence. If you would prefer others to take more leadership, you may want to sit at the side.

We often tend to sit in subgroups or teams at meetings to enhance the sense of group cohesiveness. This may prove to be a problem, however. For instance, if three disagreeing factions sit as factions, it will be extremely difficult to get them to agree on solutions that are a win for all three groups. In this case, you may want to assign seats, possibly with name tents, so that the groups do not behave as coalitions.

Where you sit when meeting with another person may also influence the outcome. Sitting directly across from one another is more likely to engender conflict; sitting side by side at the corner of a table is more likely to bring about cooperation. If you are meeting with someone with whom you have had conflicts in the past and you would like to change the relationship, don't sit across from the person!

Nearness to power tends to breed power. You may want to assess which of the power brokers you are or are not located near. Also consider if there are strategic moves that you can make to increase your proximity to power. Moving offices is often impractical, but "stopping by" on an informal and regular basis may do the trick.

Having a shared territory can also affect whether a group sees itself as a team and functions as a team. Those individuals located in proximity to each other will often behave as a team, whether they are or not. If your office is in the medical building across the street, it may be difficult for you to function as a full member of the executive team.

Reach out and touch someone. We communicate a great deal through our tactile sense. As with other nonverbal cues we send, the tactile message is often culturally based and "invisible." A study was conducted assessing the number of touches that occur in an hour between two people sitting in a restaurant or cafe. The data were gathered in San Juan, Puerto Rico; Paris; Gainesville, Florida; and London. The study measured how often, on the average, two individuals touched in an hour. In San Juan, the average number of touches per hour was 180; in Paris, 110; Gainesville, 2; and in London, 0. So imagine someone from San Juan having lunch with someone from London. They know they're very uncomfortable but often can't tell why.[6]

We also communicate power through touch. We have an unwritten rule in our culture that we can only touch people of equal or lower power than ourselves. Frequently, it can be very illuminating to assess who touches you and who you touch. Of course, you may want to alter the present touching relationships in an attempt to alter the perception of power between you and another.

Touch can also positively affect how others see us. A study on the impact of a fleeting touch was conducted in a university library.[7] Students were chosen at random to receive a fleeting touch from the person checking out their books. This fleeting touch took place as the student's library card was returned. All students as they exited the library were given a survey asking questions such as "Do you like studying in the library?," "Does the library have the books you need?," "Are the librarians helpful?," and "Were you touched while you were in the library?" Students did not remember being touched, but those who had been touched liked studying in the library more, thought it had more books that were useful, that the librarians were more helpful, and the like. We are just beginning to understand the significant impact touch can have on our perceptions of others.

Section II. The Content of Management

A physician told me that when he was in medical school, a similar study was conducted. Certain patients were chosen at random to receive a fleeting touch from the physician during the patient interview. The patient interviews were exactly seven minutes in length. As patients exited the interview, they were given a survey asking a number of questions including, "How long did the doctor spend with you?" Those that had not been touched on the average estimated 7 minutes, the exact amount of time. Those that had been touched guessed 15 minutes! Amazed at these results, the researchers replicated the study, this time sending the questionnaire to the patients' homes. They speculated that the time lag would cause more accurate estimates from respondents. In the replication, 7 minutes were still perceived to be 15 by the patients who were touched.

Hellos and goodbyes. People are much more likely to believe what we do rather than what we say. The executive who says, "I have an open door policy" but signals nonverbally when you show up that your presence is not desired is sending one of those mixed messages.

We communicate that we are open to interaction with others primarily in two ways: by open body posture and by eye contact. If you are wondering why others don't seem to come to you to ask questions, share ideas, and the like, you may want to assess the accessibility cues communicated in your posture.

On the flip side, when we are getting ready to end an interaction, we also send signals to the other person. It is our way of not surprising him or her that the end of the interaction is at hand. For instance, at the end of a discussion you may find yourself saying, "Well, it's been nice seeing you. We'll have to get together some time. I'll give you a call. OK? See you around. Goodbye." If you were to observe your body during this leave-taking rite, what you would probably see is a series of nonverbal cues including: stepping back, turning your body axis away, bowing, gestures that "push away" from the other, and breaking eye contact. All this is to prepare the other person for your exit and not catch them off guard.

These leave-taking rites are like a dance. If I begin with the first cue or step in the dance, the other person typically responds in kind. If you have wondered how to terminate a discussion with someone in a graceful manner, try initiating the leave-taking rite. If your interaction with someone is ending on an unsettling note, ensure that the leave-taking rite is used. (This is particularly important with patients. The patient is surprised when the physician leaves the examining room without leave-taking rites and feels that the physician has been "abrupt" or "hurried" or "didn't spend any time.")

Most of us do not consciously think about what we communicate nonverbally. It is an invisible process. Yet what we say to people may be

New Leadership in Health Care Management

shaded or totally disregarded if our nonverbal cues tell them something else.

Up to this point, we have been focusing on the specifics of the process of influencing others through communication (barriers, words, and nonverbal cues). Now we will look at a communication strategy that allows one to build the power base necessary to have influence across an organization. It is based on chips.

Chip Theory

Imagine you are going to work one day, and you see me in the parking lot. You say, "Hi Pat. How ya been? Haven't seen you in awhile. How have you been lately?" I simply say, "Okay," and keep on walking. A few days later, you see me in the hallway at work and say, "Hi Pat, how are you?" Again, I reply, "Okay" and keep on walking.

If you are like most people, I can rather easily predict that eventually you will probably ignore me when you see me. The reason this is predictable is that you have given me a good amount of recognition, attention, caring, and the like. We'll arbitrarily call these "chips." I have given you virtually nothing in return. The way we humans respond in such a case is to always make it equal in the end. We exchange chips through interacting with others--give and take--and keep a close eye on our accounts to cut our losses.

We are all, to some degree or another, born with chips. These chips come in the form of talent, looks, a wealthy family, intelligence, height, personality, and many more. Some of us are brought into the world with a wealth of chips and others of us are not.

We can also actively acquire chips as we go through life. You may acquire the money you were not born with, or you may acquire education, connections, experience, skills, knowledge, etc. Today it is relatively common to even acquire looks if you weren't born with them.

Chips are very important, because, whether consciously or unconsciously, they play a significant part in all our relationships. For instance, our close friends tend to have roughly the same "chip value" that we do. Not necessarily the same kind of chips, but, overall, roughly equal chip value. Furthermore, we tend to marry people who have roughly equal chip value.

Chips are profoundly important when it comes to influencing others. Strategically assessing one's chips and deploying them when appropriate can make all the difference in whether an influence effort is successful. Success is based on the following premises:

Everyone is an accountant. Throughout a given day, you are being

Section II. The Content of Management

watched. The more influential you are, the more closely you are watched. You are constantly gaining chips and losing chips. The kinds of things others might say as a result of their dealings with you are, "He spent half the morning explaining the change to him. He merely mentioned it to me in the hallway" (you'll lose chips on this one). Or, "I was really stuck on what to do about that problem and she just jumped in and helped me out" (you'll gain some chips here). The more influential your position, the more others assess the chips that they gain or lose in dealing with you.

Supply and demand. As with other forms of currency, there is a component of supply and demand with chips. For instance, when I was a university professor, we had a department secretary named Loretta. She worked in a windowless cubicle by herself all day long. It was quite evident to me that the chips that Loretta highly valued were interaction chips. So when I would see her, I'd ask about the kids, comment on the new hairdo, ask what was new in the department, etc.

One day I was working with my boss when Loretta brought me some typing. After she left, the boss asked when I had given Loretta the typing, and I replied, "This morning." Then she asked if Loretta always brought the typing when she had finished, and I told her that Loretta usually did. At this point the boss angrily pointed out that she had given Loretta typing three days ago and not only did it take days to get it back but Loretta never brought the typing when she was finished with it. The problem was that the boss never paid Loretta her "interaction chips." Certainly the boss had a right to say that she didn't hire Loretta to pay her interaction chips. But logic is not the issue. Loretta was still going to make it equal.

One of the mistakes we can make with chips is thinking that everyone values similar chips. I used to work in an engineering organization. In general, engineers do not highly value interaction. I could easily have made the mistake of giving the engineers the same interaction chips that worked so well with Loretta. This would have cost me chips. The chip an engineer usually values is being left alone to do work.

We also make the mistake of thinking that others value the same chips that we do. Not so. In assessing which chips to provide another person you must look at what the other individual values, not what you value.

Surplus account. It is a good idea to build a supply of surplus chips with those individuals who are critical to your success. We all have times when everything seems to go wrong at once. If you have a surplus account, you will be able to get the assistance you need. For instance, others will stay late or come in on the weekend, get it done sooner than they normally do, warn you when you are about to step on a political land mine, and the like if you have a surplus account of chips.

In fact, you have probably known someone who can get anything done under the table, without all the signatures, in half the time, without going through the appropriate channels. This is someone who has built up his or her chip surplus throughout the organization. The flip-side of this surplus account is chip deficit.

Chip deficit. Even the dullest person becomes a creative genius when it comes to "making it equal in the end." Employees are particularly adept at this. They will do such things as call in sick on the day you need them most, lose messages, lose files, work slower, talk behind your back, be abrupt with patients, and much more. One of the most interesting strategies for getting even is doing exactly what you ask.

The following story was told to me by the perpetrator (he's now a probation officer). He was in the navy on a ship. The captain of this ship was in deep chip deficit with almost everyone on the ship. The propeller of the ship was broken. It had been removed and placed on the top deck for repair. The captain came by, did not like the propeller being in the way, and said, "Get rid of it." The entire propeller was thrown in the Pacific Ocean, *exactly* what he said.

John was another individual who did not understand chips. He was hired into an organization where I worked and his office was next to mine, although our functions were not related. John managed a group of about 25 individuals who traveled on company business to highly undesirable locations. In this company, you were allowed a "safe arrival call" when traveling to let the family know you had arrived safely. Apparently there was a dollar limit on this call.

After John had been in his job about two weeks, he came in my office and told me that he had found out that his employees, prior to his working there, had been exceeding their dollar limit on safe arrival calls by 25 cents to $1.00. John was hot on their trails. He told me that he was going to make them pay back the money. I pointed out to John that it might cost him more than it was worth. He said it wasn't going to cost him anything, because it was going to come out of their pockets. I had been talking chips, and he only saw the money issue. John went around and collected pennies from his new employees.

In my opinion, John's group had not been a high-energy group prior to this. But suddenly you could feel the energy as you walked through the area. The team building that occurred was stunning. Of course, the team's agenda was: Destroy John. John never quite understood what happened. After the money had been collected, John had all kinds of problems. It seemed the wrong employee was always showing up to do the wrong work with the wrong equipment on the wrong day. He'd get that straightened out and something would happen elsewhere. John did not last in that position much more than six months. He did not understand the profound effect of chips.

Section II.   The Content of Management

Chips drive cooperation, support, and assistance. If you are in a position of influence, chips can make or break your success. For instance, the administrator is an important person to have on your team. Simendinger and Moore found four factors that are key to physician/administrator relations: Honesty, enthusiasm, competence, and nonadversarial behavior. Their research indicates that when these conditions are present, they significantly enhance cooperation between the physician and the administrator.[8] You can also think of these as qualities with high chip value. When they are absent, there is a need to "make it even."

In general, each and every executive must have a chip strategy to be successful. First, it is important to identify those whose support you need, those whom you need on your team. And be cautious about only looking at the formal hierarchy. Secretaries have been known to do significant damage in order to make it equal. The next step is to identify which chips those individuals value and provide the chips. You may want to build a chip surplus with key individuals or groups. Of course, always avoid chip deficit, especially with those who matter.

Whatever your goal, chips may determine your success. One cannot be influential without chips, and chips have brought down many good ideas and bright individuals who did not attend to their chip strategy.

Summary

There are few activities in our lives that we have had as much experience with as we have with communication. For the most part communication issues are difficult for us because we can't see the dynamics between us and the persons with whom we are communicating. Some of the key points of communication are:

- Have a vision for the future, and communicate it repeatedly through a variety of channels.

- Be aware of the common barriers in communication and identify situations in which those barriers may hinder effective communication with others.

- Communicate in words that make sense to the *listener*, and recognize differences in knowledge levels.

- Be aware of how power, or lack of power, may be communicated nonverbally.

- Know how team-building may be enhanced or diminished through nonverbal cues.

- Manage your chips strategically. Identify the key members of your team, establish your surplus accounts, and avoid chip deficit, especially in critical areas.

References

1. Bennis, W., and Nanus, B. *Leaders: Three Strategies for Taking Charge.* New York: Harper and Row, 1985.

2. Bettner, M., and Collins, F. "Physicians and Administrators: Introducing Collaboration." *Hospital and Health Services Administration* 32(2):151-60, May 1987.

3. Zunin, L., and Zunin, N. *Contact: The First Four Minutes.* New York: Ballantine Books Paperback, 1975.

4. *Verbatim, the Language Quarterly,* Spring 1982.

5. Anderson, J. "Burger's Highhandedness." *Buffalo Courier Express*, July 6, 1971.

6. Jourard, S. "An Exploratory Study of Body Accessibility." *British Journal of Social-Clinical Psychology,* 5(3):221-31, Sept. 1966.

7. Hesslin, D. "A Touch of Sensitivity." A *Nova* Presentation, 1980.

8. Simendinger, E., and Moore, T. "The Formation and Destruction of Physician-Administrator Cooperation." Michigan Hospitals, 22(4):25-9, April, 1986.

Further Reading

Burns, J. *Leadership.* New York: Harper Torchbooks, 1978.

Kanter, R. *The Change Masters.* New York: Simon and Schuster, 1983.

Kinzer, D. "Constructive Tension: Hospital/Medical Staff Relations." *Physician Executive* 12(1):7-9, Jan.-Feb. 1986.

Palleschi, P., and Heim, P. "The Hidden Barriers To Team Building." *Training and Development Journal* 34(7):14-18, July 1980.

Pascale, R., and Athos, A. *The Art of Japanese Management.* New York: Simon and Schuster, 1981.

Peters, T., and Waterman, Jr., R. *In Search of Excellence.* New York: Harper and Row, 1982.

Watzlawick, P., and others. *Pragmatics of Human Communication.* New York: W. W. Norton and Company, 1967.

Pat Heim, PhD, is a Principal of Heim & Associates, a management training and consulting firm in Pacific Palisades, Calif.

Section II.   The Content of Management

CHAPTER 18

Hiring and Firing

by Marilyn Moats Kennedy, MSJ

I s any decision more risky than hiring someone? Think of the potential problems. You might hire the wrong person. Later, that person might not agree he or she was wrong for the job. When, for you, firing is the only answer, the victim might sue. How do you make informed and lasting choices? It's a question of establishing and then following a step-by-step procedure to reduce the risks of making the wrong choice.

Checklist on Job Specifications

Before you fill out a job requisition, place an employment advertisement, or call a recruiter, you need to consider the following:

- What is the salary range for the person I propose to hire? Have I checked to see if it matches current offers of other organizations? Can I buy the package of skills I need for that amount? Salary must be considered first, because if you try to get someone for less than market, you'll find that the outstanding candidates won't consider the job and the poor ones will refuse to be discouraged. The latter realize you'll have to settle for one of them unless you raise the ante.

- What will the job require in terms of education, experience, technical/ special expertise, interpersonal skills, and mangerial or supervisory skills? What's your minimum in each area? When you are hiring physicians, don't forget that 50 percent of all the physicians now practicing--and the nurses, technicians, etc.--graduated in the lower 50 percent of their classes. What exactly does it prove, ten years out, to have graduated in the top 10 percent unless the person is in research? Don't get trapped in the past.

- How much training are you willing--more important, able--to give the new hire? How much training or orientation will others provide? How much specialized training, if any, is necessary before the new hire becomes fully productive? This issue is often the beginning of the end with a new employee. Unless you can answer these questions with a specific number of hours, you're not ready to begin a search. Don't underestimate the break-in time. It's probably going to be twice as long as you'd like--or anticipated.

- Are set working hours crucial? Does the person form a link in a chain such that his or her hours must be set? This can be very important in recruiting. For instance, a desirable physician or insurance clerk might be available at odd hours. Is 8 to 5 really crucial?

- What is the work flow of the job? Will there be frantically busy times bordered by lulls? Are there periods of extraordinary stress? Don't kid yourself--much less a candidate--about this. Painting the picture a bit blacker than your view of reality means that the new hire will feel he or she is doing well when things aren't quite as hectic as you said they would be.

- How much information on policies/procedures will this person need to store mentally? The more that must be stored, the longer the break-in period. Some people work best from written instructions. Do you have most policies and procedures in writing for easy access?

- Do co-workers have any preconceptions about the kind of person who should be hired? Are these preconceptions important? If they are not addressed, could co-workers create political problems within the organization? A clinic we know decided that the way to reduce nursing turnover was to hire only "mature" nurses. These nurses, when confronting younger physicians, did not hesitate to indicate that they had more practical knowledge than the physicians. Sometimes they did, but the resulting political warfare was destructive.

- Is there enough work for a full-time person, or would two people sharing the job be more effective? Could this be a half-time or two-thirds time job? If hiring the wrong person into a job is terrible, boring an outstanding hire is even worse. There should be 60 hours work in a forty-hour-per-week job.

- What are your priorities for this person? Do you have a clear idea of what is crucial to success and satisfaction in the job?

Once you have your job specifications, you're ready to write a job description--or revise an existing one. It's important not to view a written job description as more than a fence around turf. That is, a job description must be a living, changing document, a map to the territory, not a prison. Most organizations can't revise job descriptions as quickly as jobs change. This is particularly true in health care. Consequently, hiring a new person must be preceded by a look at the job. With job description and specs in hand, you're now ready for resume reviews.

Section II.   The Content of Management

Reviewing Resumes

The best source of candidates is current employees, your opposite number at another health care provider, the personnel department, or recruiters. The names you get will be prescreened. Solicit the people for resumes, or try to determine each individual's willingness to change jobs. If you can't get good candidates from these sources, use help wanted advertisements. Ads will pose more screening problems and produce fewer stars than any other method. The cost of a want ad is cheap compared to the cost of processing and responding to candidates. (Only an organization with no ethics or style would not respond to each candidate. A form letter is acceptable.) Blind want ads should not be used, because they signal the good people in the market that you have something to hide or are behaving unethically, e.g., someone is in the job you propose to fill and you don't want the employee to know it.

The best way to choose those to be interviewed is to make three piles of resumes: 1) to be interviewed, 2) definite no's, and 3) maybe's. After the first pass, review the "maybe's until you have put each one in either of the other two piles. Finally, go through the people you'd like to interview and pick 6 to 10. If there are only 5, so much the better. Return the rest of the resumes to whomever is sending out rejection letters. Why not keep all the rest in case your first few choices don't pan out? Because if you didn't like them the first time around, you're kidding yourself if you think they'll look better later. If they do, you've succumbed to panic or to unseemly haste in filling the job.

Interviewing

Once you're ready to interview, schedule as many as you can in one day. It isn't true that the first person or the last person to be interviewed has the best shot at the job. If you see people serially, it's easier to make comparisons than if they are strung out, one a day, for weeks.

There are two types of interviews:

- *Initial.* This is usually done by the personnel department or a recruiter. It screens out people whose resumes were all right but who, when interviewed, turn out to be unqualified. This interview also verifies data on the resume or application and seeks to ascertain the applicant's interest in the job. All this can be wrapped into the next step if there are few candidates and no personnel department. Initial interviews can be done by telephone.

- *Evaluation.* This is a thorough oral review of the candidate's qualifications. By talking one-on-one with a candidate, the interviewer can decide if he or she is a "possible" or an "improbable." The meeting usually lasts a minimum of 60 minutes. The average is about two hours. Obviously, at any point the applicant may cut the interview off.

The interviewer needs to be very careful so the applicant doesn't decide he or she wasn't given a fair shake and is a victim of discrimination.

There are four parts to an effective evaluation interview.

- *Rapport building.* This includes about two minutes of general discussion designed to help the candidate catch his or her breath and relax a bit. Caution: this chitchat is where lawyers tell us many people make illegal statements. Confine yourself, as Henry Higgins told Eliza, "to the weather and the state of everybody's health."

- *Q&A.* This is the body of the interview and includes all the questions that will verify or amplify information on the resume. It also includes a concise description of the job, its sociopolitical context, a breakdown of percentages of time to be spent on different tasks, and some information about the style of the organization--how it does things.

The applicant should participate freely with any questions he or she has. If the applicant doesn't ask the right questions, answer the ones he or she is supposed to ask. "When was my predecessor promoted?" "What is the career path for this job?" "Describe a typical day." "What personal qualities, other than skills/experience, are important to success in this job?" Note: When you're interviewed for a job always ask these questions.

- *Applicant response.* At some time during the interview, you must give the applicant a chance to tell you why you should hire him or her. You can ask, "Do you have anything you'd like us to know about you?" or "Is there anything you want to highlight about your work?" or you might simply stop talking. The applicant can introduce any topic he or she feels is important. It is the applicant's responsibility to sell you at this point.

- *Close.* This is the time when you tell the applicant when he or she will hear from you. Explain that you are interviewing several candidates. Don't say "I was impressed with your background" unless you were. Within two weeks, you need to contact each candidate again and give him or her a status report. Useful questions to ask in the close are why the applicant wants to work with your organization and does the applicant feel he or she understands the style and culture of your organization or department. Don't get into discussion of why the candidate won't be considered. You could slip here and say something you'd regret. Friendly neutral interest is best.

Others may also do evaluation interviews. It's common for candidates to have as many as seven interviews with different people or, as is more common in health care, a group interview.

Section II.   The Content of Management

Group interviews, an interesting form of torture because they torture both candidate and interviewers, must be managed carefully. Before you bring in a candidate, he or she must be briefed on the group process. Say, "It's very important that you give equal eye contact to everyone at the table. They'll all be involved in the decision." More good candidates are lost because they alienate people while trying to burn a hole, laser-like, into people they believe will make the decision, thus alienating everyone else, than for any other reason.

Warn candidates that the group will undoubtedly ask questions you've already asked. Suggest that the applicant simply repeat the original answer.

You control the seating at the group interview. Instead of sitting next to the candidate, which means you'd be giving no positive eye contact, you should sit across from the candidate. Put the more difficult people on either side of the candidate so he or she won't have eye contact with them. Arrange the seating by putting name labels on file folders in which you've put the candidate's resume.

Tips for successful interviewing

- Prepare the questions in advance and try them on the employees you're happiest with. If these paragons can't answer or react unfavorably, change the questions. Remember that questions reflect your values and style and give clues to the organizational culture. Do the ones you've prepared convey the message you want to give?

- Take careful notes even if it slows the interview.

- Avoid curiosity questions that may be illegal. Questions about marital status or children are two such questions.

- Focus on the why and how. "Why have you decided to apply here?" not "Why did you decide to become a physician, nurse, secretary, etc.?" "What influenced you to seek this kind of position with us?" "Were you referred to us?" "Do you know us by reputation?"

- If you don't understand an applicant's answer or if the answer isn't complete, rephrase your question and come at it again. Let something drop, and you may have to interview a second time.

- Listen intently to the applicant's answers, not only the content but the phrasing.

- If you feel you need more information, reinterview.

The Selection Process

Go through your serious candidates and rate each on a scale of one to 10 points on the following criteria:

- Skills/experience for the job.

- Fit with the organization, including personality/style.

- Your gut response to the candidate, as in like/dislike. Yes, that's legal.

- Input from others--every interviewer should rate candidates on the same scale.

- Probable longevity in the job, if that's important.

- Other important factors.

Add up the points and decide if the total reflects your overall gut response. It is almost always fatal to hire someone you're not keen on but seems to be a perfect fit, or to hire someone with a string of job failures who "needs a chance." Charity begins at home--and ought to stay there.

Offers and Contracts

All offers of employment should be in writing. An oral offer may bind you negatively, i.e., the candidate may say you offered the job when you were really only questioning availability. If you're offering a contract, here are the elements it will need to contain:

- Crystal clear details of your compensation package, including all perks. Don't assume anything. Spell out the fringe benefits, especially nontaxable ones, such as medical, life, disability, dental, optical, legal insurance, expense account, and stock options, as applicable.

- Terms of agreement. How long does the contract run? What are the results you expect the person to achieve? Can he or she be fired at will with/without cause, or does he or she have some job security? The grounds for termination should be spelled out, as well as what the termination package will be. How much severance will be given? If a contract can be broken for cause, the possible causes on both sides should be spelled out.

- References. Specify what information the organization will report in a reference check.

- Noncompete agreements. If the new hire leaves the organization, can he or she work for a competitor?

- Confidential information. The courts are likely to uphold an employee's duty not to divulge confidential information, but you must specify in the contract what is confidential.

- Attorney's fees. If either party has to sue under the contract, the winner of the suit gets money plus attorney's fees. This promotes great reasonableness.

- Location of work unit. Where will the employee be based? Can you reassign to a distant unit, or must this be negotiated?

- Successor provision. What happens if the organization is sold or merged? Does the person's contract go to the next owner?

Orientation

Your offer is accepted and now it's time to play the new person in. Here's the best approach:

Day One. Plan to spend almost the entire day with the new hire if he or she is your direct report. Even though the person has recently been through the interviewing process, go over the job description in detail. See that the employee meets everyone in the immediate work unit. If you have coffee breaks, invite others to join the two of you. Provide a tour and begin explaining policies and procedures.

Day Two. Ask for questions that the person may have after the first day. Assign three/four hours of substantive work. Then meet for a mini-appraisal. How did things go? More questions.

Day Three. Arrange for the new hire to meet with all those with whom he or she will interact to get a feel for those individuals' expectations. Ask for feedback on these meetings.

Day Four. Lunch with top management (depending on the level of the new hire) or with your boss if it's a lower level hire. Go over the telephone directory and who does what.

Day Five. Spend an hour or so with the new hire talking about the job as a whole. Beginning on day six, he or she will be doing it all, with you available but not standing by. Emphasize how important it is to ask questions now.

Here's the rule: The more time you spend up front with the individual--and we know five days is excruciatingly long--the less time you will spend later. You are buying your way out of a mess of retraining three months from now. If you abdicate the training function, the people you least admire in the work unit will fill the void. They'll "orient" the new person in ways it will take you months to change. Protect your investment.

Early Warning Signals

You've reached this point and, just when you thought everything was under control (by the way, why did you think that?), your gut begins to tell you that your new hire isn't going to work out. Your instinct is to batter the messenger and deny the message. As Rosie said in "The African Queen," "Human nature is what we're put here to rise above." So it is in management. The first whisper that all is not well should be leapt on pronto. Call in the new hire and say, "Joe, I understand there are some problems in OB/GYN." This is a neutral opener and gives Joe a chance to say anything he wants to. The worst response, from your point of view, would be Joe saying that there are no problems. If he were aware of them, they might be easier to solve.

Use the grapevine. Most people haven't the sense of urgency or the courage to complain directly about someone's performance when that person has only been there a few weeks or months. This is a pity because the person is still new enough to be changed. If the vine is picking up a lot of negatives, you should listen. Begin taking notes. Start asking the sources of the rumors if they're true. Don't wait until someone comes to you.

Meet with the person once a week and explain what problems you're seeing/hearing about. Don't ask the person if he or she did, or failed to do, something. Instead, say, "This is how we need it done. Can you do it?" It's better to ask this question too often than not often enough. If the person says, "No, I can't live with it," you've just been handed a resignation. You won't like it particularly, but it beats having to fire someone.

Termination

There are any number of valid reasons to fire an employee, but it's rare that skills failure is the only one. The reasons that cause most terminations include inability to work well within a team framework, inability to adjust to the organization's style (with physicians this may be entrepreneurial zeal), or inflexibility, i.e., "I am medically state-of-the-art, and I must do it my way."

It is much better for the organization and the individual if you handle the termination in the following way. We assume here that you've been going over the person's performance defects, whether technical or interpersonal, so that there's little chance of his or her being surprised when you initiate the warning/suspension process. Surprised people tend to sue. Don't surprise anyone. Likewise, "Things may not work

Section II. The Content of Management

out around here" is an observation apropos of nothing, not a warning.

Step one.

Verbal warning. At the person's work station you say, "You are not seeing the appropriate number of patients. This is what you need to do," or "Five patient complaints about your care per week are too many. You must deliver and maintain a service that does not generate more than one complaint a month." Then you ask the same fateful question: "Can you do this?" If the person says, "No, I can't," you are two-thirds of the way to a resignation. Stating that he or she can't perform the job means that the person has little choice but to leave.

Step two.

Two written warnings, accepted and signed by the employee. Why two? Because it's more than one. There is no set standard, but five written warnings takes the teeth out of the warning process. Warnings begin to look like traffic tickets.

You should insist that the individual sign the warning. Understand that this doesn't mean he or she agrees with the warning, only that he or she has read it. If the person doesn't understand that is what his or her signature means, explain it. If the employee still refuses to sign, get a witness that the warning was indeed presented.

Step three.

Termination. Because firing is the organizational equivalent of taking someone off life support, death to follow, there is a tremendous, natural reluctance to fire. This is doubly true if the employee's problem is interpersonal rather than technical. The solution is to make a decision and implement it as quickly as possible.

The alternative to firing is to keep someone who isn't performing until he or she voluntarily leaves. This is unwise and damaging to the organization. It reduces productivity in the immediate work area and reduces the willingness of co-workers to live within the organization's culture and rules. It weakens management's control and destroys any semblance of a leadership image. From a legal perspective, if you keep an unsatisfactory employee for several years and don't use the perform- ance appraisal system to set corrective procedures, and that employee also happens to be over 40, you may involve the organization in a lawsuit that any lawyer would be glad to take before a jury.

Tips on Firing Humanely

- Fire at the end of the day. Is there anything worse than "forgotten but not gone?" The longer the dearly departed hangs around, the longer it takes others to get back to work. If you're firing a physician, using a locum tenens is preferable to keeping the person on until someone is hired.

- Call the person into your office and explain the terms of departure. It's cruel to make someone ask how his or her organizational life will come out. Your explanation should include when the employee is to leave, how much severance pay will be provided, and what kind of references can be expected. Allow the employee to resign if that's possible.

- Detail what other support, if any, the organization will provide. Outplacement? Counseling? Don't offer the employee a chance to use the organization's facilities. It's embarassing for the employee and has a negative effect on general productivity.

- Don't imply that there is any possibility of reconciliation. This is FINAL. Don't talk about "things not working out as either of us expected." The other person may believe that he or she isn't being dismissed, just warned.

- Ask the employee to clean out his or her work space and turn over work in process to a specific person.

- Thank the employee for his/her contribution. Wish the person well. Do not say you are sorry to see him or her go unless it's true.

The major engine for firing humanely--even when you feel like announcing the departure with champagne all around--is the effect anything but the most humane treatment will have on the survivors. They are watching, and they are your most important constituency.

Finally, did you learn anything about the selection process from the firing? Did you learn anything about your biases for or against certain kinds of people? Ultimately, the lessons of each firing should be reflected in the hiring of future employees.

Marilyn Moats Kennedy, MSJ, is Managing Partner of Career Strategies, Inc., Wilmette, Illinois.

Section II. The Content of Management

CHAPTER 19

Recruiting the Stars

by Jennifer Grebenschikoff and David Kirschman

No manager can go long without being exposed to the recruitment process. The need to add and replace staff members is always present. For the manager new to a position, there will be the inevitable replacements for staff members who simply do not fit, for whatever reason. They may have been fine under the previous occupant of the position, but with new leadership, their faults become more glaring. Or they make career decisions that do not include remaining with the organization. The longer a manager stays in a position, or with a specific organization, the more likely, and more frequent, are trips to the well for new or replacement personnel likely to be.

There are no mysteries to the recruitment process, but as in any endeavor, there is a strong element of luck. The right person comes along at just the right time. More frequently, however, the process is characterized by hard work and careful planning. Good people don't just happen, or materialize from thin air. They must be found. And that means that the searcher must have a clear idea as to what kind of person is needed. The position has to be carefully defined, along with the characteristics of the potentially successful applicant. Then live bodies have to be judged and matched with those requirements. It takes time, and it takes patience. But failure is far more expensive than the time spent in ensuring success.

There are three areas of action that must be accomplished before even the first step in the actual search takes place. We call them "Consensus," "Budget and Financial Resources Allocations," and "Planning Your Timing." Regardless of how the effort to find applicants is organized, and for many a search committee it is the first step, the need that is to be met must be defined in detail and agreement on that definition must be reached within the organization or within the part of the organization most affected by the specific recruitment effort being undertaken.

Consensus

If a search committee has been established, its members need to work together to identify the need and set up goals and objectives. Members of the committee need to work together and get to know each other so that the personality of the committee is as one. The committee also needs to develop criteria that will allow it to function as a unit. When the committee reaches out into the community and begins to talk to candidates, it is important that everyone on the committee is saying essentially the same thing about both the position and the organization. It is important to use the committee to gather support for the recruitment process itself. If there is no consensus on the committee that the position in question is needed in the organization, there is no way that other members of the organization are going to believe that what the committee is going to do is important. The best candidate may eventually be hired and then fail because the process by which the person was brought into the organization was flawed. The organization was not conditioned to believe in the need for and importance of the position.

We recently were involved in a project in which we were asked to recruit a department chief for pediatrics. We naively believed that there was a consensus in the organization that this was a necessary position and started to refer candidates to the organization. To our horror, there were people on the search committee and in the interview loop who told candidates that neither they nor the position were needed by the organization. It is critical to work diligently with the people who will be interviewing candidates and with members of the search committee to make sure that the position is needed and that all involved are fully convinced of the need.

We believe that the consensus must be broadly based in the organization. Where individuals need not participate in the consensus, they should at the very least be made to feel a part of the recruitment process. It is easy and dangerous for organizations to slip into an attitude that discounts the importance of certain employees. Your organization is more than the professionals that it hires. It is also the receptionist, who will more than likely be the first person in the organization with whom candidates have contact. The receptionist needs to be aware that the recruitment process is taking place so that the initial encounters of candidates with the organization have the best chance of being positive. The same advice can be given for a wide range of organization employees who would not, on first glance, be thought to be a part of the recruitment process.

We can point to many instances in which our candidates for physician executive positions have spent as much time talking with competing organizations and groups in the communities where the recruiting organizations were located as they did with the organization itself. A

Section II.   The Content of Management

candidate we had presented for a hospital department chief position was returning with his wife for a second visit. Because they were quite serious about this position, they spent five days (at their own expense) looking at all aspects of the community. They visited the other hospitals, cultural organizations, realtors, schools, grocery stores (where they comparison-shopped), and individual physicians. Because the other providers in the community knew that this hospital was recruiting, they were able to help recruit this department chief. This may be a sensitive issue, but it may become worse if key organizations and people in the community don't know that you are trying to recruit. An important function of the search committee is to help not only the entire organization to get ready for the actual recruiting, but also the community. Developing these kinds of consensus can ensure that the recruitment process is smooth at all its steps.

Budget and Financial Resources Allocations

No recruitment effort is without its costs, and a well-done effort can be expensive. This is true whether the recruitment effort is conducted entirely by the organization or whether outside sources are used. The direct costs obviously are advertising expenses, interview expenses, and travel, room and board, and moving costs for the candidate. When the position involves recruiting a physician who will be both a department chairman or manager and a practitioner, there is also likely to be a need for new equipment, office space, additional support staff, etc. Direct costs are not going to be prohibitively high, but there are going to be expenses.

Indirect costs are slightly more difficult to assess. There is the staff time that is spent on written correspondence, telephone communication, and other clerical and secretarial tasks. Probably the most expensive indirect cost, however, is the time spent by staff on the interview process. There are many organizations that involve 10 or 15 people in the interview process. That is probably too many. If only one hour is spent on each interview by each participating member of the organization, the time expenditure becomes very expensive.

The table on the next page shows the cost of recruiting a physician for a multispecialty group practice. The data are for a particular group, so they may not be typical, but we believe that they are informative. The group determined that it costs $32,000 to recruit a physician when three candidates are to be interviewed. The process is conducted without the use of a recruiter. For the most part, these costs are for staff time, the majority of which is for time spent in developing the position description, deciding on a recruitment strategy, and then interviewing and screening candidates. Out-of-pocket costs are very small.

In viewing and using these data, it is important to remember the conditions under which they have been accumulated. No outside

COST OF RECRUITING A PHYSICIAN

Steps in the Recruiting Process	Time	Number of Individuals Involved	Dollar Value
Identification of Need	Variable	—	—
Development of Criteria (candidate)	3 hrs	12	$5,292
Placement of Advertising	3 hrs	1	441
Receiving Initial Screening of Applicants' CVs & Telephone Inquiries	10 hrs	3	4,410
Board Review of Primary Candidate	2 hrs	12	3,528
Recruiting Committee Review	5 hrs	5	3,675
Contacts with Top 3 Candidates to Set Up Visits	6 hrs	3	2,646
Visit with 3 Candidates & Spouses (average 1½ days each)	36 hrs	1 per hour	5,292
Contact References	3 hrs	3	1,323
Second Visit of Top Candidate (2½ days)	20 hrs	1 per hour	2,940
Negotiations with Top Candidate	8 hrs	2 hrs	2,352
Other Misc. Contacts with Candidate's Spouse, Representatives e.g. Lawyers, Accountants, etc.	4 hrs	1	588
TOTAL RECRUITING COSTS			**$32,487**

recruitment resources were used. Only three candidates were selected for interviews. And the data don't include the $10,000 to $20,000 it would cost to move the successful candidate into the organization. Further, this represents a search that has gone smoothly. Three candidates were interviewed, an offer was extended to one of them, and that candidate accepted. That is a very successful, and unusual, recruitment scenario.

Planning Your Timing

This element of the recruitment process might just as easily have been termed "patience." The recruitment of physicians and physician executives is time-consuming. If the process is well-organized and runs smoothly, it will require from 4 to 8 months between the initiation of the process and the arrival of the new employee. Generally, once the offer is made and accepted, another period is involved before the candidate begins work. Unless the successful candidate is unemployed, 60-90 days' notice will have to be given to the current employer.

Let us share a typical recruitment time schedule. Let us assume that the decision to recruit is made on May 1. It will probably take one to two months to locate candidates, screen their credentials, contact all those who respond to inquiries, check their references, and start to invite candidates for interviews. By the time you are ready for interviews, it's July. It will take another two months to interview candidates. Many organizations try to interview more than one candidate on the same day. If the organization has a large physical plant, this technique may be possible. However, we advise caution. First, it is poor technique to have candidates bumping into each other in the hallway. Also, as many as 5 or 6 current employees have to be scheduled to interview candidates, it may not be possible to get to them more often than every second week.

Typical Recruitment Time Schedule

Decision made to recruit .... **May 1**

Locate candidates, screen credentials, contact all respondents, check references, set up interviews

Start first and second interviews .... **July 1**

Extend offer to top candidate and send contract .... **September 1**

Candidate accepts offer .... **September 15**

Candidate becomes licensed and relocates

Candidate begins employment .... **December 15**

So, now it is September 1 and an offer has been made to the top candidate. That person can't be expected to respond in two days. A week to two weeks is required for the candidate to think about the offer. A contract is sent, and, by September 15th, it is known that the candidate will be joining the organization. In most organizations, medical directors must be licensed in the organization's state just to work in a clinical setting, whether they are practicing or not. That process will take time. The candidate also must find housing. It will be another two to three months before the candidate is on site.

So a process that started on May 1st is finally completed by about December 15th. It has taken about six months. And the same process would be involved whether the position involved practicing physicians, medical directors, department chairmen, vice presidents of medical affairs, or any other physician position.

What's the Candidate Worth?

Both the candidate and the organization are interested in the compensation package that will be agreed to. The candidate will want to be sure that his or her services are being fairly and adequately paid for. The organization will want to be sure that it is matching but not greatly exceeding market value for the position being filled. The most important thing to point out to a candidate is what the net economic benefit will be. In order to do that, the cost of living where the organization is located will have to be compared with that where the candidate currently resides. When a candidate says that an offer has been received that is $10,000 or $20,000 higher than your organization's, it is entirely possible that the net economic benefit of your organization's location is higher. A good source of information on cost of living differentials is Rand McNally's *Places Rated Almanac*. Its economic life profiles on 329 metropolitan areas include indexes for various costs of living. By comparing the index for your city with that of the candidate's city, you can show a candidate just what the differences in living costs will be. Also, some locales are inherently more attractive than others, so there is a differential based on the perceived geographical amenities of locations. Of course, all this is tempered by the level of costs. For instance, San Jose, California, is an extremely attractive city, but it is also very expensive. Albuquerque, New Mexico, is also desirable, and its cost level is lower. One would expect to pay higher salaries in San Jose than in Albuquerque. Duluth, Minnesota, on the other hand, while it has a low cost of living, is viewed as an undesirable location. As a result, salaries are apt to be higher there. (As a general aside, salary levels can be expected to be somewhat higher when professional recruiters are employed, just because the positions that are given to these professionals tend to be more difficult to fill.)

There is little evidence that the organizational environment has much effect on the level of compensation for physician executives. For instance, the AAMD's 1986 compensation survey shows that average base salaries for medical directors in hospitals, HMOs, and groups tend to be in the $100,000 to $120,000 range. These physician executives in groups and HMOs have slightly higher salaries because these organizations are more inclined to have bonus and other incentive programs in place. According to the AAMD survey, there also is little in the way of regional variation in salaries for physician executives. An HMO medical director in Richmond, Virginia, will probably earn about the same amount as an HMO medical director in Milwaukee, Wisconsin.

Critical Factors in the Recruitment Process

Recruitment is the business of enticement. The goal is to woo someone to a position. There are basically two kinds of candidates--voluntary and involuntary. The former candidates are actively in the job market. They answer ads and can be at your organization whenever they are needed. They'll stay with the organization no matter what it does to them. Involuntary candidates are more difficult. They may not be available. They are not looking for jobs. They are probably happy where they are. They have to be attracted to new positions.

Two factors make the difference between success and failure in recruitment--timing and attitude. The average "shelf life" of an attractive candidate is less than 30 days. Someone will reach the candidate in that period, or the candidate will reach someone. The candidate has absolutely no reason to wait, because he doesn't even know that your organization is interested in filling a position. One week can lose a good candidate.

Attitude is of equal importance to timing in influencing a candidate. When interviewing or otherwise expressing an interest in hiring a candidate, your attitude should be one of accommodating the needs of the candidate. It is not enough to rearrange schedules and make room for interviewing the candidate. In every possible way, the candidate must feel wanted, even pampered if possible. The candidate should have to do little more than arrive for the interview on a given day at a given time. All other arrangements should be taken care of by your organization. Otherwise, the candidate, through lack of familiarity with your organization and location, may make travel or housing arrangements that are unsuitable. Remember, the purpose of the recruitment process, including the interview, is to woo the candidate.

It is useful to view the recruitment process as a three-stage approach to the acquisition of employees: Sourcing, recruiting, and closing. The first two stages really involve locating prospects and then convincing them to at least visit the organization, to be interviewed. There are two objectives in the interview. One is to discover whether the candidate is attractive enough for your oragnization and the other is to sell the candidate on the opportunity. A problem with interviewing is that those are two completely mutually exclusive tasks. What most of us do is spend all of our time trying to discover whether the candidate is acceptable and none of our time trying to sell the candidate on the opportunity that the organization and the position represent. Recruitment is also the business of deal-making. So the overall goal is a deal with, ideally, the best candidate.

Sourcing

Sourcing is all about coming up with an attractive candidate. It is the art of casting a wide net so that largest possible pool of candidates is available for choice. Calling your mother-in-law and asking for a recommendation is a good example of sourcing. Putting a billboard on the highway will occasionally attract a candidate. The goal is to cast a net wide enough that, after the winnowing process, there are at least a couple of fish left in it at the end. The source with the highest probability of success is colleagues. A call to 10 colleagues for recommendations of candidates in the field in which recruitment is intended will provide at least one well-recommended, well-screened candidate at a relatively low investment of time and money.

New Leadership in Health Care Management

Next in order of probability are physicians on the organization's staff. Anyone related to the field will be of help. Of course advice has to be tempered by knowledge of these physicians' biases, but frequently the best candidates come from recommendations from those most closely associated with the environment into which the candidate is to be recruited. Professional recruiters will frequently use just this technique with great success, and at substantial cost to the organization. It's very inexpensive and very good recruiting to check inside before going outside. Again, we would be willing to bet that if you ask 10 of your own colleagues to make a couple of calls for recommendations, you would have yet another good candidate. And you are closing in on enough candidates to fill your own search.

Medical training programs near the organization can also be a source of candidates, certainly not for physician executives, but for staff physicians. But don't write a letter--call. A letter to the residency program will be posted on a bulletin board along with all the other letters that have been sent requesting residents, and no one will ever answer. A personal call to the department chairman for recommendations will usually elicit good ones. The chairman is anxious to place the program's best candidates.

National meetings of specialty societies can be an excellent source of candidates. A substantial amount of recruiting occurs at these meetings outside of the sessions. Physicians currently employed by the organization are likely to attend the meetings, and may be willing to interview candidates. In this case, a note on the bulletin board can attract some good candidates.

State medical associations are a possible source that should not be overlooked. Most of them have listings of people who would like to move into the organization's area. The technique is low cost, even if the results are somewhat unpredictable.

The remainder of the sourcing techniques are generally less productive. Residency job fairs are not recommended. There are three recruiters for every potential candidate. Given the odds for success, the technique is very high cost.

Advertising as a sourcing technique is high cost and low return, low yield. It may generate a lot of responses, but there is no screening mechanism. Anybody who chooses can answer the ad. It isn't the cost of the advertising that's so high; it's the time and costs in screening the responses. It's the professional job hunters who routinely answer ads. The satisfied candidates aren't looking for new employers, so the advertising pages don't normally attract them. Of course, some organizations may be forced to advertise for political or legal reasons. In any case, expectations of results should not be high.

Recruiters are also high cost. They require low time involvement on the organization's part and can be high yield. They can also merely be high cost. Whether a recruiter is worthwhile has a lot to do with the caliber of the recruiter. In choosing a recruiter, have representatives of the firm in for a personal interview before hiring anybody. And carefully check references. Wherever possible, attempt to check with clients whose names are not supplied by the recruiter. Networking with other managers can be especially productive at this point.

It is surprising how many physicians don't understand the value of networking. As potential candidates, which all physicians are, physicians should always be looking at the market and letting others know what they are doing, what is important to them, and what their career time frames are so that when recruiters are trying to find physician executives, they don't rely on ads. For the most part, recruiters use personal letters and personal telephone calls anyway. If they don't already know about a good prospect through networking, they can't recommend the person.

Direct mail is also high cost and it takes some special talents to do it, but the advantage that it offers is that it's targeted. Lists can be purchased from organizations such as the American Medical Association that have only those persons who meet the basic criteria for the position to be filled. In addition, screening before the list is purchased will ensure that the only potential responses are those in which the organization is interested.

Direct mail is not a high-response technique. Generally, the response rate is about one percent. Including a prepaid postcard or a tollfree telephone number for reply may help, but a one percent response is typical. More important, if list selection has been done appropriately and prescreening has been performed, the responses come from persons who match the criteria for the position to be filled.

If the organization enjoys a dominant position in the community, there is a high probability of success in recruiting locally. The approach has many advantages. Relocation time is reduced, there is greater knowledge of the person being recruited, and there is the possibility of inflicting damage on the competition. The military, government, the U.S. Public Health Service, and the Veterans Administration may also be good sources of candidates. There are about 14,000 physicians in these organizations, and about 20 percent of them will leave each year. Lists are hard to obtain, but they are worthwhile places to look.

Pre-Interview Stage

The interview stage should be approached with the same care and planning that has characterized other segments of the recruiting process. A preliminary step is important after the list of candidates to be interviewed has been determined. An indepth telephone conversation should be conducted with each candidate before interview invitations are extended. There are four questions that need to be answered:

- Why is the candidate worth spending time and money on?

- What about the candidate will make the organization want to extend an offer?

- What will it take to get the candidate to accept the position?

- Why is the candidate interested in the position?

We recommend that in the initial telephone conversation, before the candidate is invited for interviews, questions be asked about the candidate's present earnings and earnings expectations. When the time comes for an offer, this information is invaluable. The questions also are asked at a neutral point and the answers amount to little more than background information. When they are asked at the end of an interview, room for maneuverability is lost.

References

References should always be checked by telephone, not in writing. Few references will be willing to be candid in writing. Also, references should be checked in advance of interviews so that all interviewers are better prepared and will know what weaknesses and what strengths to look for. We start with three references. If we have three clean references, we stop. If we have two clean references and one bad reference, we add three more references to the pool. If one of those three is bad, the process is repeated until all three are clean.

To repeat, all reference checking is conducted by telephone. We recommend that the calls be taped so that the caller's concentration can be on the conversation and not on notes. Of course, the reference must be told that the conversation will be taped. If the taping is rejected, then don't tape the conversation. Without permission, the practice is against the law.

The health care field is unique when it comes to references. It is the only field of which we are aware in which references will tell you anything. If the right and enough questions are asked, almost any important information can be learned from references in the field. There is a caution, however, if the reference is bad. Any information that you receive that reflects poorly on a candidate must be retained in strictest confidence. Failure on this account may result in a lawsuit for passing along malicious hearsay.

After this step, the list of potential candidates should be complete and the interviewing process can begin. There is another step before actual interviews, however, that can do much to ensure the success of the interviews. A great deal of information about the candidates, as well as the interview process itself, should be disseminated to all the persons in the organization who will participate in the interviewing. Curricula vitae and references should be delivered to interviewers in advance. Ideally, a checklist will be developed that indicates which interviewers are responsible for which questions and what is expected specifically from each interviewer. The checklist details what each participant in the interviewing is expected to contribute to the process and all the steps that are to be completed so that the interviewing produces its intended results. The checklist also attempts to prevent unintended organizational fumbling by the interviewers. For any position, there may be an organizational problem that all the interviewers are aware of. If all of them make a point of discussing the problem with candidates, an unintended negative image of the organization may result and desirable candidates may be driven away. The problem area and its description can be assigned to one of the interviewers on the checklist, so that the problem does not become overblown. The remainder of the interviewing team is responsible for selling the organization and the position to candidates.

Interviews

The interview has two mutually exclusive objectives. First, the organization must determine if the candidate is someone whom it wants to hire. Second, if that is true and sometimes before it is known to be true, the organization desires to convince the candidate that the organization and the position in question are desirable. In the screening phase, the key is to listen. Only open-ended questions should be asked. Basically, the goal is a gut impression on whether the candidate fits the organization and the position. It just isn't possible in the interview to determine if the candidate is professionally qualified. The professional characteristics of a candidate should always be determined before the interview through a check of references.

A matter of concern is the type of questions that can legally be asked in the interview. Any question is allowed as long as the answer will not be the basis of the decision. If there is an interest in the age of candidates but there are no criteria on this subject in the job description for the position, the question may be asked. If there are age criteria, the question may not be asked. There are obvious questions that shouldn't be asked, such as, for female candidates, the issue of maternity. If interviewers are asking these questions, they have to be stopped immediately. To avoid this problem, the search committee should set question parameters at the beginning of the recruitment process.

While inquiries on certain topics (such as age, sex, religion, and national origin) might be considered a violation of equal employment opportunity laws, there are some other issues that pose a risk of discrimination. These include the candidate's availability to work on weekends (religious discrimination), children and child care (sex discrimination), and friends and relatives employed by the organization (racial and sex discrimination).

Of course the issue here is potential discrimination. And the litigation that the potential represents. When there is even a hint that formal discrimination of any kind can be charged, we recommend that the candidate in question be invited for an interview. An organization is allowed to make professional judgments on which candidate is the best fit for a position. So no harm is likely if the questionable candidate is rejected after an interview. In the absence of an interview, the issue of discrimination may remain unresolved.

The interview schedule should be arranged so that there is a strong person in the first slot, a block of time for finance and business in the middle, and then the medical director or other chief medical officer at the very end. The medical officer should have at least one hour and preferably two in which to obtain feedback, answer questions, and convince the candidate of the desirability of the organization and the position. Before the final interview takes place, as much as possible of the content of the previous interviews should be obtained so that the medical officer has a clear idea of the status of the interview process.

In selling the organization and position, always point out the obvious. Interviewers may know that the position, the organization, and the town are the most wonderful in the world, but there's every chance the candidate doesn't know those things. Modesty is not a virtue in the interviewing process.

A very large number of questions need to be answered during the interviews. Some of the questions that we believe need to be a part of the process are shown below. Don't try and ask any one candidate every question. There simply isn't time, and all the questions don't necessarily apply in every case anyway. If there are novice interviewers on the schedule, it might be advisable to slice the list of questions up and give all the interviewers parts. This will also ensure that several questions are not asked repeatedly. There is almost nothing worse than than having people on the interview schedule all ask the same set questions. Of course, there may be selected questions for which it is advisable to have comparison answers.

Typical Interview Questions

Experience

Tell me about your present position.

What aspects of your position do you like best?

What aspects of your position do you like least?

Name three accomplishments in your position of which you are particularly proud and provide details on what the accomplishment involved.

What have you been criticized for during the past four years? Do you agree or disagree with the criticism, and what is the reasoning behind your reaction?

What are your three greatest strengths? Weaknesses?

What would your subordinates say about you? What would they say they would like for you to do differently? Why do you think they would say this, and why didn't you make the changes?

How do you criticize your subordinates?

What would your boss/colleagues say needs improving about you? Would you agree with this assessment or not, and why?

How did you go about firing the last employee for which this step was necessary?

If an emergency arises, are you more interested in the cause or the solution of the problem?

What is the most difficult thing you ever had to do in your job?

Use three positive adjectives to describe yourself. Use three negative adjectives to describe yourself.

If you were able to choose a different career, what would you choose? Why?

How many hours are you used to working?

Recreation

How do you spend your leisure time?

What are your geographic preferences?

What town size do you prefer?

Do you have major needs/restrictions regarding the community?

Decribe your family, its needs, its activities.

Is religious affiliation important?

What is your financial condition?

How has your health been in recent years?

How did you get into this profession?

Does your spouse have a career? What is it, and will it affect your decision?

Compensation

What is your total compensation and what are its elements?

What are your fringe benefits?

Wind-Up

What else should I know about your qualifications or about you?

The job of the clean-up interviewer is to close. It is important to remember that the goal of the process is to make a deal with the candidate. At the end of the interview, some feedback should be given to the candidate. The candidate should know if his or her candidacy is active and whether the interview has been a good one.

After the feedback, the best way to recruit is to make an immediate and specific offer. There is no better moment than when the candidate is sitting across the desk. The offer should be specific. It should clearly state a desire to have the candidate join the organization and include the compensation amount and the starting date. Sometimes organizational policy does not permit an offer at this stage. While the statement cannot be an offer, all of the components of an offer can be included, with the provision that a formal offer must await whatever internal approval is required.

Post-Interview

Another critical juncture in the recruiting process is the post-interview stage. What is needed at this stage is consensus on the part of the interviewers. Consensus can be achieved more readily if the post-interview evaluations are in written rather than in oral form. We recommend that a form that all interviewers are expected to complete be developed.

The candidates should hear from the organization soon after the interviews, ideally within three days. A candidate's status should not be allowed to just sit for several weeks. Candidates are not going to be anxious to return if a second interview is required or may be disinclined to seriously consider any offer if two or three weeks are required for decisions. If there are difficulties in reaching a decision, let the candidates know. Candidates should also know how many candidates are in the running for the position. Mostly, this ongoing contact is a matter of courtesy and an effort to maintain interest on the part of persons who have been identified as serious contenders for the position. Now is not the point to lose a candidate who has potential with the organization.

Second Interviews

In hiring physicians or physician executives, second interviews are a critical point in the process. The list of candidates has probably been reduced to two or three names, and, if the process has been effective to date, one of these persons will be hired. Every detail of the return trip should be attended to with care. Presumably, the candidate's spouse is being invited for this interview. In addition to establishing a detailed agenda for the candidate's trip, a similar agenda should be put together for the spouse. A lot of detail is involved. To avoid difficulties, it may be advisable to assign the entire process to a member of the support staff and provide the person with a checklist of details that have to be accomplished. Within the return interview itself, it should be decided in advance who will make the offer, when the offer is to be made, and who will ask and who will answer what questions.

Now comes the time for decision-making, for both the organization and the candidates who have been interviewed. Frequently, candidates are slow to indicate their decisions on offers. Responses just aren't forthcoming. The wait for a response from one candidate places the status of other candidates in jeopardy. Deadlines should be established, preferably 10 days. If the offer isn't accepted by the end of that time, it expires. There's about an 80 percent probability that a candidate will accept a position in 10 days after the interview. After that, the probabilities decrease rapidly. The candidate who can't give an answer doesn't want the job. Three weeks later, the candidate may come back and accept the position, but not because it's a first choice.

If the recruitment process is done well, if all of the details have been carefully attended to, the result is hiring the best candidate, both for the position and for the organization. Recruiting high-quality people to your organization is hard work, but if your organization is committed to the recruitment process, you will be able to attract and hire the candidates you want.

Jennifer Grebenschikoff is Vice President and David Kirschman is President of the Physician Executive Management Center, the recruitment and counseling affiliate of the American Academy of Medical Directors.

CHAPTER 20

The Physician Executive and the Law

by Miles J. Zaremski and David J. Schwartz

H istorically, a hospital had only the responsibility to provide room and board for patients, facilities for operations, and attendants to assist physicians in patient care. Because attending physicians were not employees of the hospital, liability for injury resulting from a physician's negligent patient care did not pass through to the hospital; only the physician who caused the injury bore responsibility. Consequently, legal issues concerning health care institution management were relatively simple.

Today, hospitals and other health care facilities find themselves the dominant force in administering patient care within their respective facilities. The judicial system, reacting accordingly, now places a great deal of legal responsibility on the health care institution itself for the quality of overall patient care. A hospital's ultimate responsibility for quality care, combined with the litigious nature of American society, makes it imperative that the physician executive be aware of some of the more common legal issues that a health care institution may confront.

Legal issues a hospital is most likely to confront are liability to a patient for negligent injury and liability to a health professional for granting or withholding medical staff privileges. As institutional responsibility includes the use of reasonable care in selecting, retaining, and monitoring medical staff, a close look will be taken at the Health Care Quality Control Act, a new federal law that mandates centralized reporting of potentially substandard medical conduct.

Enhanced hospital responsibility for patient care means that an institution must continually review and evaluate the quality of care rendered by its staff. The predictable result is that some practitioners will have privileges denied or terminated. As a physician's livelihood often depends on hospital privileges, the denial or termination of privileges may have dire financial consequences on the physician's ability to maintain or develop a practice. Therefore, a conflict may develop between the hospital's interests in firm internal control and careful screening and

Section II.   The Content of Management

the practitioner's interest in broad freedom to practice his or her trade. The result may be a lawsuit with the allegation that the denial or termination of staff privileges constitutes an unlawful restraint of trade that violates antitrust laws. Although hospitals tend to be on the winning side in these disputes, an understanding of the legal concepts involved is very important.

As exposure to civil liability increases, a hospital must undertake effective risk management techniques that require the maintenance of firm control over the quality of health care administered within its walls. However, an institution that holds the reins too tightly may face a legal doctrine mandating that only licensed persons, not corporations, be allowed to practice medicine. This places the institution in an awkward position. The fulcrum that determines what constitutes the "practice" of medicine is control. Thus, while a hospital is responsible for overall patient care and must exercise firm control to maintain high-quality care, an overzealous hospital administrator may expose the institution to the charge of unlawfully practicing medicine.

Furthermore, in order to protect the institution from various forms of liability exposure, an effective risk protection program is mandatory. However, insurance increasingly is unavailable or unaffordable. Consequently, risk managers now look to alternative risk protection mechanisms.

When all else fails and a lawsuit commences, the physician executive should be familiar with rules that govern a plaintiff's right to discover data produced by the institution, such as peer review records and risk management documents.

Hospital Liability for Negligence

Upon initiation of treatment or admission of a patient into a hospital, a duty arises requiring the rendering of patient care services that meet the legally required standard of care determined by reference to hospital bylaws, regulations, and JCAH standards. When a hospital or other health care facility breaches this standard of care, liability may result pursuant to two primary legal doctrines: respondeat superior and corporate negligence.

Historically, hospitals were not responsible for the negligent acts of physicians using their facilities. Hospitals were, in effect, administrative shells providing the framework within which doctors practiced. While a hospital could be liable if it failed to provide an adequate environment, the facility was not directly responsible, nor could it be held directly accountable, for the quality of care itself.

Respondeat Superior

Under general rules of agency law, an employer may be liable for the acts or omissions of an employee who committed them while acting within the scope of employment. This doctrine, know as *Respondeat Superior* (Let the Master Answer), means that a health care facility may be held indirectly accountable for the negligence of its employees. Thus, although a hospital may have breached no direct duty to a patient, if someone within the hospital's control, such as a physician on the hospital's payroll, is responsible for patient injury, the hospital will be held accountable too.

The only wrinkle in the above analysis is that, traditionally, physicians with staff privileges, other than residents and interns, have not been treated by the courts as hospital employees. In order to maintain physician control over patient care, courts historically precluded physicians from dividing their responsibility and accountability between patient and employer. Thus, the hospital was treated as the administrative shell within which physicians, as independent contractors and not as hospital employees, were allowed to practice.

While hospitals have often escaped liability for the negligence of physicians acting as independent contractors, certain individuals, such as residents, nurses, or full-time salaried physicians, are undeniably hospital employees for whom the rule of *respondeat superior* will apply. However, a second legal doctrine, that of the borrowed servant, sometimes serves to protect the hospital from liability even for the negligence of its direct employees. If a hospital's actual right to direct and control the activities of an employee are delegated to an independent staff physician, such as when a surgeon instructs a nurse in the details of a specific act, the doctor, rather than the hospital, will be liable for the negligence of that employee. The doctrine of *respondeat superior* still applies, but in this instance the independent contractor is deemed to have borrowed the employee from the hospital and, therefore, is treated as the employer.

Although the borrowed servant doctrine protects the hospital from certain accountability it would otherwise confront, a third rule of agency law may subject a health care entity to liability it normally would not face. If an independent contractor holds himself or herself out as, or is reasonably perceived to be, a facility's employee, and a patient relies on that perception to his or her detriment, the hospital will be judicially precluded from denying the agency relationship. In this instance, under the doctrine of apparent or ostensible agency, the hospital may be treated as the employer.[1]

Corporate Negligence

Throughout the years, the hospital was not considered to be directly

Section II.   The Content of Management

responsible for the quality of patient care. If liability attached at all, it was derivative as a result of employee negligence. However, the 1965 Illinois Supreme Court case, *Darling v. Charleston Community Memorial Hospital*,[2] was the genesis for the concept of direct hospital accountability in the corporate boardroom for patient injury. This judicially recognized doctrine, known as "corporate negligence," reflects the public perception and expectancy of the modern hospital as a multifaceted health care facility responsible for the total quality of medical care and treatment rendered.

The *Darling* decision recognized a hospital's obligation to provide overall surveillance of the quality of care a patient receives and rejected the notion of the hospital as an administrative shell in which independent practitioners render patient care. *Darling* and its progeny hold that a hospital has a duty to establish a mechanism to evaluate the quality of medical care provided by the hospital and its staff and to act to avoid unreasonable risk of patient harm. Thus, a hospital has an independent and direct duty to oversee patient care within its four walls, to exercise care to ensure that physicians selected as members of the medical staff are competent, and to continually review and delineate staff privileges so that incompetent staff members are not retained. The quality of care required is determined by reference to accreditation standards, medical staff bylaws, and licensing regulations.

In the 1980 Wisconsin case, *Johnson v. Misericordia Community Hospital*,[3] the hospital failed to adhere to established procedures for checking a particular physician's credentials prior to granting him staff privileges. While on the staff, that physician negligently injured a patient. Had the hospital adhered to established procedures, it would have discovered that several other hospitals had investigated him and either denied or restricted his privileges. The court stated, "Misericordia's failure to adhere to established procedures with regard to the 'credentials process' involved a breach of the separate and distinct duty owed to potential patients and, therefore, created a foreseeable and unreasonable risk of harm to such patients."

In a 1986 Illinois Appellate Court decision,[4] a newborn was injured after being overoxygenated. The Board of Health regulations required there be one registered professional nurse trained in the care of newborn and premature infants. The hospital's failure to have a specialty trained nurse on duty at the time of injury was found to be a breach of a direct duty owed by the hospital to the newborn. Consequently, the hospital was held liable for the injury.

Although the doctrine of corporate negligence creates a direct duty between hospital and patient, it does not mean that a hospital is liable for individual acts of negligence occurring under its roof. The hospital is not a guarantor of adequate medical care. Isolated acts of negligence by an otherwise competent physician are that physician's sole responsibility. However, if the qualification or competency of the hospital staff or overall hospital monitoring system becomes an issue (i.e., but for the physician being on staff, the negligent act would not have taken place), the hospital may be held liable for violating an independent duty of care owed the patient.

Finally, while the screening, monitoring, and reviewing function may be delegated on a day-to-day basis to the medical staff, the duty and responsibility for those functions are nondelegable. The medical staff that performs the oversight function acts as the agent of the governing board, which, under the doctrine of *respondeat superior*, remains fully accountable.

Health Care Quality Improvement Act of 1986

On November 19, 1986, President Reagan signed into law the Health Care Quality Improvement Act of 1986.[5] This statute was premised on the finding by Congress that medical malpractice and the need to improve the quality of medical care are problems requiring intervention and monitoring on the federal level. Also, a need was found to restrict the ability of incompetent physicians to move from one state to another without disclosure or discovery of prior incompetent performance and to develop an effective professional peer review system.

The new federal law mandates that every entity that makes a payment under an insurance policy (including self-insurance), or in partial or full satisfaction or settlement of a judgment, must report the following information to the Secretary of Health and Human Services (HHS) or to an appropriate private or public agency as the Secretary designates:

- The name of any physician or licensed health care practitioner for whose benefit the payment is made.

- The amount of payment.

- The name (if known) of any hospital with which the physician or practitioner is affiliated or associated.

- A description of the acts or omissions and injuries or illnesses upon which the action or claim was based.

- Such other information as the Secretary determines is required for appropriate interpretation of information reported under this section.

The above information must also be reported to the appropriate state licensing board. Any entity that fails to report information of a payment required by the Act is subject to a $10,000 fine for each payment involved.

Section II.   The Content of Management

Next, the Act requires that a Board of Medical Examiners that takes adverse action against a physician for reasons relating to a physician's professional conduct or competence must report the name of the physician involved to HHS along with a description of the acts or omissions that led to the adverse action and other information HHS deems appropriate.

Third, a health care entity or professional society of physicians that follows a formal peer review process that takes action adversely affecting the clinical privileges of a physician for longer than 30 days, or accepts a physician's surrender of clinical privileges, must report to the Board of Medical Examiners the name of the physician involved and the reasons for the action taken. A health care entity that fails to substantially meet the reporting requirement will not be protected under the provisions of the Act that prevent liability for professional review actions.

Fourth, on the following occasions, it is the duty of each hospital to request information reported under this law from HHS:

- At the time a physician or a licensed health care practitioner applies to be on the medical staff or for clinical privileges at the hospital.

- Once every 2 years for any physician or practitioner who is on the medical staff or has been granted clinical privileges at the hospital. A hospital also may request this information at other times.

If the hospital does not request the information as required by this Act, it will be presumed to have had knowledge of any information reported under this law with respect to a physician or practitioner. Additionally, a hospital may rely upon information provided under this law and will not be held liable, in the absence of the hospital's knowledge that the information provided was false.

The Act also provides that the Secretary of HHS must, upon request, provide information requested under the Act to state licensing boards, to hospitals, and to other health care entities (including HMOs) that have entered, or may be entering, into an employment or affiliation relationship with a physician who has applied for clinical privileges or appointment to the medical staff.

The Act further requires confidentiality of disclosed information, provides penalties for breach of confidentiality, and contains a provision protecting the review body or its members from liability.

Antitrust and the Hospital

With the emergence of for-profit health care facilities and alternative health care organizations, general legal principles of competition have become an increasing concern for health care management. Various forms of joint venture, mergers, and consolidations may result in exposure to allegations of antitrust violations.

One of the more common areas of antitrust exposure that is unique to the health care industry involves staff membership, privileges, and credentialing decisions. When a doctor's privileges are terminated or denied, the physician's practice no doubt will suffer direct economic harm. Given the fact that a successful antitrust suit can result in the award of triple damages, it is not uncommon for the injured physician to attempt an antitrust action.

There are several federal and state statutes that provide the underpinning of a health care professional's antitrust suit, although state rules generally parallel federal statutes. With reference to staffing issues, the primary federal law is the Sherman Act, which prohibits "every contract, combination...or conspiracy in restraint of trade or commerce." Section 1 of the Sherman Act applies to combinations and conspiracies to fix prices, allocate markets, and engage in group boycotts; it also covers tying and exclusive dealing arrangements.

Conspiracy, by definition, must involve an agreement between two or more entities. In view of the multiple layers of relationships in hospital care and administration, it seems that identifying two conspiring entities would be fairly straightforward. However, such is not the case. A basic rule of law states that a single entity cannot conspire with itself.[6] Therefore, if a hospital and its medical staff or peer review committee are treated as a single entity, there can be no antitrust violation. The claim of single identity is often the first line of defense asserted in an antitrust action. Depending on specific facts, some courts have accepted this defense while others have not.

Where individual members of an organization have a personal interest in the exclusion of the complaining party, a court is more likely to find the existence of separate and distinct entities. However, the court's acceptance of two entities is only one step in the analysis of an antitrust lawsuit. It does not mean that the plaintiff will prevail. A very recent case provides an example.

In a 1987 decision, *Mosby v. American Medical International*,[7] a federal court dismissed a lawsuit by a radiologist who alleged that the hospital and a second radiologist conspired to prevent him from maintaining his practice at the hospital. The plaintiff, a staff radiologist, was listed on the hospital's on-call roster of radiologists. The hospital contracted with the second radiologist to provide continuous radiology services for the physicians practicing at the hospital. The contracting radiologist used the on-call roster for referrals in order to meet his obligation to provide services during evening and weekend hours. However, he later decided to hire a full-time assistant and ceased using

Section II.   The Content of Management

the on-call roster. The plaintiff applied for, but was denied, the assistant position. He later filed a lawsuit.[8]

Although it was clear the hospital and the contracting radiologist were two entities that were capable of conspiring, the court did not find evidence of an unreasonable restraint of trade. As the contracting radiologist could have concluded he could better control the quality of services provided under the contract by hiring an assistant, the court determined the alleged restraint had justifications that outweighed possible anticompetitive effects.

Had the above case involved an agreement among competitors, such as among several doctors, the court would not have treated the case so lightly. Agreements among competitors have traditionally been treated more strictly by the courts than agreements among noncompeting entities. An allegation that several doctors are engaging in a concerted refusal to deal with a practitioner outside their group has a greater chance of success than an allegation that a hospital and a physicians' group are refusing to deal with another physician.

The difference in judicial treatment lies in the difference between the *per se* rule and the "rule of reason." Agreements among competitors, also known as horizontal restraints, have traditionally been subject to *per se* analysis. Under this reasoning, proof that the alleged conduct occurred is sufficient; the act itself is conclusively presumed to have an anticompetitive effect and is, therefore, illegal *per se*.

In *Arizona v. Maricopa County Medical Society*,[9] competing physicians who were members of a foundation for medical care agreed upon minimum prices as full payment for medical services rendered to policy-holders of approved insurance programs. Finding that the physicians' conduct constituted horizontal price fixing, the court ruled it to be a *per se* violation of the Sherman Act. It was unnecessary for the court to receive evidence concerning the actual effect of the restraint.

Similarly, in *Weiss v. York Hospital*,[10] the court applied the *per se* rule to a horizontal group boycott. In *Weiss*, members of the medical staff agreed to disallow staff privileges to all osteopathic physicians. The court held that such concerted action automatically is presumed to have an anticompetitive effect in the marketplace.

In contrast to the *per se* rule, rule of reason analysis imposes a much more difficult burden on the complaining party. Not only must the plaintiff prove the alleged conduct occurred, but also that such conduct constitutes an *unreasonable* restraint of trade. In other words, rule of reason analysis allows the defendant to justify the challenged conduct and requires the court to balance anticompetitive effects against the claimed justifications. Only then can the court determine if the restraint was unreasonable.

Generally, a defendant hospital's pro-competitive justifications for excluding a plaintiff physician from the staff are accepted if the justifications foster legitimate hospital objectives. Pro-competitive justifications may include maintaining or improving the quality of care, efficiency, or staff harmony at the institution. For example, a hospital that has a management strategy for becoming a teaching and research institution may be justified in denying privileges to a physician who evidences no interest or background in such activities. Given the broad justification for alleged trade restraint that courts find acceptable, it should be no surprise that when rule of reason analysis is used in antitrust cases based on denial of privileges, the defendant invariably prevails.

There are several reasons for the health care institution's succeeding in denial of staff privileges lawsuits. First, as most state laws create some role for a hospital in establishing or overseeing staffing patterns and decisions, hospitals are invariably named as defendants. The net effect of this is to create an alleged vertical, rather than horizontal, restraint for which the rule of reason analysis generally applies. (A vertical restraint involves an agreement among noncompeting entities, such as between a hospital and a physicians' group.) Under the rule of reason test, the plaintiff will have great difficulty establishing more than minimal anticompetitive restraint. Conversely, much weight is given to justifications such as increased quality of care or efficiency in the delivery of health care services. Attainment of these objectives may improve the reputation of the hospital and, hence, improve its competitive position in the relevant market.

Another common situation involving denial of privileges that satisfies the conspiracy or combination requirement of the Sherman Act arises when a hospital enters into an exclusive contract with a group of physicians to supply specific services to the hospital. A physician who is denied staff privileges on the basis of not being a member of the exclusive contracting group may allege an antitrust violation under an "exclusive dealing" theory. If no other allegation accompanies that charge, courts very likely will treat the case as a vertical combination to which the "rule of reason" analysis applies. As indicated, defendant hospitals almost always prevail when this test is applied to such facts.

In an effort to persuade the court to apply the *per se* rule, plaintiffs will often claim a horizontal restraint in the form of a tying arrangement charge. A tying arrangement occurs when an entity or person sells a product, called the tying product, only on condition that the buyer purchase a second product, the tied product. Although all tying arrangements are horizontal restraints, not all tying arrangements are unreasonable *per se*. For the *per se* rule to apply, the plaintiff must demonstrate that the seller has sufficient market control over the tying product to force the buyer to purchase the tied product, which is not necessarily desired nor price/quality competitive on the free market. For example, if a seller controls 70 percent of the apple market, but

Section II.   The Content of Management

conditions the sale of an apple on the simultaneous purchase of a pear, an unlawful tying arrangement exists. If the seller does not possess sufficient market power over the tying product (i.e. the buyer can get his apples elsewhere), the arrangement will be subject to the rule of reason rather than *per se* analysis.

The seminal case involving a tying agreement and exclusive dealing contract in the context of medical staff privileges is the 1984 United States Supreme Court case, *Jefferson Parish Hospital v. Hyde*.[11] In *Hyde*, the plaintiff, an anesthesiologist denied privileges at the defendant hospital, alleged that an exclusive contract between the hospital and an anesthesiology group practice was an illegal tying arrangement because it required that every patient admitted for surgery use the services of one of four anesthesiologists in the group practice.

The court commenced its analysis by finding that two distinct services existed. It concluded that the operating room services were tied to the anesthesiology services, as a patient using the former automatically received the latter. Next, the court inquired whether the hospital had sufficient market control over operating room facilities to force patients to purchase the services of the anesthesiology group practice. The Supreme Court accepted the lower court's finding that the defendant hospital had a 30 percent market share, which the Court determined was insufficient to force patients to purchase the anesthesiology services provided at the hospital: patients always had the option to use another hospital. Therefore, the *per se* rule did not apply. After engaging in the rule of reason analysis, the Court found that the exclusive contract had no actual adverse effect on competition, and, therefore, the linkage in services did not violate antitrust prohibitions.

Subsequent cases have followed *Hyde* and held that exclusive dealing contracts between hospitals and physicians are not *per se* illegal, and, in most instances, are not illegal at all. The physician executive should be aware, however, that if the hospital in question is the only health care facility in the region, or offers unique services, the requisite market power may be found to exist.

Corporate Practice of Medicine

Although a hospital or other health care corporation has the duty to ensure that high-quality medicine is practiced under its roof, corporate entities, including hospitals, traditionally have not been permitted to "practice" medicine. The prohibition against the corporate practice of medicine is rooted in state laws that permit only natural persons to receive medical licenses. Underlying these laws is a public policy that requires that a physician's fiduciary duty to his or her patient remain paramount. If a physician were employed by a corporation, the physician would have loyalties divided between the best interests of the patient and those of the corporation, which is driven by profit motives.

Concomitantly, lay control over medical decision-making and the possible corporate shield from malpractice actions would lower the standard of professionalism and, therefore, has been perceived as dangerous to the patient.

Every profession maintains its status because of the personal responsibility and integrity involved in it. Despite the foregoing, given the legal recognition that health care facilities are, in fact, responsible for the quality of care a patient receives (see, for example, the Health Care Quality Improvement Act of 1986), exceptions to the prohibition against the corporate practice of medicine doctrine have developed.

Almost all states take the position that if a corporation hires a practitioner to service the general public, the corporation is practicing medicine. However, as very few jurisdictions actually take the time to investigate or prosecute these acts, most medical practitioners pay little attention to, if in fact they are aware of, the prohibitions. Nonetheless, the risks a physician confronts upon accepting employment with a corporation include potential loss of licensure and denial of coverage by an insurance company if this employment association is thought to violate the state's medical practice act.

An Attorney General Opinion from South Carolina, dated September 8, 1982, provides a synopsis of various state court positions on the corporate practice of medicine doctrine. There, a corporation undertook to offer paramedical services, including occupational therapy, to the general public. The corporation stated that it intended to hire an occupational therapist. The issue was whether the corporation, which could not itself be licensed, would be unlawfully practicing occupational therapy by using individuals who were licensed.

After examining the laws of various jurisdictions, the Attorney General's Opinion concluded that the critical test is whether or not the licensed individual is subject to the corporation's direction or control. Key factors that determine control are "whether the corporation maintains the office of the practitioner, owns the equipment utilized, pays the operating expenses of the licensed practitioner, receives fees or a major portion thereof that are submitted to the practitioner, and especially whether the practitioner receives a salary paid by the corporation. Other factors that often demonstrate actual practice by the corporation, through its licensed agents, are whether the corporation advertises the practice under the corporate name and has posted the names of its employee-practitioners." The Attorney General concluded that the corporation would be practicing occupational therapy without a license, as the therapist would be an employee of the corporation and thus under its control.

If the practitioner maintains control of his or her professional decision making and is not influenced by the dictates of the corporation, courts

Section II.   The Content of Management

generally allow "employment" relationships to stand. Factors a court will consider include whether the practitioner sets and collects his own fees, keeps his or her own books, and retains substantially the same relationship with and responsibility to the patient, irrespective of the existence of a contract with the corporation. Other evidence of independence from the corporation includes whether the practitioner controls his or her professional activities, conducts examinations in his own manner, and orders supplies from whomever he chooses. If such independence is established, the fact that a physician's rental consideration is tied to a certain percentage of total net fees does not render the agreement illegal.

Although the laws of all jurisdictions very clearly prohibit the corporate practice of medicine, many states have created numerous exceptions to the rule. The most common examples include hospital relationships, HMOs, professional corporations (as opposed to business corporations), independent contractors, and private industrial clinics or ambulatory care centers.

Hospitals

Most states have specific statutory exceptions permitting hospitals to employ physicians. These statutes allow hospitals to hire physicians as long as there is no interference by the hospital in the practitioner's exercise of professional judgment. Some jurisdictions distinguish between hospitals that are for-profit or not-for-profit, public or private, teaching or nonteaching, and emergency or general services facilities.

HMOs

The Health Maintenance Organization Act of 1973 provides that HMOs may do business in the corporate form and employ physicians. Additionally, some states have enacted HMO statutes that allow physician employment. However, the mere fact that a state authorizes HMOs does not necessarily mean that HMOs may circumvent the general corporate practice proscription. For example, in Texas there are statutes that provide for HMOs but that do not allow them to "employ or contract with physicians...in any manner which is prohibited by any licensing law...under which physicians...are licensed."[12]

Professional Corporations

A physician may practice in the corporate form pursuant to individual state professional corporation statutes. These acts preserve the professional's individual responsibility to patients by providing that the professional will be liable for professional services rendered despite the corporate shareholder or employee status. However, the corporate form shields the practitioner from liability for nonprofessional service debts, such as a contract to purchase equipment. Only persons licensed to practice in the particular profession can be shareholders in a professional corporation.

Independent Contractors

Often a physician's "employment" contract states that the physician is acting in the capacity of an independent contractor (see section on hospital contracts, page 291). In order to avoid the charge that the professional is in fact an employee, the contract must state very clearly that the physician maintains complete control and responsibility over, and for the benefit of, the patients. The 1982 South Carolina Attorney General Opinion discussed earlier outlines the factors that a court will consider in determining whether a practitioner is an employee or independent contractor.

Private Industrial Clinics

Some states permit corporations to hire physicians to treat their employees. For example, a Colorado statute provides that, "Any licensee...may accept employment from any person, partnership, association, or corporation to examine and treat the employees of such person, partnership, association, or corporation."[13]

Although there are many exceptions to the rule against the corporate practice of medicine, and it is an antiquated concept that has outlived the purposes for which it was created, the general prohibition still exists. The physician executive should be aware of this prohibition and the potential threat it still poses to employment relationships between physicians and health care facilities.

Insurability/Alternative Risk Protection Mechanisms

A key area of concern for the physician executive is how to best protect the health care organization from exposure to financial loss emanating from liability lawsuits. Until fairly recently, the primary method a hospital used to protect itself was to purchase commercial insurance. As premiums soared and availability of malpractice coverage plummeted, many health care institutions turned to alternative funding and risk management methods. In addition to the inadvisable option of going bare (that is, maintaining no insurance), an institution has two basic choices: funding a self-insurance program or trust on a single- or multihospital basis or the formation of a captive insurance company, also known as a limited purpose insurance company.

Funded self-insurance is a mechanism that collects and disburses funds to cover liability losses. The trust amount is actuarially determined and is managed by a qualified trustee. Generally, a self-insurance trust on a single hospital basis will not constitute the conduct of the business of insurance. The formation and operation of the trust is relatively simple,

Section II.   The Content of Management

as it will not be governed by the applicable state insurance code. However, if the trust is formed for multihospital protection, compliance with a state's applicable insurance code may be required. Consequently, individual state laws must be consulted to determine precisely what activity constitutes the business of insurance. Self-insurance trusts are often considered attractive because they eliminate the profit element of commercial insurance, investment returns remain in the trust, and claims administration and loss prevention are controlled by the health care institution itself. Of course, risk spreading, which commercial insurance is best equipped to do, is minimized.

The second alternative risk protection mechanism is the creation of a limited purpose liability company, referred to as a captive insurance company because its owners are the ones protected by its coverage. A captive insurance company is essentially a self-insurance program organized under the insurance code of a particular state. The company is in all respects a distinct insurance company that is wholly owned by its insureds. All the formalities required by the applicable insurance code must be complied with to form this type of entity. Generally, this includes capitalization, reporting, and reserve requirements, as well as limitations on risks that can be undertaken.

A bill allowing the formation of a Risk Retention Group was passed by Congress in October 1986.[14] This new law expanded a 1981 version of the law that only allowed Risk Retention Groups to insure against product liability claims. The new law allows coverage for any kind of liability and has generated a great deal of interest around the country. Consequently, it deserves more detailed treatment here.

To qualify as a Risk Retention Group, a group must be exclusively owned by persons who are insureds of the company; the group must consist of similar or related businesses. Once a group is chartered under the law of any state in accordance with the provisions of the Risk Retention Act, it may do business nationally subject only to minimal restrictions. These restrictions include certain administrative requirements, such as requiring the group to submit to each state in which it proposes to do business a copy of a feasibility study prepared for the group, a copy of certified financial statements, and a copy of an opinion of a qualified loss reserve specialist on the Group's loss and loss adjustment expense reserves. In addition, state insurance commissioners retain authority to prevent companies operating in an unsound manner from doing business in their states.

The Act provides numerous incentives for the formation of Risk Retention Groups. Once a group satisfies the regulatory requirements of its chartering state, it is virtually free to do business anywhere in the United States. This obviates the need for companies to obtain prior rate and policy form approvals in all 50 states and the need either to become licensed as an admitted insurer in all 50 states or to utilize a fronting insurer. Second, the Act facilitates the Company's ability to raise capital by providing an exemption from state securities laws and from the registration requirements of the federal securities laws. Thus, the Company may readily raise capital without incurring the substantial costs associated with a registered public offering. Third, the Act exempts Risk Retention Groups from any state law requiring such groups to utilize a broker or agent resident in the state to countersign insurance policies.

A Group will most likely be formed under the laws of the state of Delaware, although other states, such as Illinois, have recently authorized the formation of Risk Retention Groups. There are numerous advantages associated with incorporating in Delaware. First, Delaware has a positive business climate. It was the first state to incorporate a Risk Retention Group and is widely respected by insurance commissioners as a state with experience in the formation and regulation of Risk Retention Groups and other complex businesses. Second, Delaware has recently enacted legislation to substantially broaden permissible director indemnification and to limit director liability. Because the company's board will most likely comprise owner/insureds who will direct the operations of the company, this additional protection is highly desirable.

The Act is potentially a tremendous boon to the medical and health care industry, which has suffered from the unavailability of adequate insurance at reasonable cost. However, the Act is no panacea. Given the recent adoption of the Act, many questions remain as to how individual state commissioners may interpret some of its provisions. As previously mentioned, individual states in which the group plans to do business retain some discretion in regulating the capitalization of Risk Retention Groups. Although antithetical to the intent of the Act, a state commissioner may, for example, refuse to fully recognize assets represented by letters of credit as admitted assets of the group. Questions over conflicting state interpretations of the Act's provisions pertaining to purchasing groups have recently been raised by Commerce Department officials in Washington, D.C.

Although it will take time to determine how individual states interpret the Act, the right to form Risk Retention Groups within the health care industry portends a substantial increase in the availability and affordability of malpractice insurance. Because all insureds are owners and all owners are insureds, each insured has a direct incentive to employ effective risk prevention programs to minimize loss exposure. To the extent that certain insureds fall short of their responsibilities, owners of the group may redeem the shares of such insureds and thus eliminate them from the risk pool. The Risk Retention Act will not solve all insurance problems, but the physician executive should be aware of its potential and be mindful of future developments.

Section II.   The Content of Management

Civil Discovery and Risk Management

Incident reporting systems and patient care review committees are obviously an integral part of hospital risk management programs. While such programs are necessary to control and contain risk, the documents produced as a result of the programs are potential time bombs just waiting to be discovered by a plaintiff's attorney in malpractice lawsuits. Consequently, the physician executive must be aware of legal avenues available to protect the institution from unnecessary disclosure of hospital documents.

Data generated by, or for, hospital review committees may be protected against discovery by specific statutes that ensure the confidentiality of such records. For example, the Medical Studies Act of Illinois, states, in part, "All information, interviews, reports, statements, memoranda or other data...(but not the medical records pertaining to the patient) used in the course of internal quality control or of medical study for the purpose of reducing morbidity or mortality, or for improving patient care, shall be privileged, strictly confidential and shall be used only for medical research, the evaluation and improvement of quality care, or granting, limiting or revoking staff privileges...."[15]

In order to increase the likelihood that a hospital's records fall within the purview of the above act, the institution should state very clearly on each document that it has been prepared for purposes of internal quality control, for medical studies to reduce morbidity or mortality, or to improve patient care. However, labeling a document is by no means a fail-safe procedure.

The existence of a statute such as Illinois' does not guarantee that a plaintiff's attorney will not succeed in obtaining many documents, because state laws are subject to varying interpretations by the courts. For example, some state laws may only prohibit the admission of such records into evidence at trial, thereby allowing a plaintiff's attorney to review them during pretrial discovery. However, even where discovery is not prohibited by statute, some courts have prevented their disclosure on public policy grounds or have allowed a defense claim that such documents constitute privileged material.

Contracts and the Hospital[16]

Finally, hospital administrators must focus on a number of generic issues common to any type of health care contract, whether it is a service, a purchase, or some other type of contract. Although some issues, such as compensation and termination, are of utmost importance, any provision that is carelessly drafted or inadvertently deleted may result in later disputes between the parties, litigation, and loss of essential services and supplies required by the hopsital to continue to provide high-quality health care services on an uninterrupted basis.

Starting literally at the beginning of any health care contract, the identity of any parties to the agreement must be clearly and unambiguously stated. Although this might appear to be a simple and noncontroversial matter, health care administrators and their lawyers must be alert for certain problem situations. For example, shortly before the execution of one lengthy multimillion dollar hospital-vendor contract, it was discovered that the initials of the vendor, which had been assumed to stand for the company name, in fact stood for a separate subsidiary of the parent company. This discovery was significant, insofar as the parent company was a nationally known corporation with significant assets whereas its subsidiary was a newly formed entity that had been recently capitalized and held far fewer assets. In other words, the various indemnification provisions within the contract were far less meaningful when made by the subsidiary entity as opposed to the parent with whom the client thought it was negotiating.

Another example for the health care executive is to obtain additional information when negotiating a contract with a "partnership" as opposed to a corporate entity. The health care executive must be careful to ensure that the party negotiating on behalf of the partnership has the authority to enter into the agreement and to commit the partnership to providing the services or goods specified in the contract and that the terms of the proposed agreement do not in some way violate the terms of that partnership agreement. For this reason, when negotiating with a partnership, the actual partnership agreement should be reviewed in advance. Furthermore, a provision should be included within the contract wherein the other party warrants and covenants that he or she is obligated to enter into the agreement on behalf of the partnership and that the terms of the contract do not exceed the powers of the partnership's organizational documents.

If a hospital is going to be providing services of a type that it will provide to other parties, the terms of the contract should make clear that the contract is being entered into on a "nonexclusive" basis. Conversely, if you are obtaining services from a party on an exclusive basis, it should be so stated in the agreement. For example, when hiring a full-time medical director, the hospital manager should specify that that person will provide such services on an "exclusive" basis. In that type of situation, the hospital administrator should consider incorporating additional safeguards, such as specifying the period during which the medical director must be on the premises performing the responsibilities specified in the contract.

In any situation where hospital administration is providing services of some type for another health care provider or business, the hospital should be indemnified from liability for the acts or omissions of the other party. For example, if a hospital contracts to provide the inpatient component of services for a local or national HMO, the hospital should be held harmless and indemnified from any and all risks of

Section II.   The Content of Management

liabilities, claims, and judgments (including reasonable attorneys' fees) related to the HMO's discharge of its responsibilities under the agreement or its provision of patient care services. Additionally, the hospital should be listed as a named-insured on the HMO's professional liability policy, which, in itself, should be for adequate amounts. Those amounts would be determined by the nature and scope of services to be delivered by the hospital and the general demographics (i.e., age and health condition) of the HMO's patients.

Provisions regarding compensation are usually one of the two most important areas of any health care contract. After all, if it weren't for compensation, at least one of the parties would certainly not be entering into the contract. For that reason, it is essential that the contract clearly state how, when, and in what amounts compensation will be made, particularly in those instances where it is the hospital that will be receiving payment for providing services. Additionally, the contract should state what, if any, penalties may be assessed for late payments. Typically, a hospital that is not paid on a timely basis will be entitled to assess penalties in an amount not in excess of that allowed by applicable law. In many states, however, "penalty" provisions are largely unenforceable and must be included as an added payment needed to defray administrative expenses caused by the late payment. This avoids prohibition of payments otherwise described as "penalties."

In order to protect a hospital's long-term interests, any contract should require the other party to discharge its responsibilities in accordance with state and federal law, particularly regulations applicable to hospitals. For example, in contracts for goods or services costing in excess of $10,000 over a 12-month period, the vendor should be required to provide access to its books and records to the Secretary of the Department of Health and Human Services or the Comptroller General, or their designates, as may be needed by the federal government to audit those services furnished or goods supplied by the vendor. The hospital, under applicable federal regulations of the Department of Health and Human Services, is required to include this type of provision in any such contract. As a general rule, if the hospital fails to comply with federal statutes and regulations, such as the one described here, it could fall out of compliance with Medicare's Conditions of Participation or suffer adverse reimbursement determinations by state and federal regulators and payers.

Given the rapid evolution in the delivery of health care services and the various statutes and regulations applicable to hospitals and health care providers, contracts should generally provide what will happen if the law or reimbursement regulations should change during the term of the agreement. If the hospital would be seriously affected by a change in law or regulation, the facility should have the right to demand a renegotiation of the contract or to terminate the agreement. Absent such safeguards, the hospital could not only lose the benefit of an agreement, but could actually suffer very serious financial losses if it were obligated to continue to discharge its responsibilities under an agreement for which it could no longer continue to be reimbursed.

Hospital clients frequently inquire whether it is advisable to include an arbitration provision of some type in agreements. As a general rule, arbitration provisions usually benefit the party that has less leverage and is less likely to be able to afford protracted litigation and costly legal fees. Whether or not an arbitration provision should be included within a particular contract will depend on factual circumstances and can only be made on a case-by-case basis. However, in those situations where an arbitration provision is deemed suitable by the parties, an informal dispute mechanism should be drafted whereby a neutral third party will review oral and/or written briefs and make a determination based upon what he or she believes is just and equitable within 20 days of the commencement of the informal dispute mechanism. A dispute mechanism of this type is generally quick, inexpensive (for both parties), and draws less attention than if a dispute had to be litigated in a court of law.

Alternatively, parties may agree to arbitrate disputes pursuant to the rules of the American Arbitration Association (AAA) and to use an arbitrator approved by the AAA. Additionally, state law in many jurisdictions provides for arbitration procedures that may be specified to govern any dispute arising between the parties.

In order to minimize, if not completely avoid, liability by somehow being deemed to be "in business" with the other party to the contract, health care contracts should generally specify that the parties are acting as "independent contractors," and not as partners or joint venturers, for the purpose of carrying out the terms of the agreement. Further, such contracts should generally specify that one party is not acting as the agent or representative of the other party.

Additionally, in those cases where hospital management may be contracting with an individual, such as a medical director, on an independent contractor basis even though the individual would traditionally be deemed an "employee" of the facility, the hospital should obtain separate written assurances from the individual wherein he or she covenants that he or she will pay his or her income taxes in full on a timely basis. Such separate written assurances will serve to protect the hospital's financial interests in the event that the administrator or other like contracting party subsequently fails to pay his or her income taxes, in which case the hospital could be liable for those payments plus interest and possible penalties.

The second (many would say the most) important provision within any health care contract is the termination provision. Parties usually are far more acrimonious when an agreement is prematurely terminated than when it is initially negotiated. For this reason, it is critical that the duties

Section II.   The Content of Management

and responsibilities of the parties related to a contract's termination be clearly articulated within the document. For example, if one party terminates the agreement resulting from the breach of the other party, the agreement might define what constitutes "breach" within the meaning of the agreement. The contract should explicitly state which responsibilities of each party will continue following termination. For example, if the hospital is to receive payments on the the fifteenth day of each month for services provided during the immediately preceding month, then the hospital should be guaranteed payment for services provided during the last month of the agreement even though such payment may not be made until after the contract's termination.

As a general rule, hospitals should not enter into agreements wherein the term of the agreement is self-extending unless terminated upon 30 days' written notice prior to an anniversary date of the agreement. The danger of such self-extending agreements is that if the hospital should fail inadvertently to give the required notice within the required 30-day "window," it may be unable to terminate the agreement for an additional 12 months. Obviously, hospitals should avoid this situation and can be certain to prevent themselves from being locked into an automatic renewal if the term of the contract is not self-extending.

Caveat: Hospital executives should treat exhibits as seriously as the actual terms of the agreements to which they affix their signatures. Exhibits frequently contain key terms of the mutual agreement of the parties. Accordingly, never under any circumstances should an agreement be signed unless all exhibits are attached and agreed upon by the parties. Should it be necessary to execute an agreement before all exhibits are completed, at a minimum, a contract provision should be included that states that the agreement will take effect only upon completion and execution by the parties of specified attachments.

Health care executives may be familiar with the term "time is of the essence" within a contract. This phrase has an exact legal meaning and should generally not be included within a health care contract. More specifically, a contract that makes "time of essence" means that either party will have breached the contract as a matter of law should it fail to perform each and every term and duty delegated to it thereunder on a timely basis and as fully specified within the agreement. In other words, if the hospital were obligated to make a payment on the first day of the month during the term of the agreement, the hospital would be in breach of that contract if it were to submit such payment one minute late, i.e., at 12:01 a.m. on the 2nd of the month. Thereupon, the nonbreaching party would be entitled to all of its rights specified thereunder resulting from the hospital's technical failure to make timely payments. In order to avoid severe repercussions for failing to comply strictly with a contract's terms, time should not be made "of the essence."

Last, goods and services being purchased by a hospital or those to be discharged by the institution must always be carefully and unambiguously articulated within the contract so as to avoid future disputes with respect to the actual duties and responsibilities of the parties under the agreement.

Each situation will present parties negotiating a contract with different difficulties and problems requiring creative solutions designed to accommodate the special interests and factual circumstances of those parties. However, as described above, most agreements will generally have certain key points regardless of the factual circumstances. Health care executives and other health professionals and personnel with a health care facility should, however, be alert to carefully negotiate those terms. If those terms are negotiated to the satisfaction and advantage of the hospital, the contract should generally be one that will protect the institution during the term of the agreement and, perhaps more important, upon its termination.

Conclusion

Hospital liability has undergone expansive growth since the days when the hospital's only responsibility was to provide facilities in which independent health care practitioners plied their trade. Today, if a health care institution does not exercise effective control over how care is provided and who provides it, it runs the risk of liability for patient injury. Conversely, if the institution exercises too much control, it runs the risk of violating laws prohibiting the corporate practice of medicine as well as liability to practitioners for restraint of trade. The answer to this "Catch-22" is a simple prescription--knowledge and moderation. As long as the physician executive is aware of the legal environment in which he or she operates, an effective but not overly restrictive risk management course may be charted.

References

1. See, Phoenix, "Hospital Liability for the Acts of Independent Contractors: The Ostensible Agency Doctrine," 30 *St. Louis U.L.J.* 875-93 (1985-1986); Note, "Hospital Liability May Be Based on Either Doctrine of Ostensible Agency or Doctrine of Corporate Negligence," 17 St. *Mary's L.J.* 551-578 (1986).

2. 33 Ill. 2d 326, 211 N.E. 2d 253 (1965). See Zaremski and Spitz, "Liability of a Hospital as an Institution; Are the Walls of Jericho Tumbling?" *Forum* 16 (2): 225, Fall 1980; Zaremski, "Hospital Corporate Liability: The Walls Continue to Tumble," *Medicolegal News* 9(2): 13, April 1981.

3. 97 Wis. 2d 521, 294 N.W. 2d 501

4. *Northern Trust Co. v. Louis A. Weiss*, 493 N.E. 2d 6 (Ill. App. 1st, 1986).

Section II.   The Content of Management

5. 42 U.S.C., Sec. 1101 et. seq.

6. *Copperweld Corporation, et. al. v. Independence Tube Corporation,* 467 US 752 (1984)

7. 656 F. Supp. 601 (S.D. Tx 1987)

8. Because the hospital had an open staff policy that permitted physicians to request the services of any staff radiologist, the plaintiff retained full staff privileges at the hospital and continued to receive referrals. Under this open staff policy, the radiology contract was not an exclusive services contract; the contracting radiologist took only those cases where the attending physician did not designate a preference for a particular radiologist.

9. 457 US 332, 73 L. Ed. 2d 48 (1982)

10. 745 F. 2d 786 (3d Cir. 1984)

11. 104 S. Ct. 1551 (1984)

12. Tex. Ins. Code Ann., Art 20(A).0693

13. C.R.S. sec. 12-12-117(m)

14. Risk Retention Act, 15 U.S.C., Sec. 3901 et. seq.

15. Ill. Rev Stat, ch. 110, sec. 2101. The statute reads in full: "All information, interviews, reports, statements, memoranda or other data of the Illinois Department of Public Health, the Illinois Department of Mental Health and Developmental Disabilities Medical Review Board, Illinois State Medical Society, allied medical societies, health maintenance organizations and medical organizations under contract with health maintenance organizations, physician-owned inter-insurance exchanges and their agents, or committees of licensed or accredited hospitals or their medical staffs, including Patient Care Audit Committees, Medical Care Evaluation Committees and Executive Committees, Medical Care Evaluation Committees, Utilization Review Committees, Credential Committees and Executive Committees (but not the medical records pertaining to the patient) used in the course of internal quality control or of medical study for the purpose of reducing morbidity or mortality, or for improving patient care, shall be privileged, strictly confidential and shall be used only for medical research, the evaluation and improvement of quality care, or granting, limiting or revoking staff privileges, or in any judicial review thereof, the claim of confidentiality shall not be invoked to deny such physician access to or use of data upon which such a decision was based."

16. Acknowledgement is made for the assistance of Michael Roth in the preparation of the material on hospital contracts.

Miles J. Zaremski is a Senior Partner with Arnstein, Gluck, Lehr & Milligan, Chicago, Illinois, and West Palm Beach, Florida. David J. Schwartz is a member of the Illinois Bar, Chicago, Illinois.